Peripheral and Cerebrovascular Intervention

CONTEMPORARY CARDIOLOGY

CHRISTOPHER P. CANNON, MD
SERIES EDITOR

For further volumes:
http://www.springer.com/series/7677

Peripheral and Cerebrovascular Intervention

Edited by
Deepak L. Bhatt

Chief of Cardiology, VA Boston Healthcare System;
Director, Integrated Interventional Cardiovascular Program,
Brigham and Women's Hospital & VA Boston Healthcare System;
Associate Professor of Medicine, Harvard Medical School;
Senior Investigator, TIMI Study Group, Boston, Massachusetts, USA

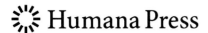

Editor
Deepak L. Bhatt, MD, MPH, FACC, FAHA, FSCAI, FESC
Department of Cardiovascular Medicine
VA Boston Healthcare System, Brigham
and Women's Hospital, and Harvard Medical School
75 Francis Street, Boston, MA 02115, USA
DLBHATTMD@post.harvard.edu

ISBN 978-1-60327-964-2   e-ISBN 978-1-60327-965-9
DOI 10.1007/978-1-60327-965-9
Springer New York Dordrecht Heidelberg London

Library of Congress Control Number: 2011941122

© Springer Science+Business Media, LLC 2012
All rights reserved. This work may not be translated or copied in whole or in part without the written permission of the publisher (Humana Press, 999 Riverview Drive, Suite 208, Totowa, NJ 07512 USA), except for brief excerpts in connection with reviews or scholarly analysis. Use in connection with any form of information storage and retrieval, electronic adaptation, computer software, or by similar or dissimilar methodology now known or hereafter developed is forbidden.
The use in this publication of trade names, trademarks, service marks, and similar terms, even if they are not identified as such, is not to be taken as an expression of opinion as to whether or not they are subject to proprietary rights.
While the advice and information in this book are believed to be true and accurate at the date of going to press, neither the authors nor the editors nor the publisher can accept any legal responsibility for any errors or omissions that may be made. The publisher makes no warranty, express or implied, with respect to the material contained herein.

Printed on acid-free paper

Humana Press is part of Springer Science+Business Media (www.springer.com)

Dedication

To my parents, for setting me on the path of education, and to my wife Shanthala and to my sons Vinayak, Arjun, Ram, and Raj for their continual support, encouragement, and understanding of my various professional endeavors.

Deepak L. Bhatt, MD, MPH

Contents

Contributors		ix
1	Peripheral and Cerebrovascular Disease *Vijay Nambi and Deepak L. Bhatt*	1
2	Lower Extremity Intervention *Samir K. Shah and Daniel G. Clair*	19
3	Critical Limb Ischemia *Raghotham Patlola and Craig Walker*	41
4	Renal and Mesenteric Intervention *Ramy A. Badawi and Christopher J. White*	79
5	Subclavian and Upper Extremity Interventions *Khung Keong Yeo and John R. Laird*	99
6	Carotid and Vertebral Intervention *Douglas E. Drachman, Nicholas J. Ruggiero II, and Kenneth Rosenfield*	115
7	Intracranial Intervention *Muhammad Shazam Hussain and Rishi Gupta*	141
8	Abdominal and Thoracic Aortic Aneurysms *Aravinda Nanjundappa, Bryant Nguyen, Robert S. Dieter, John J. Lopez, and Akhilesh Jain*	159
9	Venous Intervention *Andrew B. McCann and Robert M. Schainfeld*	191
Index		229

Contributors

Ramy A. Badawi, MD • *Department of Cardiovascular Disease, Ochsner Foundation Hospital, New Orleans, LA, USA*

Deepak L. Bhatt, MD, MPH • *Department of Cardiology, VA Boston Healthcare System, Boston, MA, USA; Department of Cardiovascular Medicine, Brigham and Women's Hospital, Boston, MA, USA; Harvard Medical School, Boston, MA, USA; TIMI Study Group, Boston, MA, USA*

Daniel G. Clair, MD • *Department of Vascular Surgery, The Cleveland Clinic, Cleveland, OH, USA; CWRU Lerner College of Medicine, Cleveland, OH, USA*

Robert S. Dieter, MD, RVT • *Division of Cardiology, Loyola University, Chicago Illinois, USA*

Douglas E. Drachman, MD • *Cardiology Division, Massachusetts General Hospital, Harvard Medical School, Boston, MA, USA*

Rishi Gupta, MD • *Emory University School of Medicine, Atlanta, GA, USA*

Muhammad Shazam Hussain, MD, FRCP(C) • *Cleveland Clinic, Cerebrovascular Section, Vascular Neurology, Endovascular Surgical Neuroradiology, Cleveland, OH, USA*

Akhilesh Jain, MD • *Division of Surgery, Yale School of Medicine, Connecticut*

John R. Laird, MD • *The Vascular Center and Division of Cardiovascular Medicine, University of California Medical System, Sacramento, CA, USA*

John J. Lopez, MD • *Department of Medicine, Loyola University, Stritch School of Medicine and Hines VA, Maywood, IL, USA*

Andrew B. McCann, MBBS • *Department of Vascular Medicine, Princess Alexandra Hospital, Brisbane, QLD, Australia*

Vijay Nambi, MD • *Department of Medicine, Section of Atherosclerosis and Vascular Medicine, Baylor College of Medicine, Houston, TX, USA*

Aravinda Nanjundappa, MD • *Division of Vascular Surgery, West Virginia University, Charleston, WV, USA*

Bryant Nguyen, MD • *Department of Internal Medicine, Division of Cardiology, Loyola University, Chicago, Illinois, USA*

Raghotham Patlola, MD • *Cardiovascular Institute of the South, Lafayette, LA, USA*

Kenneth Rosenfield, MD • *Vascular Medicine and Intervention, Department of Cardiology, Massachusetts General Hospital, Boston, MA, USA*

Nicholas J. Ruggiero II, MD • *Structural Heart Disease and Non-Coronary Interventions, Thomas Jefferson University Hospital, Philadelphia, PA, USA*

ROBERT M. SCHAINFELD, DO • *Division of Cardiology, Vascular Medicine Section, Harvard Medical School, Massachusetts General Hospital, Boston, MA, USA*
SAMIR K. SHAH, MD • *Cleveland Clinic, Cleveland, OH, USA*
CHRISTOPHER J. WHITE, MD • *Department of Cardiovascular Diseases, Ochsner Foundation Hospital, New Orleans, LA, USA*
CRAIG WALKER, MD • *Cardiovascular Institute of the South, Houma, LA, USA*
KHUNG KEONG YEO, MBBS • *The Vascular Center and Division of Cardiovascular Medicine, University of California Medical System, Sacramento, CA, USA*

1 Peripheral and Cerebrovascular Disease

Vijay Nambi, MD, *and Deepak L. Bhatt,* MD, MPH

CONTENTS

INTRODUCTION
PREVALENCE OF ATHEROSCLEROSIS
   OF NONCORONARY ARTERIES
PREVALENCE OF "POLYVASCULAR ATHEROSCLEROSIS"
   OR "MULTIBED ATHEROSCLEROSIS"
OUTCOMES OF INDIVIDUALS WITH
   PERIPHERAL ARTERIAL DISEASE
SCREENING FOR PAD
SCREENING WITH CAROTID INTIMA MEDIA THICKNESS
IMPACT OF MEASURES OF LEAD AND CAROTID
   ATHEROSCLEROSIS IN CHD RISK PREDICTION
MANAGEMENT OF INDIVIDUALS WITH LEAD AND CAROTID
   ATHEROSCLEROSIS
POTENTIAL ROLE OF REVASCULARIZATION IN IMPROVING
   THE QUALITY OF LIFE
MANAGEMENT OF CAROTID ATHEROSCLEROSIS
PERFORMANCE MEASURES
SUMMARY
REFERENCES

INTRODUCTION

"Atherogenesis" is a ubiquitous process in humans and almost no artery is spared of its development. Although atherosclerosis of the coronary arteries receives the most attention due to its potentially devastating complications, the presence of atherosclerosis in other vascular beds or "peripheral arterial disease" (PAD) very often connotes a worse prognosis than coronary artery disease alone. Below, we review the "peripheral" manifestations of atherosclerosis with respect to their prevalence and outcomes, highlighting the current deficiencies in their management.

From: *Peripheral and Cerebrovascular Intervention*, Contemporary Cardiology
Edited by: D. L. Bhatt, DOI 10.1007/978-1-60327-965-9_1
© Springer Science+Business Media, LLC 2012

For the purposes of this chapter, PAD refers to all noncoronary forms of atherosclerosis including carotid and cerebrovascular arteries, abdominal arteries (renal, celiac, and mesenteric), and arteries of the extremities (lower and upper extremities).

PREVALENCE OF ATHEROSCLEROSIS OF NONCORONARY ARTERIES

The true prevalence of atherosclerosis of noncoronary arteries is probably difficult to discern since routine evaluation for atherosclerosis in the various arterial beds other than coronary arteries in asymptomatic individuals is seldom performed. However, screening of the carotid arteries and lower extremity arteries have been performed in several epidemiological studies giving us a reasonable estimate of the prevalence of asymptomatic atherosclerosis in these arterial beds.

The prevalence of *lower extremity arterial disease (LEAD)* increases with age (Fig. 1). In the Framingham Heart Study, the annual incidence of LEAD increased from 6 per 10,000 men and 3 per 10,000 women in the 30- to 44-year-old age group to 61 per 10,000 men and 54 per 10,000 women in the 65- to 74-year-old age group *(1)*. Overall, the prevalence of asymptomatic LEAD ranges from 3 to 10%. It increases to 15–20% in those aged >70 years *(1–3)*. On the other hand, the prevalence of symptomatic LEAD (intermittent claudication) is likely between 3% in those aged 40 years and 6% in those aged 60 years of age *(4)*. Although, all the traditional cardiovascular risk factors are associated with LEAD as well, smokers and individuals with diabetes tend to have an increased prevalence/incidence of LEAD. Additionally, LEAD is more common in men and in non-Hispanic Blacks when compared with Whites *(3)*.

Atherosclerosis of the major arterial branches of the abdominal aorta is also common. With respect to the "intestinal arteries," namely the celiac and mesenteric vessels, atherosclerotic stenosis is most often asymptomatic due to their extensive interconnections. Symptoms (intestinal ischemia) are more likely to occur only when two of the three arteries are occluded or stenotic. Chronic intestinal ischemia, which occurs more

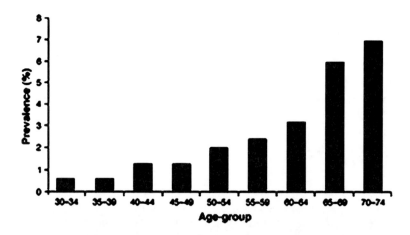

Fig. 1. Weighted mean prevalence of intermittent claudication (symptomatic PAD) in large population-based studies (4). PAD = Peripheral Arterial Disease/lower extremity arterial disease (Reprinted from Journal of Vascular Surgery, Vol. 45, 2007, S5–67 with the permission of Elsevier).

commonly in women, is more likely in individuals with a history of cardiovascular disease (CVD) and in those who have had previous coronary or lower extremity bypass surgeries *(5, 6)*.

The prevalence of *renal arterial stenosis* in the general population has not been well described. Minimal data exists related to its prevalence in individuals >65 years of age. Hansen et al. reported that in a population-based cohort, 834 participants from the Cardiovascular Health Study (a study of CVD risk factors, morbidity and mortality in adults aged >65 years), the overall prevalence of renal artery stenosis >60 was 6.8% (5.5% in women, 9.1% in men, and 6.7% of Black and 6.9% of White participants) *(7)*. On the other hand, the prevalence of renal artery stenosis in "at-risk" populations such as those with coronary artery disease or LEAD is far greater with prevalence rates of 30% in those undergoing coronary angiography with 11–18% having significant (>50% stenosis) disease *(8–10)*, and 22–59% in those with LEAD *(11–21)*.

Finally, data about the prevalence of *carotid atherosclerosis* comes from several population-based epidemiological studies that have performed carotid artery ultrasounds to measure carotid intima media thickness (C-IMT). The intima media thickness (IMT), or thickness of the arterial walls, increases (presumably in relation to atherosclerosis) as one ages. However, for the purpose of this discussion, we will use the mere presence of definite areas of carotid plaque to define the prevalence of carotid atherosclerosis. In the ARIC study, the prevalence of carotid plaque (defined on the basis of IMT greater than 1.5 mm), shape (protrusion into the lumen, loss of alignment with adjacent arterial boundary, roughness of the arterial boundary), or texture (brighter echoes than adjacent boundaries) in 45–64-year-old White and Black individuals was noted to be ~34% *(22)*. Men were noted to have plaques more frequently than women (40.1 vs. 28.3%) while Whites were noted to have plaques more frequently than Blacks (34.4 vs. 31.4%). The prevalence of plaque also increased with age with the prevalence increasing from 21.5% in individuals between 45 and 49 years of age to 47.1% in individuals 60–64 years of age *(23)*. In the Rotterdam Study *(24)*, another prospective population-based cohort study of men and women age ≥55 years, the overall prevalence of plaque was reported to be 57.8 with 24% having plaque in ≥3 carotid artery segments.

The prevalence of significant carotid artery stenosis on the other hand is much lesser. In a meta-analysis of 29 studies, de Weerd et al. reported that the pooled prevalence of moderate (≥50%) stenosis was ~4.2%, while the pooled prevalence of significant stenosis (>70%) was 1.7% *(25)*. As expected, the prevalence of moderate stenosis was higher in men and in older ages with men >70 years having a prevalence of ~10.7% while women in the same age group having a prevalence of 5.8%. In men and women <70 years of age, the prevalence was 4.8 and 2.2% in men and women, respectively.

However, in selected populations, the prevalence of significant carotid artery atherosclerosis may be enriched. For example, Kurvers et al. *(26)* reported that in 2,274 patients with atherosclerotic vascular disease (LEAD, stroke or transient ischemic attack, abdominal aortic aneurysm, and angina or myocardial infarction (MI)) or with risk factors for atherosclerotic vascular disease (diabetes, hypertension, or hyperlipidemia), the prevalence of significant (>70%) internal carotid stenosis increased along a continuum as follows: 1.8–2.3% in those with risk factors for atherosclerosis to 3.1% in those with angina or MI to 8.5% in those with abdominal aortic aneurysms to 12.5% in those with LEAD. Therefore, one may predict that "atherosclerosis begets atherosclerosis."

PREVALENCE OF "POLYVASCULAR ATHEROSCLEROSIS" OR "MULTIBED ATHEROSCLEROSIS"

Presence of atherosclerosis in one arterial bed has been associated with higher concomitant presence of atherosclerosis in other arterial beds. In the REACH registry, an international, prospective, observational registry of 67,888 individuals >45 years old with established CAD, LEAD, cerebrovascular disease, or at least three atherosclerosis-related risk factors, two-thirds (66%) of those with LEAD also had concomitant coronary or cerebrovascular disease, while two-fifths (40%) of those with carotid atherosclerosis and one-quarter (25%) of those with CAD also had concomitant atherosclerosis of other arterial beds (27, 28) (Fig. 2). Several other studies have examined the concomitant prevalence of atherosclerosis in multiple beds as well. The CAD prevalence in patients with LEAD has been varied depending on the method used to identify the presence of CAD. It has been reported that ~33–50% of LEAD patients have CAD based by clinical history or by ECG, while 66% have CAD based by stress testing (29). On the other hand, Hertzer et al. (30) reported that in patients who were preoperative for symptomatic LEAD, the incidence of CAD at cardiac catheterization was 90%, with 28% having severe three-vessel disease.

With respect to the prevalence of carotid artery stenosis among those with LEAD, carotid stenosis >30% has been described in ~51–72% of individuals with LEAD, while stenosis >70% has been reported in ~12–25% of the individuals (26–31). Finally, renal artery stenosis has been reported in 23–42% of the individuals with PAD compared to ~3% of the individuals in a general population with hypertension (4).

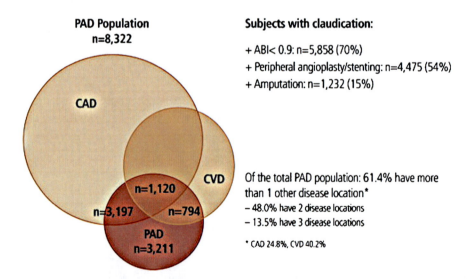

Fig. 2. Distribution of atherosclerosis in patients with lower extremity arterial disease (77). CAD = Coronary Artery Disease, CVD = Cerebrovascular Disease, PAD = Peripheral Artery Disease/lower extremity arterial disease (Reprinted with the permission of Elsevier).

OUTCOMES OF INDIVIDUALS WITH PERIPHERAL ARTERIAL DISEASE

Individuals with LEAD have a higher incidence of CVD mortality and morbidity compared with men and women of the same age without LEAD *(32–34)*. Reports have suggested a 20–60% increase in the risk of MI and a two- to sixfold increase in the risk of death due to coronary heart disease (CHD) *(33, 35–39)*. The ARIC study reported that men (but not women) with LEAD have a 4–5 times more likelihood of having a stroke or transient ischemic attack when compared to those without LEAD *(40)*, and the Edinburgh study *(36)* confirmed this association. Finally, evidence suggests that the annual mortality from LEAD is in the order of 4–5% per year *(29)*. It is therefore not surprising that the 5-year mortality associated with LEAD is worse than that associated with several malignancies including breast cancer *(41)* (Fig. 3).

More recently, the Reduction of Atherothrombosis for Continued Health (REACH) Registry was initiated to study the global prevalence of atherosclerosis of the various arterial beds and to study the clinical outcomes of these individuals over a 24-month time period. In all, of 67,888 patients in whom data were available, 8,273 (12.2%) patients had LEAD, 18,843 (27.8%) had CVD, 40,258 (59.3%) had CAD, and 12,389 (18.2%) had ≥3 risk factors for atherosclerosis. Of 64,977 participants who had one-year outcomes data *(28)*, the presence of LEAD was associated with a 5.35% incidence of cardiovascular death, stroke, or MI, while presence of CAD or cerebrovascular disease (asymptomatic carotid artery stenosis >70%) was associated with one-year incidences of 4.52 and 6.47%, respectively. The 1-year incidence of cardiovascular death, stroke, MI, or hospitalizations for atherothrombotic events in individuals with LEAD, CAD, and cerebrovascular disease were 21.1, 15.2, and 14.5%, respectively. As expected, individuals with multibed atherosclerosis had the highest event rates with

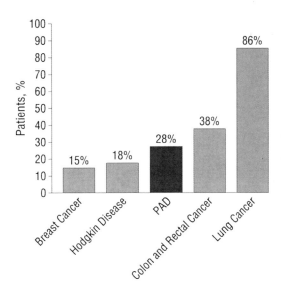

Fig. 3. The 5-year mortality rates for lower extremity arterial disease in comparison with malignancies *(41)*. PAD = Peripheral Artery Disease/lower extremity arterial disease (Reprinted with the permission of the American Medical Association).

rates for cardiovascular death, stroke, MI, or hospitalizations increasing from 5.31% in patients with risk factors only to 12.58, 21.14, and 26.27% in those with 1, 2, or 3 arterial beds being involved ($P<0.001$ for trend).

In individuals with carotid artery stenosis, the risk of stroke seems to increase with increasing degrees of stenosis and presence (increase risk) or absence (decreases risk) of symptoms. In one study, asymptomatic patients with carotid artery stenosis >75%, the annual incidence of stroke was reported to be 5.3%, and the combined rate of transient ischemic attacks and stroke was 10.5% and the rate of cardiac ischemia and vascular death was 9.9%. On the other hand, the annual incidence of stroke in individuals with carotid artery stenosis <75 was 1.3% *(42)*. In the North American Symptomatic Carotid Endarterectomy Trial (NASCET) study, which randomized symptomatic individuals with carotid artery stenosis to medical or surgical endarterectomy, in individuals with stenosis >70%, the cumulative risk of any ipsilateral stroke at two years was 26 and 9% in the medically and surgically treated patients, respectively, while the rates for a major or fatal ipsilateral stroke were 13.1 and 2.5%, respectively *(43)*. Similarly, the European Carotid Surgery study suggested that the Kaplan–Meier estimate of the frequency of a major stroke or death at 3 years was 26.5% in the medically managed group with >80% stenosis *(44)*. However, the Asymptomatic Carotid Atherosclerosis Study (ACAS) *(45)* recruited 1,662 asymptomatic individuals with ≥60% reduction in carotid artery diameter randomizing them to medical therapy or carotid endarterectomy, and at a median follow-up of 2.7 years, the overall rate of ipsilateral stroke, perioperative stroke, or death was 11.0% in the medically managed patients compared with 5.0% in the carotid endarterectomy patients. Other features that have been associated with increased risk of stroke include the presence of echolucent or heterogeneous plaques which are associated with increased lipid content, intra-plaque hemorrhage, and ulceration *(46)*.

Presence of renal artery stenosis has also been associated with increased risk of adverse events. In a series of ~4,000 individuals who were undergoing coronary angiography, the 4-year survival for those with renal artery stenosis was 57%, while for those without renal artery stenosis, it was 89%. The mortality was also noted to increase with increasing degree of renal artery stenosis, bilateral vs. unilateral renal artery stenosis (4-year survival 47 vs. 59% for bilateral and unilateral disease, respectively) and was found to be independent of the presence of CAD *(29, 47)*. There are insufficient data with respect to the cardiovascular outcomes in individuals with atherosclerosis of the abdominal arteries.

In summary, the presence of atherosclerosis in noncoronary vascular beds, whether it has become manifest or is subclinical, seems to be associated with a higher risk for the prevalence or incidence of CVD.

SCREENING FOR PAD

Given the association between the presence of subclinical atherosclerosis and CVD, screening for PAD, especially LEAD and carotid atherosclerosis, may have value.

Screening for LEAD can be easily achieved with an ankle brachial index (ABI). In simple terms, this describes the ratio of the ankle systolic pressure to the brachial systolic pressure. Briefly after a 10-min rest, the systolic blood pressure from both brachial arteries and from both the dorsalis pedis and posterior tibial arteries should be measured in a supine position. The higher right and left ankle pressure divided by the higher arm pressure will provide one with the ABI for the right and left side, respectively. An ABI <0.9 has been shown to have a sensitivity of 90% and specificity of 100% in the identification of LEAD when compared with angiography *(48)* and is far more sensitive than other routinely used screening tests such as pap smears, fecal occult blood testing, and mammography *(41)*. However, recent data has suggested that a "J-shaped" association exists between ABI and death with individuals in the "low normal" ABI or an ABI of 0.9–1.1. Those with ABI >1.4 also have higher cardiovascular mortality though not to the same degree as those with ABI <0.9 *(49)*. An ABI of 1.1–1.4 seems to identify those with the lowest risk for cardiovascular mortality. While it has been known that individuals with ABI >1.4 have a higher likelihood of noncompressible (i.e., calcified) vessels *(50, 51)* and are therefore more likely to have a higher prevalence of atherosclerosis, the group with ABI between 0.9 and 1.1 is more interesting. It is possible that several of these individuals have subclinical LEAD which may manifest only with exercise.

The appropriate population to screen for the presence of LEAD with ABI has been described. Individuals 49 years of age and younger with a history of diabetes and one other risk factor, 50–69 years of age with a history of smoking or diabetes, 70 years of age and older, those with an abnormal lower extremity pulse examination, and individuals with known atherosclerotic coronary, carotid, or renal artery disease seem to have the highest risk for the presence of LEAD. Although office-based measurements are not reimbursed at this time point, ABI measurements done in a vascular laboratory have procedural terminology codes available *(52)*. The American Diabetes Association in their consensus statement has endorsed the use of ABI to screen for LEAD in all individuals with diabetes who are aged 50 and older, in diabetic individuals younger than age 50 who have other atherosclerosis risk factors, and in individuals with diabetes of more than 10 years duration *(52)*.

SCREENING WITH CAROTID INTIMA MEDIA THICKNESS

The measurement of the carotid intima media thickness (C-IMT) is achieved through the performance of a carotid artery ultrasound examination, but the procedure is exacting and requires sonographers with experience. Ideally, the scan is performed at a depth of 4 cm in standardized angles of interrogation. The study should include sweeps of the common carotid artery, carotid bifurcation, and internal carotid artery for the presence or absence of plaque. Measurements may include mean and maximum, near and far wall (more reliable) IMT measurements of 1-cm segments of the common carotid, bulb, and internal carotid arteries of both the right and left carotid arteries. Recommended scanning protocols have been described in the American Society of Echocardiography consensus statement *(53)*.

The American Heart Association Prevention Conference V, in 2000, stated that C-IMT "can now be considered for further clarification of CHD risk assessment at the request of a physician," *(54)* while the National Cholesterol Education Program (NCEP) Adult Treatment Panel III guidelines *(55)* identified C-IMT as a potential marker for use as adjunct in CHD risk stratification. In all, ~7 guidelines have recommended the use of C-IMT as an adjunct in cardiovascular risk prediction *(53)*. The above recommendations were based on the consistent association seen between C-IMT and coronary heart disease in several studies. However, in a recent report, the US Preventive Task Force *(56)* recommended against the use of C-IMT in CHD risk prediction as they said that there was insufficient data, with respect to the ability of C-IMT, to reclassify risk, especially in the intermediate-risk groups. This has, however, been addressed in a subsequent paper which showed that adding C-IMT and plaque satisfied all statistical metrics required to show that a marker can improve risk prediction (*see* below) *(57)*.

The American Society of Echocardiography, in their consensus statement *(53)* suggested that C-IMT could be used to help in the stratification of CHD risk in intermediate-risk (6–20% estimated 10-year CHD risk) individuals and in those with family history of premature CVD (men <55 years age, women <65 years age) in a first-degree relative, individuals younger than 60 years old with significant abnormalities of a single risk factor who otherwise would not be candidates for pharmacotherapy or women younger than 60 years old with at least two cardiovascular risk factors. The United States Centers for Medicare and Medicaid has established a Current Procedural Terminology code (0126T) for C-IMT testing, but it must be noted that in general, insurance companies do not cover for this testing except in the state of Texas where recent legislation has identified groups in which insurance companies should cover for the testing.

IMPACT OF MEASURES OF LEAD AND CAROTID ATHEROSCLEROSIS IN CHD RISK PREDICTION

Both ABI and carotid atherosclerosis identify individuals at higher risk for incident coronary heart disease events. In a recent meta-analyses of 16 population-based studies which included 480,325 person-years of follow-up of 24,955 men and 23,339 women, the addition of ABI information to traditional risk factors reclassified risk in ~19% of the men and ~36% of women. Fowkes et al. *(49)* showed that the addition of ABI information to the Framingham risk score (FRS) increased the area under the receiver operator characteristics curve (AUC) from 0.646 (95% CI, 0.643–0.657) to 0.655 (95% CI, 0.643–0.666) in men and from 0.605 (95% CI, 0.590–0.619) to 0.658 (95% CI, 0.644–0.672) in women, respectively. Furthermore this study identified an ABI between 1.11 and 1.40 as the "normal" or reference value. Those with an ABI <0.9 (the current cut point for the diagnosis of LEAD) had the highest risk for incident cardiovascular events, while those with an ABI between 0.90 and 1.1 and those with an ABI >1.40 had a slightly higher risk than the reference group. Overall, it is thought that there is a 20–60% increase in risk of MI and a two- to sixfold increased risk of CHD death in individuals with LEAD *(33, 35–39)*. Similarly, LEAD has been associated with increased risk of stroke as well, although this relationship is weaker than the relationship with CHD *(31, 58)*. A graded association between LEAD severity and mortality has also been described *(33, 59)*. It is of no surprise that the majority of individuals with LEAD die from CHD (40–60%) or stroke (10–20%).

Similarly C-IMT and presence of carotid artery plaque have been associated with prevalent and incident CHD and stroke *(53, 60)*. In fact, the presence of plaque has been shown to be associated with CHD independent of C-IMT *(22, 61)*. In a recent analysis from the ARIC study, a sex-specific C-IMT >75th percentile and plaque information significantly improved CHD risk prediction when added to traditional risk factors *(57)*. Presence of a thicker C-IMT and plaque was associated with an increased incidence of coronary heart disease events in all traditional risk groups (0–5%, 5–10%, 10–20%, and >20% 10-year estimated risk). In all, it was reported that ~35–40% of individuals in the intermediate CHD risk group will be reclassified by adding C-IMT and plaque to traditional risk factors, and the net reclassification index was comparable to other markers that have been used as adjuncts in risk prediction such as C-reactive protein. A screening strategy based on the use of C-IMT and plaque in addition to traditional risk factors was found to be superior to one that used traditional risk factors alone.

Hence screening for the presence of subclinical vascular disease can significantly improve our ability to predict incident CVD. However, while identifying and treating these higher risk individuals by identifying presence of subclinical atherosclerosis sounds logical, the strategy has not been tested prospectively.

MANAGEMENT OF INDIVIDUALS WITH LEAD AND CAROTID ATHEROSCLEROSIS

Control of cardiovascular risk factors remains the key in the management of individuals with atherosclerosis of the peripheral arteries with a goal of preventing major adverse cardiovascular events. In the management of patients with LEAD, there are two aspects to consider: prevention of CHD and stroke and care of the diseased limb.

With respect to CVD prevention, individuals with LEAD are considered to be "coronary artery disease" risk equivalents and all therapies/goals that would be applicable in the care of individuals with CAD should be considered. Briefly, the low-density lipoprotein cholesterol (LDL-c) goal is <100 mg/dL, and this should be achieved with the use of a hydroxymethyl glutaryl (HMG) coenzyme-A reductase inhibitor (statin) medication if possible (Class I recommendation) and a LDL-c of <70 mg/dL is reasonable for patients at high risk for ischemic events (Class IIA recommendation). Incidentally, treatment with statins has also been shown to improve intermittent claudication and has been associated with a lesser 1-year decline in 6-min walk *(62–64)*. The blood pressure goals are similar to that for any other individual with a goal <140/90 mmHg for nondiabetics and <130/80 mmHg for patients with diabetes. Similarly the goal in the care of an individual with LEAD who has diabetes is similar to that of any other individual with diabetes with a goal hemoglobin A1C of <7%. Antiplatelet therapy with aspirin or clopidogrel (in the aspirin-intolerant individual) is also important in the prevention of cardiovascular events. Finally, smoking cessation is critical in the care of an individual with LEAD. For the treatment of claudication, exercise is the most important therapy. A supervised exercise program of at least 30–45 min for at least 3 times a week is recommended. Among medications that have been evaluated for use in the treatment of claudication, cilostazol, a phosphodiesterase type 3 inhibitor, is the only one that has reasonable evidence to show improvement in claudication symptoms and walking time. However, cilostazol should not be used in patients with congestive heart failure.

Lower extremity revascularization is primarily performed for limb salvage or symptom relief and is reviewed elsewhere in the textbook. However, an important aspect that must be considered is the potential impact of revascularization in the quality of life.

POTENTIAL ROLE OF REVASCULARIZATION IN IMPROVING THE QUALITY OF LIFE

Individuals with LEAD have increased rates of functional decline especially with respect to walking distances and time and physical activity levels as well as increased prevalence of depressive symptoms *(65–67)*. Although individuals with lower ABI clearly have more annual decreases in walking distances, even asymptomatic individuals with LEAD have a risk of functional decline when compared to those without LEAD *(65)*. Revascularization, if successful, can improve the functional ability of a given individual, and therefore is considered in those with lifestyle-limiting claudication. However, the risk of the procedure must always be weighed against the benefit. Furthermore, the durability of the benefit must also be considered. Studies comparing revascularization to exercise therapy have reported mixed results. In one study *(68)* which compared angioplasty with supervised exercise, angioplasty improved the ABI, but supervised exercise improved walking distance and claudication. In another study, however, angioplasty resulted at 6 months in significantly improved walking times, ABI, symptoms, and pain scores, but the improvement did not persist at 2 years *(69, 70)*. Angioplasty and surgical revascularization have been shown to be significantly better than conservative treatment when 18-month walking distance, functional status, and pain scores were evaluated in another prospective cohort study of 18 months *(71)*.

MANAGEMENT OF CAROTID ATHEROSCLEROSIS

Carotid artery stenosis >50% is considered to be a CAD risk equivalent and individuals with this degree of stenosis should be treated with goals as recommended for an individual with a high CHD risk. Although cholesterol levels are not as strong a risk factor for stroke as for CAD, statin therapy has also been shown to decrease strokes and hence is considered a first-line therapy in the prevention of stroke. In patients with carotid atherosclerosis, blood pressure, diabetes, smoking cessation, and weight targets are similar to that of all individuals without carotid stenosis. As far as LDL-c, a target of <100 mg/dL with an optional target of <70 mg/dL is recommended. With respect to revascularization, there are now two established options, namely, carotid endarterectomy and carotid artery stenting, and the indications/choice for each procedure is discussed elsewhere in this book.

Based on several randomized controlled trials *(43, 44)*, clear benefit with revascularization has been shown in individuals with symptomatic carotid stenosis. However, revascularization in the "asymptomatic" patient with carotid stenosis has been a little more controversial. The Veterans Administration Asymptomatic Carotid Stenosis Study *(72)* enrolled individuals with angiographic carotid stenosis >50% and reported that carotid endarterectomy resulted in significant decreases in ipsilateral strokes, transient ischemic attacks, and transient monocular blindness, but there was no significant differences when all strokes and death were considered. The Asymptomatic Carotid Atherosclerosis Study *(45)*, which enrolled individuals with carotid stenosis >60% reported that the risk of ipsilateral stroke, perioperative stroke, and death for patients with asymptomatic carotid stenosis was significantly decreased by carotid endarterectomy. Finally, the Asymptomatic Carotid Surgery Trial *(73)* evaluated individuals with carotid stenosis >60% who were asymptomatic for at least 6 months and reported significant reductions in stroke for the carotid endarterectomy group. However, it identified asymptomatic individuals with carotid stenosis >70% to benefit the most. Taken together, carotid endarterectomy is generally recommended for all symptomatic patients and those asymptomatic patients with stenosis >80%.

Table 1
Prevalence of antiplatelet and lipid lowering medication use in the REACH registry (27)

	Total (n = 67,888)	CAD (n = 40,258)	CVD (n = 18,843)	PAD (n = 8,273)	>3 risk factors (n = 12,389)
Antiplatelet therapy					
At least one antiplatelet therapy	78.6	85.6	81.8	81.7	53.9
Acetylsalicylic acid	67.4	76.2	62.1	62.5	49.8
Other antiplatelet agents	24.7	26.1	36.5	34.5	6.3
Any two antiplatelet agents	13.2	16.6	16.6	14.9	2.1
Lipid-lowering therapy					
At least one agent	75.2	80.9	61.3	70	81.3
Statin	69.4	76.2	56.4	64.2	71.6
Other lipid-lowering agents	12	12.2	9	11.5	16.1

CAD coronary artery disease; *CVD* cerebrovascular disease; *PAD* peripheral artery disease/lower extremity arterial disease (Reprinted with permission of the American Medical Association).

PERFORMANCE MEASURES

Although data clearly suggest that LEAD is associated with similar or higher risk of adverse cardiovascular events when compared to CAD or CVD, the perception or attention given to it is not the same. Several studies have documented physicians' under-recognition of the elevated risk in patients with PAD and consequent under-treatment of them (Table 1) *(74, 75)*.

McDermott et al. conducted a national physician survey to determine practice behavior among physicians with respect to PAD. Physicians (internists, family practitioners, cardiologists, and vascular surgeons) were randomized to one of three questionnaires that described a 55–65-year-old patient with PAD or CAD or no clinically evident atherosclerosis. Physicians were found to be less likely to prescribe antiplatelet therapy to LEAD patients when compared to CAD patients. Similarly, they reported that physicians felt that antiplatelet and lipid-lowering therapy was more important for CAD patients when compared to PAD patients *(75)*.

The PAD Awareness, Risk, and Treatment: New Resources for Survival (PARTNERS) program was a cross sectional multicity, multicenter study designed partly to evaluate patient and physician awareness of PAD and included 6,979 individuals. Interestingly, while 83% of patients with prevalent PAD were aware of their diagnosis, only 49% of their physicians were aware of the same. Hypertension and hyperlipidemia were treated less frequently in those with PAD and antiplatelet therapy prescribed less frequently when compared to those with CVD *(76)* (Table 2).

More recently, in the REACH registry *(77)*, patients with LEAD were shown to have significantly less control of all risk factors (systolic and diastolic blood pressure, smoking

Table 2
Prevalence of Atherosclerosis Risk Factors in the PARTNERS Survey (76)

| Variables | Reference Group | All atherosclerotic disease clinical groups ||||||| Reference groups vs. all atherosclerotic disease groups |
| | | PAD only ||| CVD only* | PAD and CVD ||| |
		New	Prior	P value		New PAD	Prior PAD	
Current and former smoking	1,499 (50)	274 (60)	235 (64)	0.25	816 (53)	215 (59)	449 (67)	<0.001
Proportion treated	607 (41)	146 (53)	120 (51)	0.62	288 (35)	78 (36)	188 (42)	0.66
Diabetes	1,025 (34)	150 (33)	161 (44)	0.001	572 (38)	155 (42)	304 (45)	<0.001
Proportion treated	874 (85)	122 (81)	137 (85)	0.38	467 (82)	128 (83)	257 (85)	0.10
Hyperlipidemia	1,672 (69)	243 (74)	225 (77)	0.38	1,059 (82)	264 (86)	482 (86)	<0.001
Proportion treated	714 (43)	106 (44)	127 (56)	0.006	768 (73)	174 (66)	366 (76)	<0.001
Hypertension	2,108 (70)	371 (81)	304 (83)	0.60	1315 (86)	335 (92)	618 (92)	<0.001
Proportion treated	1,772 (84)	312 (84)	267 (88)	0.17	1,244 (95)	325 (97)	594 (96)	<0.001
Postmenopausal	1,537 (87)	261 (89)	174 (86)	0.05	565 (91)	154 (89)	250 (90)	0.08
Proportion treated	612 (40)	88 (34)	58 (33)	0.98	187 (33)	36 (23)	73 (29)	<0.001
Antiplatelet medication use	1,043 (34)	151 (33)	199 (54)	<0.001	1076 (71)	263 (71)	510 (74)	<0.001

All values are expressed as numbers (percentages). The proportion treated represents the fraction of those with each risk factor who were receiving treatment for that risk factor (Reprinted with permission of the American Medical Association).

PAD peripheral artery disease/lower extremity arterial disease; CVD cardiovascular disease.

*$P<0.01$ for those with prior peripheral arterial disease (PAD) alone vs. those with cardiovascular disease (CVD) alone.

cessation, diabetes, and cholesterol) when compared to individuals without LEAD. In fact, there were very few patients (5%) with optimal control of all risk factors. Interestingly, it was patients with LEAD who had concomitant CAD, had a lower extremity angioplasty, or was under the care of a general practitioner, internist, or cardiologist who had better risk factor control. Patients with "LEAD only" were less likely to be on a statin (50.2 vs. 73%), ACE-inhibitor (33 vs. 49.4%), antiplatelet agent (76.3 vs. 84.6%), beta-blocker (22.8 vs. 51.3%), or an antidiabetic drug (34.5 vs. 42.8%) when compared to those with a polyvascular LEAD (i.e., LEAD+CAD and/or CVD). However, LEAD-only patients were more likely to get an anticlaudication medication (32.2 vs. 26.9%). Most importantly, the authors reported that good or improved risk factor control was associated with better outcomes when compared to those with poor risk factor control.

There may be several factors associated with this under-recognition and under-treatment of LEAD, including physician or patient lack of knowledge. In one study, McDermott et al. reported that compared to individuals without any manifest atherosclerosis and individuals with CAD, patients with LEAD underestimated the high risk of adverse cardiovascular events associated with LEAD, and in fact, all three groups of individuals (normal controls, individuals with CAD, and individuals with LEAD) felt that the risk for MI, stroke, or death was higher for an individual with CAD when compared to those with LEAD *(78)*. Another potential contributor is that patients with LEAD are more frequently referred to vascular surgeons who are not as comfortable in managing traditional atherosclerotic risk factors and that the primary care physicians do not follow up on the same. Furthermore, it is possible that physicians do not recognize that LEAD is associated with worse outcomes. Whatever the cause may be, it is clear that physicians need to perform significantly better in the care of individuals with LEAD.

SUMMARY

Atherosclerosis of noncoronary arteries receives less attention in general than atherosclerosis of the coronary arteries, yet it is of considerable importance. There is clear evidence to suggest that the concomitant presence of atherosclerosis of multiple arteries significantly worsens outcomes. LEAD is most frequently associated with atherosclerosis in other arterial beds. However, the risk associated with having peripheral artery disease is under-appreciated by both patient and physician. Identification of subclinical atherosclerosis and early identification of at-risk patients will likely be critical in implementing preventive strategies and improving quality of life in patients with atherosclerosis involving noncoronary arterial beds, though such a strategy does need to be validated prospectively.

REFERENCES

1. Criqui MH, Fronek A, Barrett-Connor E, Klauber MR, Gabriel S, Goodman D. The prevalence of peripheral arterial disease in a defined population. *Circulation.* 1985;71:510–515.
2. Hiatt WR, Hoag S, Hamman RF. Effect of diagnostic criteria on the prevalence of peripheral arterial disease. The San Luis Valley Diabetes Study. *Circulation.* 1995;91:1472–1479.
3. Selvin E, Erlinger TP. Prevalence of and risk factors for peripheral arterial disease in the United States: results from the National Health and Nutrition Examination Survey, 1999–2000. *Circulation.* 2004;110:738–743.

4. Norgren L, Hiatt WR, Dormandy JA, Nehler MR, Harris KA, Fowkes FG. Inter-Society Consensus for the Management of Peripheral Arterial Disease (TASC II). *J Vasc Surg.* 2007;45(Suppl S):S5-S67.
5. Hollier LH, Bernatz PE, Pairolero PC, Payne WS, Osmundson PJ. Surgical management of chronic intestinal ischemia: a reappraisal. *Surgery.* 1981;90:940–946.
6. Johnston KW, Lindsay TF, Walker PM, Kalman PG. Mesenteric arterial bypass grafts: early and late results and suggested surgical approach for chronic and acute mesenteric ischemia. *Surgery.* 1995;118:1–7.
7. Hansen KJ, Edwards MS, Craven TE, et al. Prevalence of renovascular disease in the elderly: a population-based study. *J Vasc Surg.* 2002;36:443–451.
8. Harding MB, Smith LR, Himmelstein SI, et al. Renal artery stenosis: prevalence and associated risk factors in patients undergoing routine cardiac catheterization. *J Am Soc Nephrol.* 1992;2:1608–1616.
9. Weber-Mzell D, Kotanko P, Schumacher M, Klein W, Skrabal F. Coronary anatomy predicts presence or absence of renal artery stenosis. A prospective study in patients undergoing cardiac catheterization for suspected coronary artery disease. *Eur Heart J.* 2002;23:1684–1691.
10. Jean WJ, al-Bitar I, Zwicke DL, Port SC, Schmidt DH, Bajwa TK. High incidence of renal artery stenosis in patients with coronary artery disease. *Cathet Cardiovasc Diagn.* 1994;32:8–10.
11. Wilms G, Marchal G, Peene P, Baert AL. The angiographic incidence of renal artery stenosis in the arteriosclerotic population. *Eur J Radiol.* 1990;10:195–197.
12. Choudhri AH, Cleland JG, Rowlands PC, Tran TL, McCarty M, Al-Kutoubi MA. Unsuspected renal artery stenosis in peripheral vascular disease. *BMJ.* 1990;301:1197–1198.
13. Swartbol P, Thorvinger BO, Parsson H, Norgren L. Renal artery stenosis in patients with peripheral vascular disease and its correlation to hypertension. A retrospective study. *Int Angiol.* 1992;11:195–199.
14. Missouris CG, Papavassiliou MB, Khaw K, et al. High prevalence of carotid artery disease in patients with atheromatous renal artery stenosis. *Nephrol Dial Transplant.* 1998;13:945–948.
15. Missouris CG, Buckenham T, Cappuccio FP, MacGregor GA. Renal artery stenosis: a common and important problem in patients with peripheral vascular disease. *Am J Med.* 1994;96:10–14.
16. Olin JW, Melia M, Young JR, Graor RA, Risius B. Prevalence of atherosclerotic renal artery stenosis in patients with atherosclerosis elsewhere. *Am J Med.* 1990;88:46 N-51 N.
17. Louie J, Isaacson JA, Zierler RE, Bergelin RO, Strandness DE Jr. Prevalence of carotid and lower extremity arterial disease in patients with renal artery stenosis. *Am J Hypertens.* 1994;7:436–439.
18. Zierler RE, Bergelin RO, Polissar NL, et al. Carotid and lower extremity arterial disease in patients with renal artery atherosclerosis. *Arch Intern Med.* 1998;158:761–767.
19. Rossi GP, Rossi A, Zanin L, et al. Excess prevalence of extracranial carotid artery lesions in renovascular hypertension. *Am J Hypertens.* 1992;5:8–15.
20. Metcalfe W, Reid AW, Geddes CC. Prevalence of angiographic atherosclerotic renal artery disease and its relationship to the anatomical extent of peripheral vascular atherosclerosis. *Nephrol Dial Transplant.* 1999;14:105–108.
21. Valentine RJ, Clagett GP, Miller GL, Myers SI, Martin JD, Chervu A. The coronary risk of unsuspected renal artery stenosis. *J Vasc Surg.* 1993;18:433–439; discussion 439–440.
22. Hunt KJ, Sharrett AR, Chambless LE, Folsom AR, Evans GW, Heiss G. Acoustic shadowing on B-mode ultrasound of the carotid artery predicts CHD. *Ultrasound Med Biol.* 2001;27:357–365.
23. Li R, Duncan BB, Metcalf PA, et al. B-mode-detected carotid artery plaque in a general population. Atherosclerosis Risk in Communities (ARIC) Study Investigators. *Stroke.* 1994;25:2377–2383.
24. van der Meer IM, Bots ML, Hofman A, del Sol AI, van der Kuip DA, Witteman JC. Predictive value of noninvasive measures of atherosclerosis for incident myocardial infarction: the Rotterdam Study. *Circulation.* 2004;109:1089–1094.
25. de Weerd M, Greving JP, de Jong AW, Buskens E, Bots ML. Prevalence of asymptomatic carotid artery stenosis according to age and sex: systematic review and metaregression analysis. *Stroke.* 2009;40:1105–1113.
26. Kurvers HA, van der Graaf Y, Blankensteijn JD, Visseren FL, Eikelboom BC. Screening for asymptomatic internal carotid artery stenosis and aneurysm of the abdominal aorta: comparing the yield between patients with manifest atherosclerosis and patients with risk factors for atherosclerosis only. *J Vasc Surg.* 2003;37:1226–1233.

27. Bhatt DL, Steg PG, Ohman EM, et al. International prevalence, recognition, and treatment of cardiovascular risk factors in outpatients with atherothrombosis. *JAMA.* 2006;295:180–189.
28. Steg PG, Bhatt DL, Wilson PW, et al. One-year cardiovascular event rates in outpatients with atherothrombosis. *JAMA.* 2007;297:1197–1206.
29. Hirsch AT, Haskal ZJ, Hertzer NR, et al. ACC/AHA 2005 Practice Guidelines for the management of patients with peripheral arterial disease (lower extremity, renal, mesenteric, and abdominal aortic): a collaborative report from the American Association for Vascular Surgery/Society for Vascular Surgery, Society for Cardiovascular Angiography and Interventions, Society for Vascular Medicine and Biology, Society of Interventional Radiology, and the ACC/AHA Task Force on Practice Guidelines (Writing Committee to Develop Guidelines for the Management of Patients With Peripheral Arterial Disease): endorsed by the American Association of Cardiovascular and Pulmonary Rehabilitation; National Heart, Lung, and Blood Institute; Society for Vascular Nursing; TransAtlantic Inter-Society Consensus; and Vascular Disease Foundation. *Circulation.* 2006;113:e463-e654.
30. Hertzer NR, Beven EG, Young JR, et al. Coronary artery disease in peripheral vascular patients: a classification of 1000 coronary angiograms and results of surgical management. *Ann Surg.* 1984;199:223–233.
31. Golomb BA, Dang TT, Criqui MH. Peripheral arterial disease: morbidity and mortality implications. *Circulation.* 2006;114:688–699.
32. Howell MA, Colgan MP, Seeger RW, Ramsey DE, Sumner DS. Relationship of severity of lower limb peripheral vascular disease to mortality and morbidity: a six-year follow-up study. *J Vasc Surg.* 1989;9:691–696; discussion 696–697.
33. Criqui MH, Langer RD, Fronek A, et al. Mortality over a period of 10 years in patients with peripheral arterial disease. *N Engl J Med.* 1992;326:381–386.
34. McKenna M, Wolfson S, Kuller L. The ratio of ankle and arm arterial pressure as an independent predictor of mortality. *Atherosclerosis.* 1991;87:119–128.
35. Smith GD, Shipley MJ, Rose G. Intermittent claudication, heart disease risk factors, and mortality. The Whitehall Study. *Circulation.* 1990;82:1925–1931.
36. Leng GC, Lee AJ, Fowkes FG, et al. Incidence, natural history and cardiovascular events in symptomatic and asymptomatic peripheral arterial disease in the general population. *Int J Epidemiol.* 1996;25:1172–1181.
37. Kornitzer M, Dramaix M, Sobolski J, Degre S, De Backer G. Ankle/arm pressure index in asymptomatic middle-aged males: an independent predictor of ten-year coronary heart disease mortality. *Angiology.* 1995;46:211–219.
38. Newman AB, Sutton-Tyrrell K, Vogt MT, Kuller LH. Morbidity and mortality in hypertensive adults with a low ankle/arm blood pressure index. *JAMA.* 1993;270:487–489.
39. Vogt MT, Cauley JA, Newman AB, Kuller LH, Hulley SB. Decreased ankle/arm blood pressure index and mortality in elderly women. *JAMA.* 1993;270:465–469.
40. Zheng ZJ, Sharrett AR, Chambless LE, et al. Associations of ankle-brachial index with clinical coronary heart disease, stroke and preclinical carotid and popliteal atherosclerosis: the Atherosclerosis Risk in Communities (ARIC) Study. *Atherosclerosis.* 1997;131:115–125.
41. Belch JJ, Topol EJ, Agnelli G, et al. Prevention of Atherothrombotic Disease Network. Critical issues in peripheral arterial disease detection and management: a call to action. *Arch Intern Med.* 2003;163:884–892.
42. Chambers BR, Norris JW. Outcome in patients with asymptomatic neck bruits. *N Engl J Med.* 1986;315:860–865.
43. North American Symptomatic Carotid Endarterectomy Trial Collaborators. Beneficial effect of carotid endarterectomy in symptomatic patients with high-grade carotid stenosis.. *N Engl J Med.* 1991;325:445–453.
44. MRC European Carotid Surgery Trial (ECST). Randomised trial of endarterectomy for recently symptomatic carotid stenosis: final results of the MRC European Carotid Surgery Trial (ECST). *Lancet.* 1998;351:1379–1387.
45. Executive Committee for the Asymptomatic Carotid Atherosclerosis Study. Endarterectomy for asymptomatic carotid artery stenosis. *JAMA.* 1995;273:1421–1428.

46. Moore WS, Barnett HJ, Beebe HG, et al. Guidelines for carotid endarterectomy. A multidisciplinary consensus statement from the Ad Hoc Committee, American Heart Association. *Circulation.* 1995;91:566–579.
47. Eisele B, Bates SR, Wissler RW. Interaction of low density lipoproteins from normal and hyperlipemic rhesus monkeys with arterial smooth muscle cells in culture. *Atherosclerosis.* 1980;36:9–24.
48. Fowkes FG. The measurement of atherosclerotic peripheral arterial disease in epidemiological surveys. *Int J Epidemiol.* 1988;17:248–254.
49. Fowkes FG, Murray GD, Butcher I, et al. Ankle brachial index combined with Framingham Risk Score to predict cardiovascular events and mortality: a meta-analysis. *JAMA.* 2008;300:197–208.
50. Everhart JE, Pettitt DJ, Knowler WC, Rose FA, Bennett PH. Medial arterial calcification and its association with mortality and complications of diabetes. *Diabetologia.* 1988;31:16–23.
51. McDermott MM. The magnitude of the problem of peripheral arterial disease: epidemiology and clinical significance. *Cleve Clin J Med.* 2006;73 Suppl 4:S2-S7.
52. American Diabetes Association Consensus Group. Peripheral arterial disease in people with diabetes. *Diabetes Care.* 2003;26:3333–3341.
53. Stein JH, Korcarz CE, Hurst RT, et al. Use of carotid ultrasound to identify subclinical vascular disease and evaluate cardiovascular disease risk: a consensus statement from the American Society of Echocardiography Carotid Intima-Media Thickness Task Force. Endorsed by the Society for Vascular Medicine. *J Am Soc Echocardiogr.* 2008;21:93–111; quiz 189–190.
54. Greenland P, Abrams J, Aurigemma GP, et al. Prevention Conference V: beyond secondary prevention: identifying the high-risk patient for primary prevention: noninvasive tests of atherosclerotic burden. *Circulation.* 2000;101:e16-e22.
55. National Cholesterol Education Program. Third Report of the National Cholesterol Education Program (NCEP) Expert Panel on Detection, Evaluation, and Treatment of High Blood Cholesterol in Adults (Adult Treatment Panel III) final report. *Circulation.* 2002;106:3143–3421.
56. Helfand M, Buckley DI, Freeman M, et al. Emerging risk factors for coronary heart disease: a summary of systematic reviews conducted for the U.S. Preventive Services Task Force. *Ann Intern Med.* 2009;151:496–507.
57. Nambi V, Chambless L, Folsom AR, et al. Carotid intima-media thickness and presence or absence of plaque improves prediction of coronary heart disease risk: the ARIC (Atherosclerosis Risk In Communities) study. *J Am Coll Cardiol.*55:1600–1607.
58. Leng GC, Fowkes FG, Lee AJ, Dunbar J, Housley E, Ruckley CV. Use of ankle brachial pressure index to predict cardiovascular events and death: a cohort study. *BMJ.* 1996;313:1440–1444.
59. McDermott MM, Feinglass J, Slavensky R, Pearce WH. The ankle-brachial index as a predictor of survival in patients with peripheral vascular disease. *J Gen Intern Med.* 1994;9:445–449.
60. O'Leary DH, Polak JF, Kronmal RA, Manolio TA, Burke GL, Wolfson SK Jr. Cardiovascular Health Study Collaborative Research Group. Carotid-artery intima and media thickness as a risk factor for myocardial infarction and stroke in older adults. *N Engl J Med.* 1999;340:14–22.
61. Wyman RA, Mays ME, McBride PE, Stein JH. Ultrasound-detected carotid plaque as a predictor of cardiovascular events. *Vasc Med.* 2006;11:123–130.
62. Pedersen TR, Kjekshus J, Pyorala K, et al. Effect of simvastatin on ischemic signs and symptoms in the Scandinavian simvastatin survival study (4 S). *Am J Cardiol.* 1998;81:333–335.
63. Mohler ER 3 rd, Hiatt WR, Creager MA. Cholesterol reduction with atorvastatin improves walking distance in patients with peripheral arterial disease. *Circulation.* 2003;108:1481–1486.
64. Giri J, McDermott MM, Greenland P, et al. Statin use and functional decline in patients with and without peripheral arterial disease. *J Am Coll Cardiol.* 2006;47:998–1004.
65. McDermott MM, Liu K, Greenland P, et al. Functional decline in peripheral arterial disease: associations with the ankle brachial index and leg symptoms. *JAMA.* 2004;292:453–461.
66. McDermott MM, Greenland P, Liu K, et al. The ankle brachial index is associated with leg function and physical activity: the Walking and Leg Circulation Study. *Ann Intern Med.* 2002;136:873–883.
67. Arseven A, Guralnik JM, O'Brien E, Liu K, McDermott MM. Peripheral arterial disease and depressed mood in older men and women. *Vasc Med.* 2001;6:229–234.

68. Perkins JM, Collin J, Creasy TS, Fletcher EW, Morris PJ. Exercise training versus angioplasty for stable claudication. Long and medium term results of a prospective, randomised trial. *Eur J Vasc Endovasc Surg.* 1996;11:409–413.
69. Whyman MR, Fowkes FG, Kerracher EM,et al. Randomised controlled trial of percutaneous transluminal angioplasty for intermittent claudication. *Eur J Vasc Endovasc Surg.* 1996;12:167–172.
70. Whyman MR, Fowkes FG, Kerracher EM, et al. Is intermittent claudication improved by percutaneous transluminal angioplasty? A randomized controlled trial. *J Vasc Surg.* 1997;26:551–557.
71. Feinglass J, McCarthy WJ, Slavensky R, Manheim LM, Martin GJ. Functional status and walking ability after lower extremity bypass grafting or angioplasty for intermittent claudication: results from a prospective outcomes study. *J Vasc Surg.* 2000;31:93–103.
72. Hobson RW 2nd, Weiss DG, Fields WS, et al. Efficacy of carotid endarterectomy for asymptomatic carotid stenosis. The Veterans Affairs Cooperative Study Group. *N Engl J Med.* 1993;328:221–227.
73. Halliday A, Mansfield A, Marro J, et al. Prevention of disabling and fatal strokes by successful carotid endarterectomy in patients without recent neurological symptoms: randomised controlled trial. *Lancet.* 2004;363:1491–1502.
74. Anand SS, Kundi A, Eikelboom J, Yusuf S. Low rates of preventive practices in patients with peripheral vascular disease. *Can J Cardiol.* 1999;15:1259–1263.
75. McDermott MM, Hahn EA, Greenland P, et al. Atherosclerotic risk factor reduction in peripheral arterial disease: results of a national physician survey. *J Gen Intern Med.* 2002;17:895–904.
76. Hirsch AT, Criqui MH, Treat-Jacobson D, et al. Peripheral arterial disease detection, awareness, and treatment in primary care. *JAMA.* 2001;286:1317–1324.
77. Cacoub PP, Abola MT, Baumgartner I, et al. Cardiovascular risk factor control and outcomes in peripheral artery disease patients in the Reduction of Atherothrombosis for Continued Health (REACH) Registry. *Atherosclerosis.* 2009;204:e86-e92.
78. McDermott MM, Mandapat AL, Moates A, et al. Knowledge and attitudes regarding cardiovascular disease risk and prevention in patients with coronary or peripheral arterial disease. *Arch Intern Med.* 2003;163:2157–2162.

2 Lower Extremity Intervention

Samir K. Shah, MD, *and Daniel G. Clair,* MD

CONTENTS

INTRODUCTION
INDICATIONS
ROLE OF SCREENING TESTS: WHEN ARE THEY APPROPRIATE AND IN WHOM?
CONTRAINDICATIONS
TECHNIQUES
REFERENCES

INTRODUCTION

It is significant that nearly 40 years after the introduction of angioplasty by Dotter and Judkins and ultimate streamlining of the procedure through the introduction of the angioplasty balloon by Gruentzig, that this form of treatment remains the mainstay of therapy for patients with peripheral occlusive disease affecting the aortoiliac and superficial femoral segments *(1, 2)*. In the interim, since these initial reports, numerous interventional therapies have been introduced to try and improve upon the effects of angioplasty. None of these technologies have proven effective in completely eradicating recurrent disease in these vessels. Significant advances have been made with the introduction of stents *(3–5)*, atherectomy, and manipulations of the angioplasty balloon to try and improve its efficacy. While we are clearly making progress in terms of the minimally invasive treatment of occlusive disease of the lower extremity, much needs to be done in order to enhance the effectiveness of these less morbid procedures. In the current setting, there remains a significant role for bypass surgery as a method of treatment for patients with occlusive disease as well. It is important for the interventionalist not only to understand the benefits and roles of all of the interventional options available to treat lower extremity occlusive disease, but to also understand when surgical treatment of this disease would provide a better option for the patient. Because of the investigations into alternative therapies for treating these patients, it is likely that there will be continued change over the next several years in terms of options available to patients.

From: *Peripheral and Cerebrovascular Intervention*, Contemporary Cardiology
Edited by: D. L. Bhatt, DOI 10.1007/978-1-60327-965-9_2
© Springer Science+Business Media, LLC 2012

Table 1
Therapies for Patients with Peripheral Arterial Disease

Smoking cessation
Weight reduction
Regular exercise program
Antiplatelet therapy
Lipid lowering agents
   Primarily statin therapy
Diabetes management
Blood pressure control
   ACE inhibitor therapy
Cilostazol
Percutaneous revascularization
Surgical revascularization

Hopefully these options will be critically assessed with randomized trials so that evidence-based decisions can be made regarding treatments for patients with peripheral occlusive disease (Table 1).

INDICATIONS

Indications for lower extremity intervention have not changed dramatically since the introduction of angioplasty for the treatment of occlusive disease. These indications are normally broken down into two different classification: those patients with disabling claudation and those with critical limb ischemia. The definition of disabling claudication varies widely among physicians caring for these patients, but it is more often based upon patients' impressions of their levels of disability and walking limitations. Claudication, simply put, is pain upon walking. It can have a vascular cause or in some situations other causes. Walking normally leads to an increase in oxygen demand in the muscles of the lower extremity. In normal individuals, the flow of blood increases as the need for oxygen increases. In patients with peripheral arterial disease, the ability of the flow to increase is limited because of fixed stenosis or occlusion in the blood vessels. In these individuals, the oxygen demand outstrips the blood supply. The lack of adequate oxygen supply leads to carbohydrate metabolism along anaerobic pathways leading to the production of lactic acid. The buildup of lactic acid in the muscle tissue leads to pain and ultimately, muscle failure. The patient may feel this as pain, cramping, or simply may label it fatigue. Even with normal blood pressure in the ankle at rest an individual may be unable to increase blood flow adequately during demand leading to claudication. The best test to assess for the presence of vascular disease as a cause of claudication is the exercise treadmill test with ankle-brachial pressure measurements. This test will reveal whether the patient's blood vessels in the lower extremity are able to accommodate to increase the amount of blood flow needed by the muscles of the lower extremity. In the setting in which the blood flow is fixed by the extent of disease above a dilated vascular bed, the pressure below the fixed defect will drop and the ankle-brachial index will fall with exercise. This is an important method of distinguishing vasculogenic from nonvasculogenic causes of claudication.

Critical limb ischemia refers to the situation where the ischemic threat to a patient's limb is such that the risk for limb loss is significant. Patients will either report rest pain or may have tissue loss or even gangrene of a portion of the foot. These patients will have such severe limitation of the arterial flow to the foot that the decrease in pressure generated by elevating the foot at night may be enough to lead to inadequate tissue oxygenation and subsequent lactic acidosis and pain. Often, the patient with rest pain will find relief in leaving the foot dependent. It is for this reason that some individuals with rest pain will present with significant edema, complicating the initial evaluation. For these patients, any small injury to the foot or overgrowth of fungus between the toes can lead to an infected wound and ultimately the risk of limb loss. For those patients with a wound on the foot and an ankle-brachial index below 0.4, the diagnosis of critical limb ischemia must be made. Often however, the patient will not have meaningful pressures at the ankle because of severe vascular calcification. In this situation additional testing with toe pressures or pulse volume recordings will be necessary to make the diagnosis. Patients with critical limb ischemia generally benefit from revascularization.

Therapy for the Patient with Peripheral Arterial Disease

It is important to remember that in the majority of patients with claudication in general, the progression of disease is slow and the likelihood of ultimately needing amputation is extremely small *(6, 7)*. While over the long run, these patients can develop ischemic rest pain and ischemic ulceration, there is no evidence that withholding early intervention precludes later revascularization. It is also important to remember that in these patient populations, the largest risk to the patient derives from the likelihood of systemic vascular events (e.g., myocardial infarction) and the development of malignancy *(6–8)*. As such, medical therapy for these patients must include aggressive intervention to lower their overall cardiovascular risk.

There is clear evidence that smoking cessation should be pursued aggressively in these patients to reduce the progression of their claudication and peripheral arterial disease as well as to reduce the overall risks to their health in terms of cardiovascular complications from atherosclerotic vascular disease *(9, 10)*. Whether or not the patient receives intervention, smoking cessation should be a significant part of the treatment of these patients. Beyond smoking cessation, patients should also be counseled regarding the benefits of weight reduction and regular exercise. The benefits of weight reduction include a reduction in the incidence and progression of diabetic disease and complications as well as a lower overall mortality from cardiovascular diseases *(11, 12)*.

In multiple studies, regular exercise has been proven to improve overall walking distance and pain free walking distance *(13, 14)*. In addition to improving walking ability, there is evidence that regular exercise, especially when supervised, may be helpful in improving the cardiovascular risk profile of individuals undergoing this form of therapy *(15)*

In addition to these lifestyle modifications, which can benefit patients, there is significant evidence that basic medical therapy should accompany any form of treatment of patients with peripheral arterial disease. The primary medications that should be utilized in treating these patients include some form of antiplatelet therapy, medication for cholesterol level modification and lipid lowering, aggressive therapy for control of diabetes and hypertension, along with the potential for pharmacologic therapies to improve walking distance. Of these varying therapies, the least likely to result in long-term health benefit is the medical therapy for claudication itself. For this reason, the associated medical therapies of antiplatelet treatment, diabetes and hypertension management and lipid modification, should remain as a primary form of therapy in all patients with peripheral vascular disease. The evidence for aspirin or at least some form of antiplatelet therapy has been well documented in multiple studies *(16, 17)*. While there is some evidence that clopidogrel may offer improved risk reduction in these patients it is clear that at least some form of antiplatelet therapy should be incorporated as part of the treatment of these patients *(18)*.

Diabetes in and of itself confers a markedly increased risk of developing claudication and the complications of peripheral arterial disease *(19–22)*. In those patients with diabetes, aggressive glycemic treatment has been shown to reduce diabetes-related complications. While this treatment did not result in a lowering of the risk of amputation from peripheral arterial disease, there is clearly systemic benefit in the aggressive treatment of a patient's diabetes and this should be pursued in patients with peripheral arterial disease *(23)*. As with diabetes, hypertension is associated with at least a two to threefold increased risk of atherosclerotic disease progression *(24)*. These patients with hypertension are also at significantly increased risk for progression of their PAD to that of a symptomatic stage with claudication *(19, 25, 26)*. While there is no direct evidence comparing aggressive management of hypertension in patients with peripheral arterial disease to a more lax approach to this problem, consensus still maintains that more aggressive management of blood pressure and hypertension is warranted in these patients to reduce atherosclerotic progression and overall occurrence of cardiovascular end points *(26)*. In terms of choices of therapies to treat the hypertension, there is no evidence that beta-blockers worsen claudication and these agents can be used when indicated in treating patients with hypertension; however, angiotensin converting enzyme inhibitors (ACE inhibitors) are a more appealing initial therapy in patients with peripheral arterial disease *(27)*. These agents have been shown to reduce atherosclerotic progression beyond that created solely by an antihypertensive effect and function with diminished cardiovascular complications *(28–30)*.

There is no direct evidence that aggressive lipid management in patients with peripheral arterial disease alone affects cardiovascular morbidity and mortality. Despite this, there is significant evidence that in patients with coronary artery disease, aggressive management of lipids has significant beneficial effect in cardiovascular risk reduction and reduction in symptomatic atherosclerotic disease progression *(31–33)*. There appears to be the potential for these lipid lowering agents to also have an effect on walking speed and distance as well as a lower rate of annual decline in walking ability *(34, 35)*. All of this evidence favors an aggressive posture in dealing with the management of patients with peripheral arterial disease.

All of these medical interventions should be part of the treatment plan for patients with identified peripheral arterial disease. Once the patient becomes symptomatic, however, decisions need to be made regarding potential interventions to improve the functional status or perhaps even the limb retention of the patient in question. For those patients with claudication, an exercise regimen, especially when performed in a supervised setting, can have a more significant impact than any medical therapy that has been developed to date *(13, 36)*. There are clearly benefits to pharmacologic therapies for treatment of claudication. Both pentoxifylline and cilostazol have shown benefit in randomized placebo controlled trials *(37–43)*. The benefits of these medical therapies, however, are limited. Pentoxifylline, while it has shown overall a benefit when compared with placebo, achieves limited benefit at best. Patients will not have tremendous improvement in their walking abilities with pentoxifylline alone. Cilostazol also, has shown the capacity to improve walking ability and, in one of the largest studies performed to date on this drug, the increase in walking ability was only twice that achieved with placebo given in randomized fashion to affected patients *(39)*.

Because medical therapies have proven extremely limited in treatment of patients with claudication, many patients and physicians have looked to interventional therapies to improve functional status and walking ability with revascularization techniques.

Unfortunately, there is little meaningful evidence upon which to base decision making regarding revascularization. Randomized trials comparing angioplasty with medical therapy have shown conflicting results *(44–49)*. Because of the confusing results of these trials which partly relates to the difficulties in performing this type of randomized trial, it is important in the long run to have additional data comparing the outcomes of the best medical therapy, which should include an exercise regimen, to best medical therapy with an exercise regimen and some form of revascularization procedure. In order to determine what to do with patients suffering from claudication, in each individual case, the physician will need to weigh the risks and benefits of intervention when compared with the disability caused by the peripheral arterial disease. The more significant the disability, the more likely the patient is to push the physician in the direction of interventional therapy. Additionally, for these extremely limited patients, the ability to even perform regular exercise is difficult at best. For those patients with mild claudication, initial attempts at medical therapy with an exercise regimen should be incorporated as the frontline of therapy. Failure of the medical regimen with progression of their symptoms may prompt an aggressive posture towards revascularization of the lower extremities. Conversely, in patients with severe limitation from their vascular disease, an earlier move to revascularization would be warranted not only to improve the symptoms for the patient, but to also allow the patient to begin an exercise regimen as part of their overall health maintenance.

For those patients with critical limb ischemia, which includes the patient with rest pain or tissue loss related to ischemia, there is no question that revascularization techniques have benefit in reducing the risks related to limb loss *(50–53)*. Primary amputation without revascularization in this population ranges from 10 to 40% over 6 months after the initial identification of ischemic tissue loss *(51, 52)*. It is particularly notable that in those patients with more limited flow to the foot, the amputation rates are exceedingly high. In addition, these patients carry significant risk of mortality with mortality rates from 10 to 30% per year *(51, 52)*. In these patients, the choice between percutaneous revascularization and surgical revascularization has also not been answered *(54)*. The results of the only randomized clinical trial comparing bypass with angioplasty, the BASIL trial, seem to be somewhat ambiguous *(55)*. When the outcomes were assessed at 2 years after randomization, there appeared to be no difference between an interventional first versus a bypass first revascularization strategy. Beyond this 2-year point, there appeared to be a benefit for those patients who underwent open bypass revascularization as the initial method of therapy. There are flaws with this trial that limit its applicability to the general population with critical limb ischemia. These problems include the large number of patients who were evaluated but did not meet the criteria, as well as varying definitions of suitability for interventional and surgical therapies. Furthermore, the authors examined patients with "severe leg ischemia" in contrast to critical limb ischemia, which is often more clearly defined in the literature. They did not provide any objective information regarding degree of limb ischemia such as ankle-brachial index, toe or ankle pressure, and transcutaneous oximetry. As such, the authors failed to distinguish different outcomes in the spectrum of patients that exists within the category of severe limb ischemia. For instance, although the authors did demonstrate that there was no difference in the number of patients with ankle pressures above and below 50 mmHg between the two arms, each group was individually inadequately powered. It is likely that patients with relatively higher ankle pressure may behave differently clinically in terms of overall survival and amputation-free survival, two of the primary endpoints, from those with lower pressures but the BASIL trial does not allow us to draw any easily translatable conclusions. With this said, it is fairly clear that in patients that have high risk for surgical revascularization either for medical reasons such as underlying cardiac or pulmonary disease, or for those patients who have high risk due to complicated surgical revascularization such as those patients with inadequate venous conduits, poor distal targets, and significant wound problems which would expose the bypass graft to infection, percutaneous intervention offers a reasonable initial attempt to revascularize the foot and save the limb. In fact, in many situations where surgical revascularization provides a viable option for limb salvage, percutaneous therapy may be a reasonable initial maneuver with surgical bypass reserved for those patients who fail this strategy. Until more information is collected regarding those patients who would benefit from surgical revascularization versus those who would benefit from percutaneous revascularization, the decision making will be in the hands of the physician caring for these patients. A thorough understanding of the risks and benefits associated with each form of therapy is necessary in order to make an educated decision regarding the strategy to treat each patient.

ROLE OF SCREENING TESTS: WHEN ARE THEY APPROPRIATE AND IN WHOM?

Routing screening for asymptomatic peripheral arterial disease in the general population has not proven to be cost effective and, in fact, the US Preventive Services Task Force guidelines have not recommended routine screening for peripheral arterial disease and intermittent claudication *(56, 57)*. Briefly, the task force does not recommend screening with even an ankle-brachial index to detect asymptomatic peripheral arterial disease. These recommendations are based upon the potential harms of screening that include false positive results and adverse events associated with a more aggressive diagnostic work-up including angiography and the potential contrast and intervention related complications, which could ensue. Despite this, there are at least two well-performed screening studies that assessed the feasibility of detecting peripheral arterial disease and the intensity of risk factor treatment in those patients who were identified to have peripheral arterial disease during these screening evaluations *(58, 59)*. In both of these studies, a significant percentage of the patients were identified as having undocumented asymptomatic peripheral arterial disease, and notably in this extremely high-risk group of patients, few were receiving appropriate therapy in terms of antiplatelet therapy, adequate blood pressure control, cholesterol modification, and estrogen replacement therapy. As our population ages, the need for aggressive management of cardiovascular risk factors will increase. Specifically in those patients above the age of 60–65, the risk of peripheral arterial disease continues to increase dramatically. It is not until these patients are recognized and adequately treated for their overall atherosclerotic risk, that reduction in morbidity and mortality related to cardiovascular disease can be achieved. Clearly in the group of patients with underlying alternate site atherosclerotic disease, screening for peripheral arterial disease is warranted. In these patients, an understanding of the extent of the disease and its implications for the patient are important and should be part and parcel of treating these patients.

The screening test to perform for identifying patients with PAD is simple. The most straightforward and reproducible of the screening tests is the ankle-brachial index. This test is performed by measuring the arm blood pressure in both arms and comparing it to a pressure obtained with a blood pressure cuff just above the ankle and Doppler insonation of the posterior tibial and dorsalis pedis artery. The higher of the two pressures at the ankle level is compared to the higher of the two arm pressures to give an ankle to brachial pressure ratio. An ankle-brachial index of less than 0.9 is considered to be abnormal, indicative of peripheral arterial disease. The lower the index beyond 0.9, the more significant the peripheral arterial disease, and the more significant the risk of cardiovascular events in the patient. This test can be abnormal or difficult to interpret in the diabetic patient or those with calcified vessels; however, it is extremely reproducible and reliable in the vast majority of patients evaluated in the clinician's office.

CONTRAINDICATIONS

There are few contraindications to revascularization in the individual with severe claudication or critical limb ischemia. There are clearly situations where either percutaneous therapy or surgical therapy to revascularize the limb has a distinct advantage. But especially in the patient with critical limb ischemia, the only things that should limit the progression toward revascularization of the limb are systemic comorbidities that make any form of revascularization high risk. Since these patients are at significant risk of coronary and cerebrovascular disease, patients with symptomatic carotid disease and other severe congestive heart failure or symptomatic coronary ischemic syndromes or for that matter any ischemic symptomatology that affects a critical vascular bed, the revascularization strategy should initially involve treatment of the other ischemic bed to preserve the life of the patient prior to proceeding with revascularization of the ischemic limb. Table 2 highlights some situations where preference might be given to either surgical or percutaneous revascularization to deal with the limb ischemia a patient is experiencing.

The other situation in which revascularization may be contraindicated is in the patient with such severe limb ischemia that revascularization will not allow retention of a meaningful walking surface for the patient. This can happen in the diabetic with extensive infection that can spread to the midfoot and can also occur when the ischemia has

Table 2
Intervention Factors

Factors Favoring Percutaneous Intervention
Prohibitive patient comorbidities (e.g., severe CAD, CHF, COPD, etc.)
Symmetric lesions
Noncalcified lesions
Short segment disease
Tissue loss in anatomic configuration likely to predispose to graft infection
Factors Favoring Open Surgical Intervention
Eccentric lesions
Calcified lesions
Long segment disease
Lesions across joints in association with extensive disease above or below this region
Femoral bifurcation lesions
Extensive tissue loss in the foot

been long standing and not addressed. Exposing this patient to the risk of revascularization when there is an extremely high likelihood of progressing to amputation is not a reasonable alternative. There are situations when the co-existing diseases preclude the ability to achieve adequate revascularization necessitating continued medical therapy and perhaps primary amputation. An example of this might be a patient with symptomatic congestive heart failure. In this situation, even percutaneous therapy for revascularization carries some risk and in certain instances, continued medical therapy may offer the patient the best chance for survival.

TECHNIQUES

The methods for treating peripheral arterial disease are best divided between the iliac artery system and the infra-inguinal segment. Iliac artery disease is usually a bit easier to deal with and is usually addressed first in those patients with peripheral artery disease, so the technique for treatment of these vessels will be addressed first.

Iliac artery lesions can be addressed from one of three approaches. The first of these approaches is ipsilateral femoral access with retrograde passage through the lesion. The second approach is contralateral femoral access with wire passage over the aortic bifurcation and antegrade passage of the wire through the lesion, and finally the third approach is transbrachial with retrograde access in the brachial artery and passage through the descending thoracic and abdominal aorta to achieve antegrade passage of the wire through the iliac artery from the arm. The ipsilateral approach can be combined with either of the other approaches in challenging iliac artery occlusions, but in most instances, one of these approaches will be successful. It is helpful to have some assessment of the anatomic problem ahead of time in order to plan the approach. For common iliac artery stenosis, the simplest approach is the ipsilateral femoral puncture with retrograde wire passage. In this setting, access is obtained in the common femoral artery. This access can be achieved with percutaneous puncture or utilizing ultrasound guidance, depending upon the strength of the ipsilateral pulse and the familiarity of the interventionalist with this approach. Passage through the lesion is facilitated by the use of a hydrophilic, angled guide wire, which can be rotated to assist with advancement across the lesion. Once access is achieved across the lesion, confirmation of placement in the true lumen of the vessel above the stenosis is mandatory. This is initiated by assessing for the passage of blood through a catheter passed over the wire and measuring pressures above the stenosis, by connecting the catheter to a pressure gauge, or in some instances, simply by injecting contrast through the catheter under fluoroscopic guidance to visualize the contrast within the vessel lumen. This concept of assessing the catheter position within the vessel beyond either the stenosis or the occlusion is routine and mandatory when treating these lesions. After completing the traversal, a flush catheter is advanced over a wire to within the aorta above the area of the blockage. Normally a pelvic aortogram will provide adequate images of the vasculature above the lesion and the vessels beyond the area to be treated. These images can provide a roadmap for proceeding with interventional therapy for the stenosis. The key issue of performing the intervention is achieving and maintaining wire access across the lesion. For most stenotic lesions, this can be achieved from the ipsilateral approach.

Occlusions on the other hand provide a more demanding approach and ipsilateral access may often not be the best strategy. Most plaque in the iliac arteries, especially when occurring in the common iliac arteries, originates in the aorta. In fact atherosclerotic plaque, in general, tends to become thicker and more heavily calcified the closer it is to the aortic wall. This thickening of the plaque close to the aorta makes traversing complete occlusions more challenging in the retrograde direction. In many situations, the best approach to cross these lesions will be either the contralateral femoral artery or the brachial approach. Both of these techniques allow the tip of the catheter to be lodged in the proximal "cap" of the occlusion and the wire slowly advanced into the occlusion. In most cases a rapid rotating motion, approximating a drill, with some forward pressure will allow initiation of the traversal across the cap of the lesion. This often proves the most vexing part of the recanalization process and usually, once entrance into the lesion is obtained, the wire can be advanced to the point at which it re-enters the true lumen of the vessel. This may involve subintimal passage of the wire through the arterial occlusion *(60)*. In some situations, however, the true lumen cannot be re-entered and the wire remains in a subintimal plane even after the wire has been advanced beyond the point at which the vessel has reconstituted. This is particularly problematic when the re-entry cannot be achieved cephalad to the common femoral artery. In this situation, one can attempt to enter the same plane from the ipsilateral femoral approach. In advancing the wire here, the likelihood is that one will not be able to easily pass the wire into the true lumen at the other end of the occlusion. When this occurs, with access above and below the occlusion, and wires in the subintimal plane from both approaches, the wire from one end can be snared from the other end and through-and-through wire access can be achieved through the occlusion. To assist in the process of being able to either re-enter directly or to allow enough space to be created in which to snare the wire from the other direction, a low profile balloon can be inflated in the subintimal plane in the upper or lower portion of the occlusion. This inflation will enlarge the subintimal space and in some instances may create a channel directly into the true lumen, but in nearly all circumstances, will create enough space to allow for a wire to be snared and through-and-through access to be achieved. In certain instances, access across the lesion will still remain elusive. Here one can use a re-entry device from either the arm or the groin to re-enter the true lumen at either the cephalad or caudad end of the occlusion. Using these combinations of techniques, nearly every iliac occlusion can be crossed and in most series evaluating this, at least 90% can be recanalized *(61, 62)*. While some authors do advocate the use of lytic therapy to assist with lesion crossing *(63, 64)*, this is rarely necessary to achieve access across iliac artery occlusions. Once access across the lesion has been achieved, treatment can be initiated.

In most instances, for noncomplex lesions of the iliac arteries, angioplasty of iliac lesions will provide adequate short- and long-term success rates that are comparable to primary stenting, and stenting can be reserved for those cases in which there is either recoil of the lesion, dissection or inability to achieve adequate luminal dilation.*(65)* When the lesions however are more complex, for example TASC C or D lesions (Table 3), the use of stents will likely need to be more liberal and the results are likely better with primary stenting *(66)*. The only other technique in common practice that has been reported for treating iliac artery occlusive disease is covered stent placement *(67, 68)*. There are limited data evaluating this and meaningful comparisons with uncovered stents is lacking. Situations where covered stents offer a clear advantage appear to be areas where there is extensive, irregular calcification which poses a rupture risk for dilation with balloon or uncovered stent. Additionally, in the setting of iliac rupture following initial treatment, covered stents provide the only reasonable method to avoid open surgical conversion. Results of interventional therapies for treating iliac artery occlusive disease are given in Table 4.

Determining equipment for treatment of the iliac artery lesions requires an understanding of the anatomy of this region and normal sizes of these vessels. Optimally, sizing of the interventional devices can be assisted by fluoroscopic measurement systems or intravascular ultrasound. These systems allow assessment of vessel diameters and lesion lengths. Balloon expandable stents are primarily utilized for origin stenosis of either the common iliac or in some instances the external iliac artery. These devices provide precision in placement and significant resistance to compression or crush. They tend to displace calcific lesions better and offer the ability to over-dilate the stents to an appropriate size. These stents, however, are less flexible and will often not be used in the external iliac arteries where arterial motion and flexion are common. These areas are treated with either angioplasty (Fig. 1) for noncomplex lesions or, if needed, self-expanding nitinol stents. These stents are usually oversized about 10–20% to provide adequate radial force to maintain the vessel lumen. It is important to remember that the most commonly ruptured peripheral artery undergoing interventional therapy is the external iliac artery, so caution must be used in deciding the diameter of the angioplasty balloon or stent to be used in this vessel.

Femoro-popliteal disease can be treated from one of three approaches as well. These approaches include contralateral femoral, retrograde access with treatment across the aortic bifurcation, ipsilateral femoral with antegrade femoral artery access, and finally, ipsilateral popliteal (with the patient in the prone position) and retrograde access in the popliteal artery to traverse the femoral lesion in retrograde fashion. The most commonly used of these approaches is the contralateral femoral approach with access across the

Table 3
TASC Classification (85).

TASC Classification of Iliac Disease

Type A
- Unilateral or bilateral stenosis of the common iliac artery
- Unilateral or bilateral single short (less than or equal to 3 cm) stenosis of the external iliac artery

Type B
- Short (less than or equal to 3 cm) stenosis of infrarenal aorta
- Unilateral common iliac artery occlusion
- Single or multiple stenoses totalling 3–10 cm involving the external iliac artery not extending into the common femoral artery
- Unilateral external iliac artery occlusion not involving the origins of the internal iliac or common femoral arteries

Type C
- Bilateral common iliac artery occlusions
- Bilateral external iliac artery stenoses 3–10 cm long not extending into the common femoral artery
- Unilateral external iliac artery stenosis extending into the common femoral artery
- Unilateral external iliac artery occlusion that involves the origins of the internal iliac or common femoral artery or both
- Heavily calcified unilateral external iliac artery occlusion with or without involvement of origins of the internal iliac or common femoral artery or both

Type D
- Infra-renal aortoiliac occlusion
- Diffuse disease involving the aorta and both iliac arteries requiring treatment
- Diffuse multiple stenoses involving the unilateral common iliac artery, external iliac artery, and common femoral artery
- Unilateral occlusions of both common iliac and external iliac arteries
- Bilateral occlusions of the external iliac artery
- Iliac stenoses in patients with abdominal aortic aneurysms requiring treatment and not amenable to endograft placement or other lesions requiring open aortic or iliac surgery

TASC Classification of Femoropopliteal Disease

Type A
- Single stenosis less than or equal to 10 cm in length
- Single occlusion less than or equal to 5 cm in length

Type B
- Multiple lesions (stenoses or occlusions), each less than or equal to 5 cm
- Single stenosis or occlusion less than or equal to 15 cm not involving the infrageniculate popliteal artery
- Single or multiple lesions in the absence of continuous tibial vessels to improve inflow for a distal bypass
- Heavily calcified occlusion less than or equal to 5 cm in length
- Single popliteal stenosis

Type C
- Multiple stenoses or occlusions totalling >15 cm with or without heavy calcification
- Recurrent stenoses or occlusions that need treatment after two endovascular interventions

Type D
- Chronic total occlusions of the common femoral or superficial femoral arteries (>20 cm, involving the popliteal artery)
- Chronic total occlusion of popliteal artery and proximal trifurcation vessels

(Reprinted with the permission of Elsevier.)

Table 4
Femoropopliteal interventions

			Primary Patency (Months)									
	% CLI	1	3	6	9	12	18	24	36	48	Remarks

PTA
   Conrad et al. (76) | 46 | | | | | | | 64.3 | 54.3 | | |

PTA with Stent
   Laird et al. (71)
     PTA | 0 | | | 47.4 | | 36.7 | | | | | Nitinol stent significantly superior
     PTA/S | | | | 94.2 | | 81.3 | | | | | |
   Dearing et al. (77) | 38.8 | | | | | | | | | | |
     PTA/S | TASC A/B | | | | | 79 | | 67 | 57 | | Nitinol stents
     PTA/S | TASC C/D | | | | | 52.7 | | 36 | 19 | | |
   Krankenberg et al. (78)
     PTA | 3.5 | | | | | 38.6[a] | | | | | Nitinol stent; no difference
     PTA/S | 2.5 | | | | | 31.7 | | | | | |
   Schillinger et al. (70)
     PTA | 13 | | | 43[a] | | 63[a] | | | | | Nitinol stent significantly superior
     PTA/S | 12 | | | 24[a] | | 37[a] | | | | | |

Cryoplasty
   Gonzalo et al. (79) | 100 | 100 | 91 | 91 | | 91 | | | | | |
   Laird et al. (80) | 0 | | | | 70.1 | | | | | | |

Directional Atherectomy
   McKinsey et al. (81) | 63.3 | | | | | 64.2 | 53.5 | | | | |
   Zeller et al. (82) | | | | | | 84 | 73 | | | | 56% of patients underwent PTA, 2% underwent stenting

Laser Atherectomy
   Laird et al. (83) | 100 | | | 93[b] | | | | | | | Adjuvant balloon angioplasty (96%) and stent (45%)
   Wissgott et al. (84) | 11.9 | 93.8 | | 78.2 | | 58.8 | | 42.8 | 33.6 | 26 | |

[a]Indicates restenosis rates in lieu of primary patency.
[b]Indicates limb salvage rate in lieu of primary patency.
PTA Percutaneous transluminal angioplasty; *PTA/S* Percutaneous transluminal angioplasty with stent.

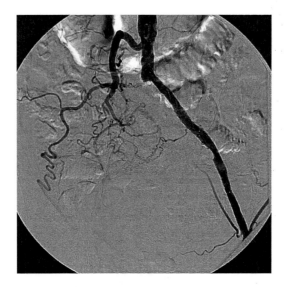

Fig. 1. Iliac occlusion images.

aortic bifurcation. Normally, after imaging the pelvis nonselectively, access with catheter across the bifurcation can be achieved and selective access to the common femoral artery above the area of stenosis is obtained. Selective angiography of the lower extremity to be treated is performed from this position to assess the anatomy of the lesion and the runoff vessels beyond the area of disease. For stenotic lesions (Fig. 2), a 0.035-in hydrophilic guide wire is advanced across the lesion and the catheter then advanced over the wire through the lesion. Confirmation of access into a patent vessel beyond the area of stenosis is performed by manual aspiration of blood through the catheter followed by angiographic injection into the vessel. After confirming passage across the lesion, treatment can be initiated. In most instances, this will involve passage of a sheath across the aortic bifurcation to assist with passage of interventional devices and to allow for imaging of the lesion while maintaining wire access across the lesion.

In the setting of femoral artery occlusions (Fig. 3), following initial imaging of the vessels of the leg to be treated, one will likely need to obtain sheath access across the aortic bifurcation. Wire access normally must be achieved beyond the common femoral artery and in most instances, the wire is advanced into the profunda femoris artery and an interventional diameter sheath is advanced over the wire. The sheaths used are typically 6–8F and normally range in length from 45 to 55 cm. These are ring reinforced sheaths to prevent collapse of the sheath in areas of bending. This sheath provides stability for the catheter and wire during attempts to manipulate across the occlusion in the femoral artery. This sheath keeps the catheter from "buckling" up the aorta and lowers the potential for loss of wire access across the lesion. With the sheath firmly in place, an angled hydrophilic wire is advanced into the "cap" of the lesion and either an attempt at drilling across the lesion or subintimal techniques are utilized to cross the lesion. The subintimal technique has been described elsewhere *(69)* but involves forming the wire tip into a "J" configuration and advancing the wire through the occlusion and allowing it to re-enter the lumen after dissecting through the subintimal plane. Confirmation of access across the lesion into patent distal vessel must be confirmed.

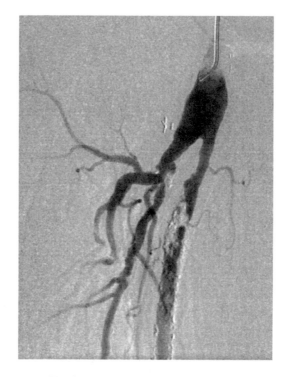

Fig. 2. Femoral artery stenosis images.

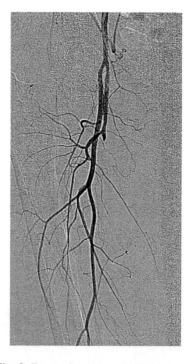

Fig. 3. Femoral artery occlusion images.

Sometimes the access from the contralateral groin will be impossible to achieve or will still limit recanalization attempts because of vessel tortuosity or buckling of sheath and catheter during attempts to cross the lesion. In these situations, the use of the ipsilateral femoral approach in antegrade fashion allows better pushability through the lesion without the concern for buckling of the access sheath. This approach, however, may be difficult with proximal superficial femoral artery (SFA) occlusions and in some situations may prove impossible to treat lesions that are high up along the path of the SFA. When alternate approaches have failed or the groin access is not useable because of infection or other issues, the patient can be placed in the prone position and access can be gained into the popliteal artery below the area of the occlusion. Surface ultrasound is routinely used to perform this access maneuver along with a lower diameter needle and wire access system for initial access into the artery. Normally forceful advancement of wire and catheter together will allow passage through the occlusion, and treatment can be initiated. Using this strategy, nearly 85% of femoral occlusive lesions will allow traversal, but there are still lesions which simply cannot be crossed with interventional therapies. As noted earlier, re-entry catheters can be utilized when the true lumen cannot be re-entered when using the subintimal technique.

Treatments for the femoro-popliteal segment are more varied related likely to the fact that the outcomes with all devices are not as successful as what is seen in the iliac arteries. Angioplasty with long, semicompliant balloons at low pressure for long periods of time (2–3 min) acts as a mainstay of therapy in this region, but there are clear advantages to stenting for occlusive lesions in this vascular bed *(70, 71)*. Unfortunately, when recurrences do occur with stents, the treatment of these is much more complex. Angioplasty and stenting results are noted in Table 5 along with results for other interventional therapies for this segment. There is currently no single best therapy and each device has some advantages, while all have the disadvantage of limited patency rates. Atherectomy has the ability to allow avoidance of stents in areas of bifurcation or in areas of extensive flexion of the vessel, such as the popliteal artery. Cryoplasty has similar advantages with decreased need for stenting with similar patency rates. No one of these approaches has proven to be the answer to all issues and interventionalists treating patients in this area should have access to and experience with all of the differing types of devices. It is likely that some form of combined therapy (atherectomy and medicated stenting, or angioplasty and atherectomy) may provide the best alternative in therapeutic options, but none of these techniques, other than angioplasty and stenting have been compared in any meaningful way.

Postprocedural Care and Follow-Up

Care of patients following intervention is similar to that utilized after coronary stenting. The access site is compressed and activity level is limited depending upon how the access site has been treated. Careful attention to the access site must be maintained especially over the first 4–6 h and either additional compression or ultrasound guided compression or perhaps even thrombin injection should be utilized early if there are concerns and hematoma or pseudoaneurysm has been identified.

Nearly all patients are initiated and maintained on antiplatelet therapy with aspirin 325 mg (once daily) and clopidogrel 75 mg (once daily) to reduce platelet adhesion and activation. This aggressive antiplatelet approach is maintained for 4–6 weeks following

Table 5
Iliac interventions

		% for CLI	Primary Patency 1 Year	2 Year	3 Year	5 Year	6–8 Year	10 Year	Remarks
AbuRahma et al. (66)	Primary Stent TASC A/B	62	100	98	98	87			No difference between selective and primary stent groups for TASC A/B with significantly superior results for primary stenting in TASC C/D
	Selective Stent TASC C/D	66	96	90	72				
Park et al. (72)	Primary Stent TASC A/B	N/A	100	93	85	85			No difference by TASC class
	TASC C/D		46	28	28				
	TASC A/B		95–96		84–85	81–85			
	TASC C/D		93–94		74–94	74–78			
Klein et al. (65)	Primary Stent	5	96	94			90		No difference in freedom from lesion revascularization
	Selective Stent	8	97	98			81		
Galaria et al. (73)	TASC A/B	23				53		24	Selective stenting in 51% without predefined criteria
Powell et al. (74)		40	61		43				Multilevel iliac disease with stenting based on surgeon preference
Tetteroo et al. (75)	Primary Stent	6		71.3					No difference
	Selective Stent			69.9					

completion of the procedure. Follow-up for these procedures varies based upon the type of revascularization performed and there remains to be proven any advantage to routine imaging following these interventions; however, most interventionalists would recommend routine follow-up to allow intervention prior to failure of the revascularization, with an initial assessment performed within 6 weeks of the revascularization.

Duplex imaging of the revascularized vessel offers the best method of assuring patency of the revascularization strategy and assessment of the degree of narrowing. For iliac interventions, this will prove more challenging than with femoral artery interventions. The velocity criteria for determining stenosis vary; however, if the peak systolic velocity is >300 cm/s, one can assume that the degree of stenosis is significant enough to warrant further evaluation either with CTA or MRA or perhaps even direct angiography.

Although there are no standard recommendations as to when to perform this assessment, for iliac interventions, this assessment is usually performed at 6-month intervals for the first 24 months and then once annually following this. For interventions below the inguinal ligament, these assessments are routinely performed every 3 months for the first 12 months, then every 6 months for the next year and then annually thereafter. This is similar to imaging strategies performed for bypass grafting performed below the inguinal ligament. These duplex images are usually accompanied by ankle-brachial indices to assess the adequacy of blood flow to the feet. Evidence of significant elevation of the velocities or decrement in the ankle-brachial index should lead to a more in-depth assessment of the vascular status of the lower extremities. This assessment will also allow for evaluation of the contralateral extremity as it remains at increased risk of developing significant ischemia as well. Maintaining a close relationship with these patients is crucial and allows the physician to identify and treat those patients who develop problems early before these progress to a point where intervention becomes difficult.

REFERENCES

1. Dotter CT, Judkins MP. Transluminal treatment of arteriosclerotic obstruction. Description of a new technique and a preliminary report of its application. *Circulation.* 1964;30:654–670.
2. Gruntzig A, Kumpe DA. Technique of percutaneous transluminal angioplasty with the Gruntzig balloon catheter. *AJR* 1979;132:547–552.
3. Sigwart U, Puel J, Mirkovitch V, Joffre F, Kappenberger L. Intravascular stents to prevent occlusion and restenosis after transluminal angioplasty. *N Engl J Med.* 1987;316:701–706.
4. Palmaz JC, Sibbitt RR, Reuter SR, Tio FO, Rice WJ. Expandable intraluminal graft: a preliminary study: work in progress. *Radiology.* 1985;156:73–77.
5. Schatz RA, Palmaz JC, Tio FO, Garcia F, Garcia O, Reuter SR. Balloon-expandable intracoronary stents in the adult dog. *Circulation.* 1987;76:450–457.
6. Taute BM, Thommes S, Taute R, Rapmund I, Lindner K, Podhaisky H. Long-term outcome of patients with mild intermittent claudication under secondary prevention. *Vasa.* 2009; 38(5):346–355.
7. Aquino R, Johnnides C, Makaroun M, et al. Natural history of claudication: Long-term serial follow-up study of 1244 claudicants. *J Vasc Surg.* 2001; 34:962–970.
8. Olin JW, Sealove BA. Peripheral artery disease: current insight into the disease and its diagnosis and management. *Mayo Clin Proc.* 2010;85(7):678–692.
9. Kannel WB, Shurtleff D. The Framingham Study: cigarettes and the development of intermittent claudication. *Geriatrics.* 1973;28(2):61–68.

10. Jonason T, Bergstrom R. Cessation of smoking in patients with intermittent claudication: effects on the risk of peripheral vascular complications, myocardial infarction and mortality. *Acta Med Scand.* 1987;221(3):253–260.
11. Kumakura G, Kanai H, Aizaki M, et al. The influence of the obesity paradox and chronic kidney disease on long-term survival in a Japanese cohort with peripheral arterial disease. *J Vasc Surg.* 2010;52(1):110–117.
12. Lavie CJ, Milani RV, Ventura HO. Obesity and cardiovascular disease: risk factor, paradox, and impact of weight loss. *J Am Coll Cardiol.* 2009;53:1925–1932.
13. Gardner AW, Poehlman ET. Exercise rehabilitation programs for the treatment of claudication pain. A meta-analysis. *JAMA.* 1995;274:975–980.
14. Regensteiner JG, Gardner A, Hiatt WR. Exercise testing and exercise rehabilitation for patients with peripheral arterial disease: status in 1997. *Vasc Med.* 1997;2:147–155.
15. Izquierdo-Porrera AM, Gardner AW, Powell CC, Katzel LI. Effects of exercise rehabailitation on cardiovascular risk factors in older patients with peripheral arterial occlusive disease. *J Vasc Surg.* 2000;31:670–677.
16. Antithrombotic Trialist Collaboration. Collaborative meta-analysis of randomized trials of antiplatelet therapy for prevention of death, myocardial infarction, and stroke in high risk patients. *BMJ.* 2002;324(7329):71–86.
17. Berger JS, Krantz MJ, Kittelson JM, Hiatt WR. Aspirin for the prevention of cardiovascular events in patients with peripheral artery disease: a meta-analysis of randomized trials. *JAMA.* 2009;301(18):1909–1919.
18. CAPRIE Steering Committee. A randomized, blinded, trial of clopidogrel versus aspirin in patients at risk of ischaemic events (CAPRIE). *Lancet.* 1996;348(9038):1329–1339.
19. Murabito JM, D'Agostino RB, Silbershatz H, Wilson WF. Intermittent claudication. A risk profile from The Gramingham Heart Study. *Circulation.* 1997;96:44–49.
20. Kannel WB, McGee DL. Update on some epidemiologic features of intermittent claudication: The Framingham Study. *J Am Geriatr Soc.* 1985;33:13–18.
21. Kannel WB, McGee D. Diabetes and cardiovascular disease. The Framingham Study. *JAMA.* 1979;241:2035–2038.
22. Kannel WB, D'Agostino RB, Wilson PW, et al. Diabetes, fibrinogen, and risk of cardiovascular disease: The Framingham experience. *Am Heart J.* 1990;120:672–676.
23. UK Prospective Diabetes Study (UKPDS) Group. Intensive blood-glucose control with sulphonylureas or insulin compared with conventional treatment and risk of complications in patients with type 2 diabetes (UKPDS 33). *Lancet.* 1998;352:837–853.
24. Sixth report of the Joint National Committee on detection, evaluation, and treatment of high blood pressure (JNC-VI). *Arch Intern Med.* 1997;157:2413–2446.
25. Vogt MT, Cauley JA, Kuller LH, Hulley SB. Prevalence and correlates of lower extremity arterial disease in elderly women. *Am J Epidemiol.* 1993;137:559–568.
26. Safar ME, Laurent S, Asmar RE, et al. Systolic hypertension in patients with arteriosclerosis obliterans of the lower limbs. *Angiology.* 1987;38:287–295.
27. Hirsch AT, Haskal ZJ, Hertzer NR, et al. ADD/AHA 2005 Practice guidelines for the management of patients with peripheral arterial disease(lower extremity, renal, mesenteric, and abdominal aortic): a collaborative report from the American Association for Vascular Surgery/Society for Vascular Surgery, Society for Cardiovascular Angiography and Interventions, Society for Vascular Medicine and Biology, Society of Interventional Radiology, and the ACC/AHA Task Force on Practice Guidelines for the Management of Patients With Peripheral Arterial Disease): endorsed by the American Association of Cardiovascular Pulmonary Rehabilitation: National Heart, Lung, and Blood Institute; Society for Vascular ; Transatlantic Inter-Society Consensus; and Vascular Disease Foundation. *Circulation.* 2006;113(11):e463–e654.
28. Radack K, Deck C. Beta-adrenergic blocker therapy does not worsen intermittent claudication in subjects with peripheral arterial disease: a meta-analysis of randomized controlled trials. *Arch Intern Med.* 1991;151(9):1769–1776.
29. Lonn E, Yusuf S, Dzavik V, et al. Effects of ramipril and vitamin E on atherosclerosis: the study to evaluate carotid ultrasound changes in patients treated with ramipril and vitamin E (SECURE). *Circulation.* 2001;103(7):919-925.

30. Yusuf S, Sleight P, Pogue J, Bosch J, Davies R, Dagenais G; Heart Outcomes Prevention Evaluation Study Investgators. Effects of an angiotensin-converting-enzyme inhibitor, ramipril, on cardiovascular events in high-risk patients. *N Engl J Med.* 2000; 342(3):145–153.
31. Fox KM. Efficacy of perindopril in reduction of cardiovascular events among patients with stable coronary artery disease: randomized, double-blind, placebo-controlled, multicentre trial (the EUROPA study). *Lancet.* 2003;262(9386):782–788.
32. Heart Protection Study Collaborative Group. MRC/BHF heart protection study of cholesterol lowering with simvastatin in 20,536 high-risk individuals: a randomized placebo-controlled trial. *Lancet.* 2002;360(9326):7–22.
33. Randomized trial of cholesterol lowering in 4444 patients with coronary heart disease: The Scandinavian Simvastatin Survival Study (4S). *Lancet.* 1994;344(8934):1383–1389.
34. Olsson AG, Ruhn G, Erikson U. The effect of serum lipid regulation on the development of femoral atherosclerosis in hyperlipidaemia: a non-randomized controlled study. *J Intern Med.* 1990;227: 381–390.
35. McDermott MM, Guralnik JM, Greenland P, et al. Statin use and leg functioning in patients with and without lower-extremity peripheral arterial disease. *Circulation.* 2003;107(5):757–761.
36. Giri J, McDermott MM, Greenland P, et al. Statin use and functional decline in patients with and without peripheral arterial disease. *J Am Coll Cardiol.* 2006;47(5):998–1004.
37. Leng GC, Fowler B, Ernst E. Exercise for intermittent claudication. *Cochrane Database Syst Rev.* 2000; (2):CD000990.
38. Hood SC, Moher D, Barber GG. Management of intermittent claudication with pentoxifylline: meta-analysis of randomized controlled trials. *Can Med Assoc J.* 1996;155:1053–1059.
39. Girolami B, Bernardi E, Prins MH, et al. Treatment of intermittent claudication with physical training, smoking cessation, pentoxifylline, or nafronyl: a meta-analysis. *Arch Intern Med.* 1999;150:337–345.
40. Regensteiner JG, Hiatt WR. Improvements in quality of life in cilostazol-treated patients with intermittent claudication. *Vasc Med.* 2000;5:198.
41. Beebe HG, Dawson GL, Cutler BS, et al. A new pharmacological treatment for intermittent claudication: results of a randomized, multicenter trial. *Arch Intern Med.* 1999;150:2041–2049.
42. Money SR, Herd JA, Isaacsohn JL, et al. Effect of cilostazol on walking distances in patients with intermittent claudication caused by peripheral vascular disease. *J Vasc Surg.* 1998;27:267–274.
43. Strandness DE Jr. Two doses of cilostazol versus placebo in the treatment of claudication: results of a randomized multicenter trial. *Circulation.* 1998;95:I–12.
44. Dawson D, Cutler BS, Hiatt WR, et al. A comparison of cilostazol and pentoxifylline for treating intermittent claudication. *Am J Med.* 2000;109:523–530.
45. Whyman MR, Ruckley CV. Should claudicants receive angioplasty or just exercise training? *Cardiovascular Surgery.* 1998;6(3):226–231.
46. Spronk S, Bosch JL, Veen HF, den Hoed PT, Hunink MGM. Intermittent claudication: functional capacity and quality of life after exercise training or percutaneous transluminal angioplasty—systematic review. *Radiology.* 2005;235:833–842.
47. Wilson S, Gelfand D, Jimenez J, Gordon I. Comparison of the results of percutaneous transluminal angioplasty and stenting with medical treatment for claudicants who have superficial femoral artery occlusive disease. *Vascular.* 2006;14(2):81–87.
48. Nylaende M, Abdelnoor M, Stranden E, et al. The Oslo Ballon Angioplasty versus Conservative Treatment Study (OBACT)—The 2-years results of a single centre, prospective, randomized study in patients with intermittent claudication. *Eur J Vasc Endovas Surg.* 2007;33:3–12.
49. The MIMIC Trial Participants. The adjuvant benefit of angioplasty in patients with mild to moderate intermittent claudication (MIMIC) managed by supervised exercise, smoking cessation advice and best medical therapy: results from tow randomized trials for stenotic femoropopliteal and aortoiliac arterial disease. *Eur J Vasc Endovas Surg.* 2008;36:680–688.
50. Mazari JAK, Gulati S, Rahman MNA, et al. Early outcomes from a randomized, controlled trial of supervised exercise, angioplasty, and combined therapy in intermittent claudication. *Ann Vasc Surg.* 2010;24:69–79.
51. Management of peripheral arterial disease(PAD). TransAtlantic Inter-Society Consensus (TASC). *J Vasc Surg.* 2000;31:S1–S206.

52. Novo S, Coppola G, Milio G. Critical limb ischemia: definition and natural history. Current Drug Targets. *Cardiovascular & Haematological Disorders.* 2004;4:219–225.
53. Slovut DP, Sullivan TM. Critical limb ischemia: medical and surgical management. *Vascular Med.* 2008;13:281–291.
54. Varu VN, Hogg ME, Kibbe MR. Critical limb ischemia *J Vasc Surg.* 2010;51:230–241.
55. Adam DJ, Beard JD, Cleveland T, et al. Bypass versus angioplasty in severe ischaemia of the leg (BASIL): multicentre, randomized controlled trial. *Lancet.* 2005;366:1925–1934.
56. Walsh JJ Jr, Cofelice M, Limpkin D, Kerstein MD. Is screening for vascular disease a valuable proposition? *J Cardiovasc Surg* 1988;29:306–309.
57. U.S. Preventive Services Task Force. *Screening for Peripheral Arterial Disease: Recommendation Statement.* AHRQ Publication No. 05-0583-A-EF. Rockville, MD: Agency for Healthcare Research and Quality. 2005. http://www.ahrq.gov/clinic/uspstf05/pad/padrs.htm
58. Hirsch AT, Criqui MH, Treat-Jacobson D, et al. Peripheral arterial disease detection, awareness, and treatment in primary care. *JAMA.* 2001;286:1317–1324.
59. Hirsch AT, Halverson SL, Treat-Jacobson D, et al. The Minnesota regional peripheral arterial disease screening program: toward a definition of community standards of care. *Vascular Med.* 201;6:87–96.
60. Bolia A, Fishwick G. Recanalization of iliac artery occlusions by subintimal dissection using the ipsilateral and the contralateral approach. *Clin Radiol.* 1997;52(9):684–687.
61. Leville CD, Kashyap VS, Clair DG, et al. Endovascular management of iliac artery occlusions: extending treatment to TransAtlantic Inter-Society Consensus class C and D patients. *J Vasc Surg.* 2006;43:32–39.
62. Gandini R, Gabiano S, Chiocchi M, Chiappa R, Simonetti G. Percutaneous treatment in iliac artery occlusion: long-term results. *Cardiovasc Intervent Radiol.* 2008;31:1069–1076.
63. Motarjeme A, Gordon GI, Bodenhagen K. Thrombolysis and angioplasty of chronic iliac artery occlusions. *JVIR.* 1995; 6:66S–72S.
64. Taddei G, Tamellini P, Niccolo F, Antonio I. Thrombolysis during the endovascular treatment of iliac artery occlusions. *Diagn Interv Radiol.* 2010;16:84–89.
65. Klein W, van der Graaf Y, Seeger J, et al. Dutch iliac stent trial; long-term results in patients randomized for primary or selective stent placement. *Radiology.* 2005;238 (2): 734–744.
66. AbuRahma AF, Hayes JD, Flaherty SK, Peery W. Primary iliac stenting versus transluminal angioplasty with selective stenting. *J Vasc Surg.* 2007;46(5):965–970.
67. Krajcer Z, Sioco G, Reynolds T. Comparison of Wallfraft and Wallstent for treatment of complex iliac artery stenosis and occlusion. *Tex Heart Inst J.* 1997;24(3):193–199.
68. Rzucidlo EM, Powell RJ, Zwolak RM, et al. Early results of stent-grafting to treat diffuse aortoiliac occlusive disease. *J Vasc Surg.* 2003;37:1175–1180.
69. Reekers JA, Bolia A. Percutaneous intentional extraluminal (subintimal) recanalization: how to do it yourself. *Eur J Radiol.* 1998;28:192–198.
70. Schillinger M, Sabeti S, Loewe C, et al. Galloon angioplasty versus implantation of nitinol stents in the superficial femoral artery. *N Engl J Med.* 2006;254(18):1879–1888.
71. Laird JR, Katzen BT, Scheinert D, et al. RESILIENT investigators. Nitinol stent implantation versus balloon angioplasty for lesions in the superficial femoral artery and proximal popliteal artery: twelve-month results from the RESILIENT randomized trial. *Circ Cardiovasc Interv.* 2010;3(3):267–276.
72. Park KB, Do YS, Kim DI, et al. The TransAtlantic InterSociety Consensus (TASC) classification system in iliac arterial stent placement: long-term patency and clinical limitations. *J Vasc Interv Radiol.* 2007;18:193–201
73. Galaria II, Davies MG. Percutaneous transluminal revascularization for iliac occlusive disease: long-term outcomes in TransAtlantic Inter-Society Consensus A and B lesions. *Ann Vasc Surg.* 2005;19:352–360
74. Powell RJ, Fillinger M, Bettmann M, et al. The durability of endovascular treatment of multisegment iliac occlusive disease. *J Vasc Surg.* 2000;31:1178–1184
75. Tetteroo E, van der Graaf Y, Bosch JL, et al. Randomised comparison of primary stent placement versus primary angioplasty followed by selective stent placement in patients with iliac-artery occlusive disease. Dutch Iliac Stent Trial Study Group. *Lancet.* 1998;351:1153–1159
76. Conrad MF, Cambria RP, Stone DH, et al. Intermediate results of percutaneous endovascular therapy of femoropopliteal occlusive disease: a contemporary series. *J Vasc Surg.* 2006;44:762–769

77. Dearing DD, Patel KR, Compoginis JM, Kamel MA, Weaver FA, Katz SG. Primary stenting of the superficial femoral and popliteal artery. *J Vasc Surg.* 2009;50:542–547.
78. Krankenberg H, Schluter M, Steinkamp HJ, et al. Nitinol stent implantation versus percutaneous transluminal angioplasty in superficial femoral artery lesions up to 10 cm in length: the femoral artery stenting trial (FAST). *Circulation.* 2007;116:285–292.
79. Gonzalo B, Solanich T, Bellmunt S, et al. Cryoplasty as endovascular treatment in the femoropopliteal region: hemodynamic results and follow-up at one year. *Ann Vasc Surg.* 2010;24:680–685.
80. Laird J, Jaff MR, Biamino G, et al. Cryoplasty for the treatment of femoropopliteal arterial disease: results of a prospective, multicenter registry. *J Vasc Interv Radiol.* 2005;16:1067–1073.
81. McKinsey JF, Goldstein L, Khan HU, et al. Novel treatment of patients with lower extremity ischemia: use of percutaneous atherectomy in 579 lesions. *Ann Surg.* 2008;248:519–528.
82. Zeller T, Rastan A, Sixt S, et al. Long-term results after directional atherectomy of femoro-popliteal lesions. *J Am Coll Cardiol.* 2006;48:1573–1578.
83. Laird JR, Zeller T, Gray BH, et al. LACI Investigators. Limb salvage following laser-assisted angioplasty for critical limb ischemia: results of the LACI multicenter trial. *J Endovasc Ther.* 2006;13:1–11
84. Wissgott C, Scheinert D, Rademaker J, Werk M, Schedel H, Steinkamp HJ. Treatment of long superficial femoral artery occlusions with excimer laser angioplasty: long-term results after 48 months. *Acta Radiol.* 2004;45:23–29.
85. Norgren L, Hiatt WR, Dormandy JA, et al. Inter-Society Consensus for the Management of Peripheral Arterial Disease (TASC II). *J Vasc Surg.* 2007;45:S5–S67.

3   Critical Limb Ischemia

Raghotham Patlola, MD, FACC,
and Craig Walker, MD, FACC

CONTENTS

INTRODUCTION
EPIDEMIOLOGY
CLINICAL PRESENTATION
TREATMENT OF CRITICAL LIMB ISCHEMIA
CASE STUDIES: ENDOVASCULAR INTERVENTIONS IN CLI
FUTURE PERSPECTIVES AND CONCLUSIONS
REFERENCES

INTRODUCTION

Critical limb ischemia (CLI) as defined by the TransAtlantic Inter-Society Consensus (TASC) is persistent recurring ischemic rest pain necessitating opiate analgesics for more than 2 weeks, ulceration or gangrene of the foot or toes, ankle-brachial index (ABI) <0.4, toe pressure <30 mmHg, systolic ankle pressure <50 mmHg, and absent pedal pulses. *(1, 2)*

CLI which has emerged as a major public health challenge remains an undertreated condition with poor outcomes, making this condition a focus of increasing interest and attention in the medical community. CLI affects 1–2% of patients with peripheral arterial disease, a serious condition affecting a growing number of patients worldwide, particularly with the increasing prevalence of diabetes mellitus. More than 250,000 amputations are performed annually as a consequence of CLI resulting in huge economic and social burden and significantly compromised quality of life. *(3–6)*.

Multivessel/Multisegment disease is the norm in patients with CLI. Small caliber, negatively remodeled vessels with heavy calcifications pose increasing challenge particularly in renal failure and diabetic patients. The untreated CLI patients have a 1-year amputation rate of 50% or greater, with associated high morbidity and mortality rates, hence early diagnosis and management of CLI are essential to optimize the chances of limb salvage.

From: *Peripheral and Cerebrovascular Intervention*, Contemporary Cardiology
Edited by: D. L. Bhatt, DOI 10.1007/978-1-60327-965-9_3
© Springer Science+Business Media, LLC 2012

Although surgical bypass has historically been the gold standard for treatment, the BASIL (Bypass Versus Angioplasty in Severe Ischemia of the Leg) trial *(7)* showed similar clinical outcomes between surgery and balloon angioplasty. Moreover, the higher surgical and anesthetic risks, secondary to numerous comorbidities, the frequent lack of venous conduits, poor distal targets, and infected distal anastamotic areas lead to notable paradigm shift in treating patients with CLI by endovascular approach. This translated to major advances in this field. Moreover, in the last several years there have been many published reports on the safety and efficacy of endovascular therapy in patients with CLI *(30, 31)*. Endovascular therapy as the first therapeutic modality in patients with CLI even if unsuccessful does not jeopardize the subsequent surgical options *(32)*. The goal of endovascular therapy in these patients is obviously long-term benefits of limb salvage, but most importantly, the immediate goal of these procedures is to alleviate symptoms, avoid tissue loss, and promote wound healing.

EPIDEMIOLOGY

The statistics revealed that at the beginning of the twentieth century, cardiovascular diseases (CVD) accounted for less than 10% of all deaths worldwide while at the beginning of the twenty-first century CVD accounts for nearly half of all deaths in the developed world and 25% in the developing world. In this context, CVD needs to be treated as an "epidemic" and consequently PAD and CLI, intrinsic to CVD, could become a global health problem. The recent literature on CLI shows great awareness. CLI has started to be defined as a global epidemic and to be discussed not only as a medical problem but as a public health problem at large medical gatherings such as the Charing Cross Symposium and the first international multidisciplinary CLI Summit.

CLI has a significant dimension in medical practice being bilateral and incurable. Unfortunately, there is lack of data regarding CLI incidence and prevalence. The literature reports a CLI incidence between 500 and 1,000 cases per million per year. The prevalence in the US is 1% in the population older than 50 years and approximately 2% in the population older than 70 years. In patients with PAD, when lesion obstruction exceeds 50% it may cause intermittent claudication; estimates of the prevalence of intermittent claudication vary by population, from 0.6% to nearly 10%. Approximately 20–25% of patients will require revascularization, while fewer than 5% will progress to CLI. The reports on amputations due to CLI reveal a number of greater than 150,000–200,000 major and minor lower extremity amputations in the US and Europe yearly. The amputation rate in the US has increased from 19 to 30 per 100,000 persons over the last two decades, primarily due to diabetes and an ageing population. In the population over 85 years of age, the amputation rate is 140 per 100,000 persons per year with a morality rate of 13–17%. When referring to CLI in diabetics, statistics show that one out of every four diabetics will face CLI within their lifetime, and those with CLI will have a 7–40 times greater risk of amputation. An amputation is a marker for death as the 3–4-year mortality postamputation is >50–60%.

CLINICAL PRESENTATION

Prompt recognition of the clinical symptoms of CLI greatly improves the outcomes. CLI typically presents as rest pain, trophic skin changes, tissue loss, ulcerations and gangrene, which left untreated or if the therapeutic modalities fail, then they quickly progress to limb loss. (Fig. 1) Rest pain in CLI is typically manifested in the distal foot and toes as a "burning" pain which is usually worse at night. This pain is aggravated by limb elevation and relieved with dependency as gravity increases the perfusion pressure in the ischemic leg. Patients with ischemic rest pain often need to dangle their legs over the side of the bed or sleep in a recliner to regain gravity-augmented blood flow and relieve the pain. This is commonly referred by patients as intense, requiring large doses of narcotic analgesics. The etiology of rest pains is from a combination of ischemia, tissue loss, and ischemic neuropathy.

The ill-perfused limb with progressive tissue hypoxemia leads to tissue ulcerations and gangrene. The necrotic tissue can serve as a nidus for infection which can progress to systemic sepsis if untreated with dire consequences. On the other hand, the gangrenous tissue shrinks, mummifies, and may undergo spontaneous amputation. (Figs. 2 and 3)

The CLI is usually associated with multiple comorbid conditions including diabetes mellitus, chronic obstructive pulmonary disease, and significant physical deconditioning – these might prevent patients from having the classic symptoms of CLI secondary to

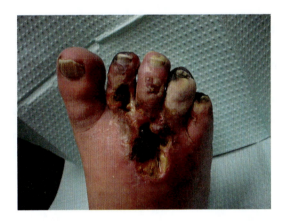

Fig. 1. A patient presenting with critical limb ischemia, nonhealing ulcerated lesions of the dorsum of the foot.

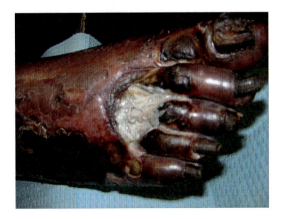

Fig. 2. Nonhealing ischemic ulcerated lesions with unhealthy granulation tissue.

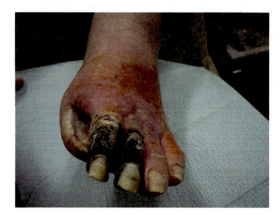

Fig. 3. Known patient with severe PAD, autoamputation of great toe, now presenting with gangrene of the toes.

poor functional status, insensate legs, and decreased ambulation. Hence a high index of suspicion of peripheral arterial disease in these subgroups of patients is strongly recommended to prevent limb loss.

Multiple sites of atherosclerotic arterial occlusion are typical in patients with CLI. Nonhealing wounds are usually found in areas of foot trauma caused by improperly fitting shoes or an injury. A wound is generally considered to be nonhealing if it fails to respond to a 4–12-week trial of conservative therapy such as regular dressing changes, avoidance of trauma, treatment of infection, and debridement of necrotic tissues. Gangrene is usually found on the toes. The risk factors for CLI are those of general atherosclerosis: cigarette smoking, diabetes mellitus, dyslipidemia, hypertension, hyperhomocysteinemia, increased fibrinogen and high level of C-reactive protein, obesity, and metabolic syndrome.

Clinical Evaluation in Critical Limb Ischemia

A good history and physical examination are the main keys to the diagnosis and evaluation of peripheral arterial disease and CLI. The battery of tests used in the diagnosis of CLI are Ankle Brachial Pressures (ABI), Toe Pressures, Pulse Volume recordings (PVR), Arterial Duplex Ultrasonograms, Computer Tomographic Angiograms, Magnetic Resonance Angiograms, and the conventional Peripheral Angiograms in the catheterization laboratory.

The CLI patient typically presents with rest pains, trophic skin changes, ulcerations and gangrene which are all very obvious on examination, but we still need noninvasive testing to determine the presence of PAD thus differentiating it from other confounding presentations, severity and location of the lesions, to plan the intervention and determine wound healing ability.

The ABI and PVR are simple, office-based inexpensive screening tools which are well validated. However, the sensitivity and predictive values are prone to being compromised in diabetic incompressible calcified arteries. Moreover, they cannot precisely localize the level of the lesion or the number of lesions and they cannot discriminate a stenosis from occlusion. Hence, for these reasons, color duplex ultrasound is used to

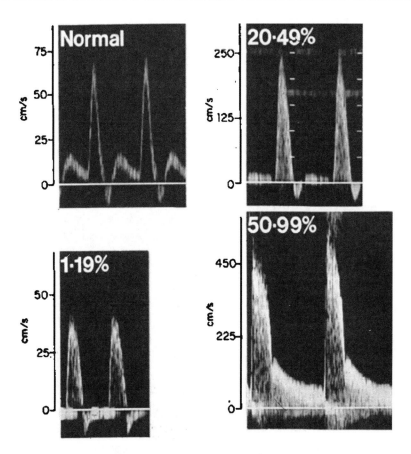

Fig. 4. Duplex: Lower extremity. Classic spectral Doppler wave patterns in patients with PAD with varying degree of severity.

augment the results of the above-mentioned indirect tests. This test helps in screening the entire arterial tree from the aorta to lower extremity or a detailed study of a segment of arterial tree, localizing the degree and the length of the lesion and it can be used as follow-up test postintervention or after surgical revascularization. The technique employed in our lab is: 5 MHZ linear array transducer (range: 3–10 MHZ); we then optimize gray scale and color Doppler parameters to the area of interest, which involves adjusting the pulse repetitive frequency to detect hemodynamic disturbances and we perform pulse Doppler in all areas and in regions of color aliasing.

The normal peripheral arterial wave form is triphasic: (Fig. 4)
Initial high velocity forward flow component
Early diastolic reversal flow component
Late diastolic forward flow component

We also look at the peak systolic velocities at each given segments. The normal peak systolic velocities range from 40 to 100 cm/sec in the lower extremities. The wave form shape, peak systolic velocities, and spectral envelope help in identifying and grading the severity of the lesion. There may be a potential to fail to localize significant arterial disease in obese individuals and to miss distal disease in small vessels. Diabetics with obese body habitus pose a significant challenge to this modality. The efficacy of this technique is proportional to the skills of the operator.

Transcutaneous oxygen tension (TcPO2) has been found in numerous studies of noninvasive lower limb perfusion to be useful – a TcPO2 of less than 30 mmHg is consistent with poor healing.

In summary, noninvasive testing provides a safe and effective means of diagnosing PAD and CLI. Appropriate application and skilled assessment provide the most effective use of these tests. All of these tests have several advantages and also disadvantages which can be overcome by invasive testing.

The invasive modalities of testing in CLI include CTA, MRA, and arterial angiography. The arterial angiography has been the gold standard for diagnosis and evaluation of PAD and CLI. With advent of lesser invasive tests such as CTA and MRA, invasive angiography is no longer employed as the initial diagnostic mode. These noninvasive imaging techniques, not only help in diagnoses but also in formulating the plan of care.

Peripheral Vascular CTA

Sixty-four slice Peripheral Vascular CTA (PV-CTA) has revolutionized not only the diagnostic but also the comprehensive clinical management and treatment of PAD. Lesion morphology assessment as permitted by this technology plays a key role in most clinical decision making, especially for endovascular interventions. Device planning during intervention is now determined before the procedure by PV-CTA lesion characteristics, such as calcification, ulceration, thrombus, dissections, soft plaque, and intimal hyperplasia (Figs. 5 and 6). This information allows appropriate tailoring of PVI

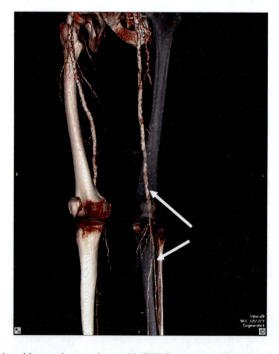

Fig. 5. 3D volume rendered image in a patient with ESRD on hemodialysis, classic depiction of heavy calcification of the vessels (*arrows*).

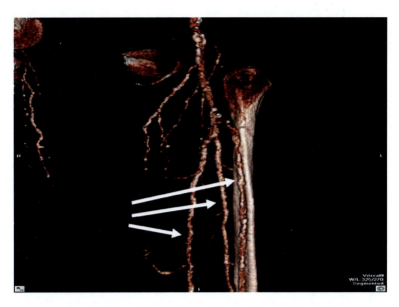

Fig. 6. ESRD CLI, Heavy calcium (*arrows*), Patent SFA, Severe infrapopliteal disease.

devices to the specific lesion or lesions to be treated. Examples of these decisions include PTA, cutting-scoring balloon PTA, laser atherectomy, plaque excision, orbital atherectomy, cryoplasty, bare-metal stents, covered stents, mechanical thrombectomy, and primary thrombolysis.

CTA of the infrainguinal and infrapopliteal arteries is particularly helpful in periprocedural planning in complex CLI patients, despite significant calcification. Using a CLI-CTA protocol with a delayed second lower extremity scan from the knees to the toes, we regularly identify patent distal infrapopliteal and pedal vessels – distal targets – that were not previously imaged during angiography. Contemporary postprocessing software allows vessel magnification, automated region growing techniques, osseous segmentation, curved planar reconstruction, maximal intensity projections, semitransparent volume rendering, vessel tracing to the foot, vessel probing with automated measurements, all as three-dimensional image reconstructive tools designed to allow maximal contrast opacification and infrapopliteal vessel identification and analysis. PV-CTA has become an integral clinical tool in our overall interventional, surgical, and medical management, and follow-up of patients with PVD.

TREATMENT OF CRITICAL LIMB ISCHEMIA

Apart from optimizing medical therapy and risk factor modification, the major modalities of therapy are minimally invasive endovascular approach and the gold standard surgical approach. These modalities aim to relieve pain, promote wound healing, and prevent amputation. Endovascular approach is largely replacing the surgical approach, there has been a dramatic increase in percutaneous revascularization procedures, escalating from 69 to 184 per 100,000 Medicare beneficiaries in the period from 1996 to 2006 with advent of newer tools in Interventional management of CLI. *(8, 9)* (Fig. 7)

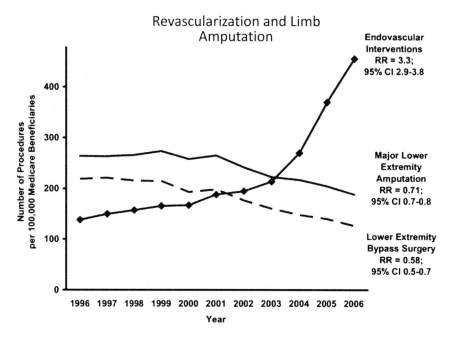

Fig. 7. Revascularization and limb amputation. In recent years, it is encouraging that there is a significant decline in major amputation rates of lower extremities, while the endovascular interventions are on a steep rise (Reprinted with permission from Elsevier from Goodney PP, Beck AW, Nagle J, Welch HG, Zwolak RM, J Vasc Surg 2009;50:54–60).

Endovascular Techniques

The application of the endovascular techniques has become common practice worldwide. Advances in endovascular techniques have allowed for improved acute and long-term success in the treatment of these anatomically complex and high-risk patients, with a significant evolution over the past two decades.

Transition from POBA to the present generation stents, atherectomy devices and CTO crossing devices have made crossing and treating long total occlusions a common practice in most institutions with skills. Most importantly, the morbidity and mortality associated with these procedures are minimal *(9)*. These procedures properly done by experienced operators do not prohibit future surgical bypass or additional endovascular interventions.

Diffuse, multilevel, calcified atherosclerotic obstructive disease is the usual norm in patients with CLI. Diabetics and patients with chronic renal failure on hemodialysis pose an even higher challenge. Chronic total occlusions are very challenging lesions to deal. In this section, we will discuss the modalities of crossing the CTOs followed by reconstruction and their outcomes.

CTO Crossing

The most popular method of crossing a CTO has been the subintimal dissection method of Bolia *(10)*. The success rate reported with this technique is nearly 90% *(11–13)*. The inability to reenter the distal true lumen has been the primary limitation to success in crossing CTOs; however, there is no major downside by trying to avoid the subintimal space for traversal. However if we are unable to reenter at this point, a reentry device can be used to renter the true lumen, which will be discussed later.

Before the procedure is started, we usually perform aortic angiography with run-off using Omniflush catheter (Angiodynamics, Latham, NY) – this gives a landscape of the disease. Majority of the cases we use a contralateral cross-over technique using a Stiff angled Glide Wire (Terumo, Somerset, NJ). Although most devices today can be placed/deployed using 6-Fr sheaths, a larger diameter sheath will provide for more support to penetrate and cross a CTO. A 90-cm sheath is commonly used from a contralateral approach to provide additional support to cross a popliteal or tibial occlusion.

Soon after the access is established and sheaths are placed – anticoagulation needs to be addressed. In our practice, we commonly use bivaliuridin (The Medicines Company, Parsippany, NJ), as most of these procedures are long and therefore consistent, reliable anticoagulation is needed without the necessity for frequent monitoring. Bleeding from perforation is a concern in these situations. If perforations occur – majority of the times they are wire or small catheter related, they can be quickly managed with prolonged balloon inflations, inflating a sphygmomanometer cuff around the calf in tibial vessel perforations and discontinuing the anticoagulation. However, covered stents should be available in the lab treating these patients with diffuse CTOs.

Crossing the CTO in the subintimal plane is best accomplished with the 0.035" Glidewire looped for 2–3 cm, with the Quick Cross (Spectranetics, Colorado Springs, Colorado, USA) catheter looped along – which is a straight tapered, supportive catheter designed for crossing occlusions (Figs. 8–11). However, angled 4-Fr Glide catheter (Terumo, Somerset, NJ, USA) can also be used for this purpose. If the directional control of the wire and catheter is not sufficient to achieve the penetration, then the sheath can be positioned very close to the occlusion to provide more direct axial force with the wire and catheter. If resistance at a point along the occlusion is felt and the loop is not advancing,

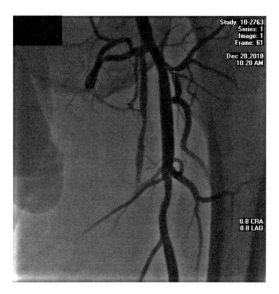

Fig. 8. Total occlusion of the left proximal superficial femoral artery.

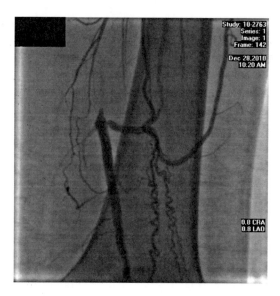

Fig. 9. Distal reconstitution of the left superficial femoral artery. This vessel was collateralized via profunda femoris artery.

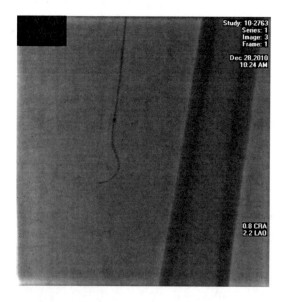

Fig. 10. 0.035" Glide wire advanced to the proximal cap of the SFA occlusion using quick cross catheter.

then manipulation of the wire back into the catheter and redirection of the wire tip within the occlusion will then allow for further progression in crossing the occlusion.

Variations in the wires and catheters for subintimal recanalization can include straight catheters and wires; tapered supported catheters are also effective and are more a personal choice. Ideally, a wire used for subintimal crossing has a hydrophilic coating to minimize drag, particularly in long occlusions. Hydrophilic coating on the supporting catheter is also useful to facilitate catheter traversal of the subintimal space.

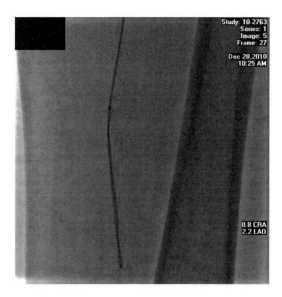

Fig. 11. Classic looping of the wire in the subintimal plane. Caution: The diameter of the loop should never be more than the diameter of the vessel.

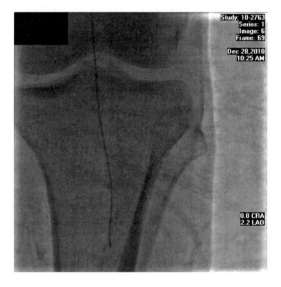

Fig. 12. The nonlooped wire advances freely into the distal true lumen without resistance.

After reaching the point of reconstitution of the vessel beyond the occlusion, the wire is again withdrawn into the catheter and advanced in a nonlooped fashion into the distal lumen (Fig. 12). Then, the support catheter is gently advanced into the distal lumen without resistance, the wire is removed and a confirmation angiography is performed to confirm the true lumen entry (Fig. 13). If the wire does not pass freely into the distal true lumen, then retraction and manipulation of the wire and catheter just proximal to the end of the occlusion may afford true lumen passage.

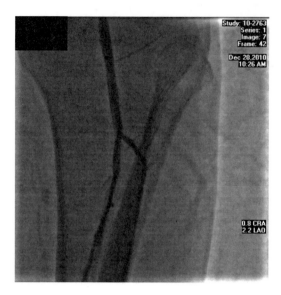

Fig. 13. Angiogram confirming the distal true lumen.

HARDWARE: (WIRES AND CATHETERS)

All the 0.014" coronary wires can be used in these patients. Our work horse wire is Choice PT extra support hydrophilic wire (Boston Scientific, Natick, Massachusetts, USA). This wire offers good support and torque with excellent ability to navigate through the long diffuse stenosis or occlusions.

CTOs of the infrapopliteal vessels do require excellent sheath/catheter support. We commonly use 90-cm sheaths to park the tip in the popliteal artery, under fluoroscopic road map we attempt to cross these lesions with use of Quick Cross support catheters. The use of wires is one's personal choice and experience, we commonly start with Choice PT extra support wire and we gradually escalate up to Asahi Miracle Bros (Abbott Vascular, Redwood City, California, USA) 3–6 g and then finally Confianza wire (Abbott Vascular, Redwood City, California, USA).

ADJUNCTIVE TOOLS FOR CTOs

CROSSER catheter (C.R. Bard, Inc. Murray Hill, NJ) is an ultrasonic energy delivery catheter that disrupts the plaque and thrombus in a CTO directly distal to the tip of the catheter, which then allows for passage of a wire through the occlusion (Fig. 14). The peripheral application of this catheter can be either monorail or over the wire, allowing for utilization of the wire of your choice. The energy is supplied by a small generator that connects to the end of the catheter. The Generator and Transducer convert AC power into high frequency mechanical vibrations which are propagated through a Nitinol core wire to the metal tip of the CROSSER Catheter, which aids in the recanalization of the CTO. We recently presented our experience with this device at TCT 2010, RESPECT trial (Traversing Peripheral Chronic Total Occlusions with the COSSER Device: The Real World Experience of 2050 CTOs) 2050 patients with CTOs, a multicenter registry. Technical success rate was 86.8% in an average CTO length of 220 mm with a total procedure time of 91 min. *(14)*

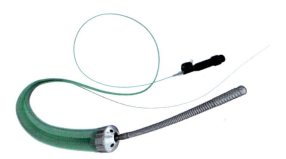

Fig. 14. CROSSER catheter (Courtesy of C.R. Bard, Inc. Murray Hill, NJ).

EXCIMER LASER (Spectranetics, Colorado) Laser catheters can be used as an energy source to allow for penetration and traversal of CTOs. The "Step Technique" of crossing occlusions with the laser involves placing the laser catheter at the proximal cap, without the wire extending out of the catheter. The laser is activated and the lesion is penetrated for a short distance of 1–2 mm with the laser, the wire is then advanced out of the end of the laser catheter a short distance until resistance is met, and the laser is then activated and advanced to the point over the wire. With further ablation of the lesion at the point of resistance, the wire is again advanced to penetrate further. This sequence is repeated in a stepwise fashion to eventually traverse the entire lesion.

FRONTRUNNER CATHETER (Cordis, Miami Lakes, Florida, USA) is a specially designed catheter for penetration and crossing CTOs. The end of the catheter has a small microdissector that can spread its jaws with the repetitive movement of a pistol grip mechanism. It is a low profile device with a crossing profile of 0.039" and comes with a 4.5 F microguide catheter for support. With actuation, the jaws open to a maximum of 2.3 mm outer diameter. In a series of 44 iliac and femoro-popliteal CTOs that had failed routine catheter wire methods for crossing, microdissection was employed, with a technical success in 40 (91%) of these lesions. *(15)*

Controlled blunt microdissection can facilitate penetration of the organized cap of a thrombotic CTO and allow for initiation of true lumen passage. The relatively delicate action of the front runner may not be adequate to cross very fibrous or calcified lesions. The frontrunner may be particularly useful for primary utilization for penetration of an occlusion in certain anatomic circumstances. These include the penetration of an occlusion that is flush at a branch point such as a proximal SFA occlusion where a dissection from subintimal passage at that level is undesirable. The frontrunner may also be useful in crossing of a proximal common iliac occlusion approached from the contralateral femoral access where the guiding catheter has less support to force penetration of the wire into and across the occlusion.

Despite the fact that many devices are now available in the armamentarium of the CLI tool box, central lumen crossing of these long segmental occlusions is a major challenge. These long, heavily calcified, fibrous capped lesions, though they are traversable majority of the times with experience and skills, there should be multiple locations in the vessel, where the hardware could be luminal and subintimal on several occasions. This leads to greater use of reentry devices and adjunctive therapies such as stents, which in these situations have a greater likelihood of stent fractures, which can eventually translate into poor clinical outcomes.

The primary indication for the use of reentry devices is failure to obtain distal true lumen entry, which is the most common cause of acute technical failure in treatment of a CTO. These devices facilitate precise access back into the true lumen, preserve the collateral flow, and limit the extent of dissection and subsequent stenting. There are two types of reentry devices presently available, fluoroscopic guided and IVUS guided.

OUTBACK LTD CATHETER (Cordis Corporation, Miami, FL) is a fluoroscopic guided 5 Fr needle reentry catheter with a retractable nitinol hypotube that has a curved needle end. The rotational orientation of the needle deployment is provided by fluoroscopic guiding marks on the catheter. Before deployment, the "L" mark is oriented to point the true lumen, and in an orthogonal view, the "T" is oriented over the true lumen. If the needle penetrates the true lumen, then the wire freely passes, which can then be advanced and used to accomplish the reconstruction. Available results suggest the Outback LTD to be useful in lesions that have failed other attempts at reentry, with a technical success rate of 88% *(8)*.

The PIONEER CATHETER (Medtronic) is an IVUS guided reentry device. The IVUS image provides an image of the vessel wall, the dissection, and the true lumen. This helps in directing the needle deployment into the true lumen. High success rates have been reported with the use of this device in both iliac and femoral arterial segments *(16, 17)*.

RECONSTRUCTION

The three modes of reconstructing the vessel after successful crossing of the CTO are: balloons, atherectomy devices, and stents.

Balloons

Plain old balloon angioplasty (POBA) is the mainstay endovascular modality of revascularization in CLI. Several studies have shown the technical success of this technique as high as 95% *(18, 19)*. In the BASIL trial, 30-day mortality rates were statistically equivalent between surgery and angioplasty groups (5% and 3%, respectively), complications were significantly less in the angioplasty arm and clinical success at 1 year was not statistically different between surgery and angioplasty (56% vs. 50%, respectively). However, POBA is frequently encountered with densely fibrotic and heavily calcified lesions in patients with CLI, and this where speciality balloons have a great role to play. These balloons include Vascutrak Balloon, Cutting Balloon, Angiosculpt Balloon, and Cryoballoon.

Speciality Balloons

VASCUTRAK (C.R. Bard, Inc. Murray Hill, NJ)

Low profile, monorail System uses Focal Force Pressure (50–400 x's pressure) Concentrates pressure along two axial dimensions providing creation of longitudinal expansion planes to overcome hoop stress thereby increasing luminal diameter with less barotrauma. Diameters – 2–7 mm Lengths – 20–300 mm. Design incorporates two wires to focus balloon inflation force. Improve acute results and long-term outcomes by controlled plaque modification through focal force technology. Use a stress concentrator to fracture plaque at low inflation pressures, before balloon is fully inflated. Reduce the rate of vessel stretching. Enhance lumen enlargement by addressing the causes of recoil and uncontrolled dissection. When a slow controlled stretching occurs, recoil and barotrauma are reduced, maximizing luminal gain.

We retrospectively reviewed 50 patients treated with VT2 and performed an interim analysis of 90-day follow-up. We obtained the limb salvage rates, case time, fluoro time, complications, and adjunctive therapy (anterior tibial – 10, posterior tibial – 5, peroneal – 9, tibioperoneal – 3). Average lesion length – 4.3 cm, 14/27 total occlusions. The technical success rate was 100%, average inflation pressure was 3 atm, and average inflation time was 2 min No complications were noted and adjunctive therapy was used in only 16% of the patients and limb salvage rate at 90 days was 88%.

Cutting Balloon

The infrapopliteal vessels deem enough respect similar to that of the coronary vessels. They are almost similar in size and diameter, clearing the indication for use of cutting balloons in the infrapopliteal vessels. This balloon is equipped with atherotomes on its surface mounted on a noncompliant balloon and when dilated causes controlled scoring of the plaque with fewer flow limiting dissections and elastic recoil. *Ansel*, reported a 1-year limb salvage rate of 85.9% with 20% adjunctive stenting for dissections and inadequate dilatation *(20)*.

Angiosculpt Balloon (Angioscore, Inc., Freemont, CA)

This is a two-component system balloon. It is an OTW or rapid exchange system with nitinol spiral cage encased around the balloon, which is thought to increase device flexibility and improve deliverability. Bosier et al. reported their data in 31 CLI patients treated with Angiosculpt balloon. One-year survival and limb salvage were 83.9% and 86.3%, respectively *(33)*.

Cryoplasty (Boston Scientific) (Fig. 15)

The PolarCath Peripheral Dilatation System (Boston Scientific) is a disposable unit which uses nitrous oxide to fill an angioplasty balloon to approximately 8 atm, cooling its surface to −10°C, the triple layered angioplasty balloon is inflated, the cold surface of the balloon cools the vascular lesion, which exerts both mechanical and biological

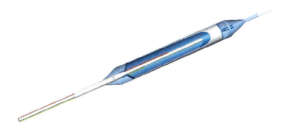

Fig. 15. The PolarCath Peripheral Dilatation System (Courtesy of Boston Scientific). Cryoplasty Procedure: (1) Liquid refrigerant travels through the lumen of the catheter to the balloon. (2) The liquid changes to a gas expanding the balloon and reducing the temperature. (3) Refrigerant flows continuously throughout the treatment cycle and the temperature is regulated. (4) The gas is evacuated and the balloon is deflated.

effects that may help prevent restenosis by the mechanism of apoptosis. The BTK-Chill trial *(21)* at 12 months follow-up revealed technical success rate of 97.3% and amputation free survival at 1 year was 85%.

Drug Eluting Balloons

In.Pact Deep (Medtronic Invatec), the paclitaxel-eluting balloon has the best available clinical data at the present time. A prospective registry data of 107 patients using this balloon on below the knee arteries was recently presented.

Mean lesion length was 174 ± 89 mm, 60.5% of patients had an occlusion, and the remaining 39.5% had stenotic disease. The follow-up included angiography after 3 months and clinical follow-up at 3, 6, and 12 months. At 3 months, an angiographic restenosis rate of more than 50% was seen in 27% of all lesions treated, with restenosis of the entire treated segment of 11%. Awaiting long-term data, the ongoing trials including EURO canal study should provide the evidence needed to prove the clinical benefit of this application in below the knee arterial segments. The combination of atherectomy followed by a drug eluting balloon in these arterial distributions makes perfect technical and clinical sense and we are looking forward for large randomized trials to be conducted to answer this question.

ATHERECTOMY DEVICES

Removal of the plaque from the diseased segments of the artery is a very attractive option. There are numerous atherectomy devices available at the present time. These devices can broadly be classified into three major groups, namely, Rotational (Diamondback –CSI, Jetsream G2 – Pathway medical), Excisional (Silverhawk – EV3), and Ablative (Excimer Laser – Spectranetics). The use of these devices is marred by increased cost, larger size sheaths, and potential for distal embolization. Moreover, there is no randomized data at the present time showing the benefit of these devices over the conventional therapy, and we do not expect them to be anytime in the near future due to several reasons. However, these devices can be used in certain special situations like infrapopliteal disease, ostial lesions, bifurcating lesions, and calcified lesions. In this section, we will briefly review the atherectomy devices and the supporting data.

Diamondback 360° (Cardiovascular Systems Inc., St. Paul, MN) (Fig. 16)

This is a rotational orbital atherectomy system which is equipped with diamond-coated crown orbits that rotates at high RPMs, preferentially sanding calcium and avoiding barotrauma. The particulate sizes as determined in lab were 2.3 μ, compared with 7 μ diameter particulate size of the conventional Rotablator system. Hence distal embolism is uncommon with use of this device and distal protection device is not needed. By removing the noncompliant components of the plaque, this device can produce excellent stand-alone result with less use of adjunctive therapy. We presented our data with the use of this device in 80 patients presenting with infrapopliteal disease comparing with conventional POBA *(22)*. The procedural success rate was higher in Diamondback group compared with POBA (94% vs. 88%) and adjunctive stenting was used in 5% vs. 45% which is consistent with the OASIS data for this outcome. *(23)*

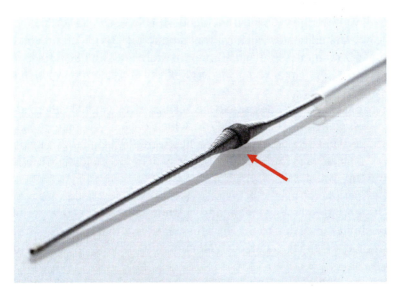

Fig. 16. Diamond coated (*arrow*) burr of orbital atherectomy system (OAS) (Courtesy of Cardiovascular Systems Inc., St. Paul, MN).

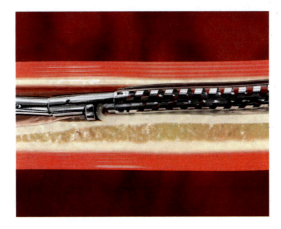

Fig. 17. Silverhawk Atherectomy device (Courtesy of (ev3 Inc., Plymouth, MN).

Of great importance was a larger luminal gain in the minimal luminal diameter with Diamondback device. In our experience, this device works extremely well in heavily calcified fem-pop and infrapopliteal vessels.

Silverhawk Plaque Excision System (ev3 Inc., Plymouth, MN). (Fig. 17)

It is a directional atherectomy device, consisting of a 110–135-cm flexible shaft designed to track over a 0.014-in. guidewire. The device can be introduced through a 6- to 8-F sheath. The carbide cutter rotating at 8,000 rpm excises the plaque that is collected into the catheter nose cone. This is the only device that is currently approved by the US Food and Drug Administration (FDA) for excisional atherectomy.

There are no randomized trial data for excisional atherectomy with the Silverhawk in CLI. The largest of the registries is the TALON (Treating Peripherals with Silverhawk:

Outcomes Collection) registry, which included 19 US centers *(24)*. The technical success was 97.6%, and adjunctive therapy was required in 21.7% of patients. The target lesion revascularization rates at 6 and 12 months were 90% and 80%, respectively. The 12-month outcomes compare favorably to angioplasty and stenting, which have reported patency rates of 61–67%.

Recently, McKinsey et al. described the results of excisional atherectomy in 275 patients (579 lesions) from 2004 to 2007 in which 63% of the patients had CLI. The 18-month primary and secondary patency rates were 49% and 70%, respectively, for CLI patients. Limb salvage rate was 92.4% per patient at 18 months. The 30-day perioperative mortality was 1.8%. *(35)*.

TurboHawk peripheral plaque excision system (ev3 Inc.) is designed for the treatment of all lesion morphologies, including calcium located in native peripheral arteries. It is very similar in design to the Silverhawk, except that it has four angled cutters that are designed to engage and cut calcium, thus making it useful for calcified vessels.

These excisional atherectomy devices work exceptionally well in eccentric and bifurcating lesions. Since this device works on the concept of excision, there is always a risk of distal embolization, hence use of embolic protection device is strongly recommended to be used in conjunction.

Excimer Laser Atherectomy (Spectranetics corporation, Colorado) (Fig. 18)

This is a cold-tipped laser that delivers bursts of ultraviolet/xenon energy (308 nm) in short pulse durations, which causes photochemical ablation. The ultraviolet light provides a direct lytic action that ablates 5 µm of tissue on contact without a rise in surrounding tissue temperature, hence there is no untoward tissue trauma. Our group has a tremendous experience with its use.

The LACI (Laser Angioplasty for CLI) *(26)* study enrolled 145 patients with CLI at 14 sites in the US and Germany and examined the excimer laser in 155 limbs and 423 lesions: 41% SFA, 15% popliteal, 41% infrapopliteal, and 70% combination of stenoses. The patients were all deemed poor surgical candidates. Straight-line flow to the foot was restored in 89% of the patients, with adjunctive PTA and stenting in 96% and 45% of cases, respectively. The 6-month limb salvage rate was 92.5% with a major amputation rate of 8%. Based on these data and with further advancements, laser therapy may play a greater role in the treatment of CLI.

This device is widely used in our practice in multiple settings including its use in heavily burdened atherothrombotic vessels. Its use in calcified lesions is limited, as the degree of tissue calcification increases, the XeCl ablation mechanism changes from a photoablative decomposition to a laser-induced plasma shock wave disruption. However, pretreating the calcified lesions with LASER will make the lesions more compliant and amenable for adjunctive therapy.

STENTS IN CLI PATIENTS

At the present time there is no randomized data supporting systematic stenting in BTK lesions. This modality is reserved for interventions with elastic recoil, flow limiting dissections, perforations, and suboptimal results. The standard teaching is to deploy balloon expandable stents in the proximal noncompressible segments and self-expanding

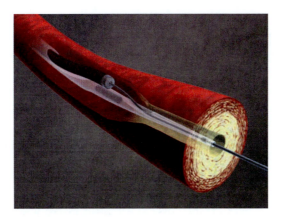

Fig. 18. Turbo Tandem Laser, with the ability to create larger lumens with four-quadrant ablation abilities (Courtesy: Spectranetics Inc).

stents in the mid-distal compressible segments of the tibial vessels which conform to the vessel wall.

Balloon Expandable Stents

The use of bare-metal stents in BTK lesions has traditionally been associated with a 6-month binary restenosis rates of over 50%. And since there are no dedicated BTK bare-metal stents, coronary stents are used in this territory which have major limitations in stent sizes and lengths. Moreover the flow dynamics in infrapopliteal vessels is much different than in the coronary circulation.

The drug-eluting stents have been a focus of interest lately to extrapolate the observations from the drug-eluting stent trials in the coronary vasculature. Katsanos et al. reported their data in 103 CLI patients treated with sirolimus eluting stent versus bare metal stents. Three-year patency rate was 60% versus 10% (HR 4.8. 95% CI 2.9–7.9; $p<0.001$)

The Paradise study investigated the efficiency and safety of balloon-expandable drug-eluting stents to prevent amputation in patients with BTK CLI. The 3-year cumulative rate of amputation was $6\%\pm2\%$, and binary restenosis occurred in 12% of the 35% of patients who underwent repeat angiography *(27)*.

Rastan et al. reported the primary use of sirolimus-eluting stents in the infrapopliteal arteries *(28)*. After 6 months and 1 year, the primary patency rates were 88.5% and 83.7%, respectively.

Lookstein et al. presented their data in 56 CLI patients, where in 101 drug eluting stents were used for bail-out in patients with suboptimal results (86 sirolimus, 13 everolimus, 2 paclitaxel). The primary patency at 6 and 24 months were 90% and 72% respectively, and freedom from amputation was 89.3% for the entire cohort *(33)*.

Self-Expanding Stents

The EXCELL study evaluated the use of self-expanding Xpert stent in BTK lesions. A total of 120 patients with varying degree of severity were enrolled. Mean stented vessel length was 7.6 cm. At 6-month follow-up in 115 patients, interim data showed that there were a total of 36 target lesion revascularizations (31.3%), of which, 21 (18.3%) were symptomatic. There were seven major amputations (6.1%), six deaths (5.2%), four target vessel revascularizations (3.5%), and one access-site complication requiring transfusion (0.9%). Wound healing data showed that 68 wounds (53.5%) were 100% healed, 43 (33.9%) had significantly decreased wound areas, and 16 (12.6%) had increased wound areas at 6-month follow-up. *(29)*

CASE STUDIES: ENDOVASCULAR INTERVENTIONS IN CLI

Case 1

History: 76-year-old female patient with history of diabetes mellitus, hypertension, coronary artery disease with 1-year history of progressively worsening claudication pains. The initial angiogram revealed 100% occlusion of right mid-SFA with distal reconstitution via large inter-arterial collaterals (Fig. 19).

Hardware Used: 6 F 42 cm contralateral cross-over sheath, 300 cm length Choice PT-extra support wire, CROSSER – 18 catheter, 2 mm OTW Spectranetics Laser catheter, Vascutrak 6×60 mm balloon, and Self-expanding 6×100 mm Nitinol Stent.

Procedure in detail: CROSSER-18 catheter with Choice PT wire support was parked at the proximal cap Fig. 20) and the catheter was activated. Total crossing time into the distal true lumen was 1.8 min. The wire was gently advanced into the distal lumen without resistance (Fig. 21). Following this, the CROSSER catheter was exchanged with Spectranetics 2 mm Laser catheter was advanced to the location of the proximal cap and the entire segment was ablated at the rate of 1 mm/sec (Fig. 22). Following which a balloon angioplasty was performed with VASCUTRAK 6×60 mm Balloon, slow inflation to 3 atm for 2 min (Fig. 23) and lastly 6×100 mm Nitinol self-expanding stent was deployed with an excellent angiographic result (Fig. 24). Patient had immediate resolution of symptoms.

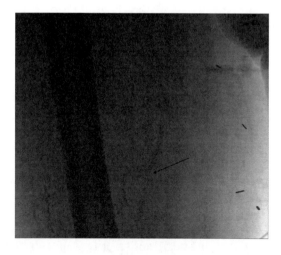

Fig. 19. 100% occluded mid-SFA with distal reconstitution (*arrow*).

Critical Limb Ischemia 61

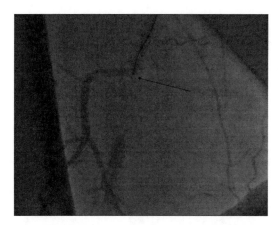

Fig. 20. CROSSER 18 catheter with 0.014 in. support parked at the proximal cap (*arrow*) and activated.

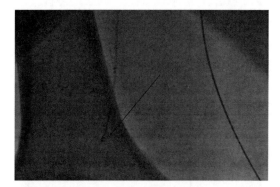

Fig. 21. Successful traversal of the CROSSER catheter into the distal true lumen (*arrow*) without resistance and 0.014-in. wire being advanced into distal lumen.

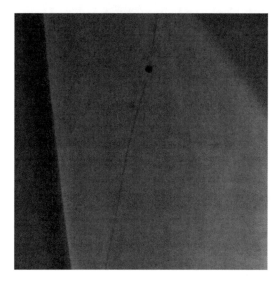

Fig. 22. LASER atherectomy with 2-mm probe.

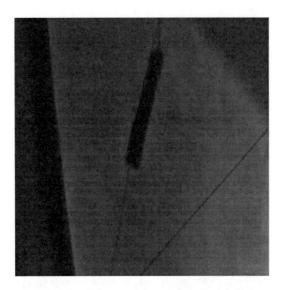

Fig. 23. Balloon angioplasty with Vascutrak 6×60 mm balloon.

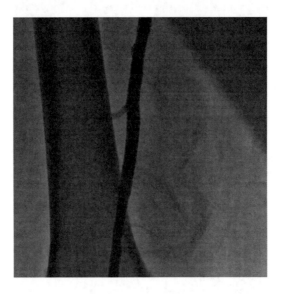

Fig. 24. Final angiogram following stenting with 6×100 self expanding Nitinol Stent. NOTE: Collaterals are still preserved.

Case 2

History: 78-year-old white female patient with long-standing history of uncontrolled diabetes mellitus and chronic active smoking referred from outside institution after failed fem-tibial bypass graft with gangrene of the toes and nonhealing ulcers on the dorsum of the foot. This patient was recommended BTK amputation at outside institution.

Hardware Used: 6 F 90 cm contralateral cross-over sheath, 300 cm length Choice PT-extra support wire, CROSSER – 14 S catheter, Vascutrak 3×100 mm balloon.

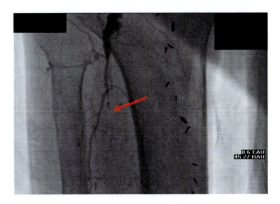

Fig. 25. Crosser 14 s, Advanced (*arrow*).

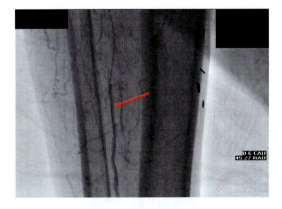

Fig. 26. Crosser advanced, peroneal wired (*arrow*).

Procedure in detail: Initial angiogram was performed through the sheath parked in the popliteal artery, which revealed total occlusions of the tibial and peroneal artery with distal reconstitution at the level of the ankle collateralizing both the tibial arteries. CROSSER-14 S catheter with Choice PT wire support was parked at the proximal cap of the peroneal artery (Fig. 25) and the catheter was activated. Total crossing time into the distal true lumen was 2.2 min. The wire was gently advanced into the distal lumen without resistance (Fig. 26). Following this, the CROSSER catheter was exchanged with VASCUTRAK 3×100 mm Balloon, slow inflation to 3 atm for 4 min was performed (Fig. 27) and excellent angiographic results were obtained without the need for any further adjunctive therapy (Fig. 28). Patient went onto have trans-metatarsal amputation and flapped stump healed in 1 month. This intervention has greatly averted an otherwise aggressive amputation to relatively smaller one.

Case 3

History: 82-year-old black male patient with history of diabetes mellitus and chronic smoking, severe COPD with continuous oxygen dependence and multiple lower extremity endovascular interventions, S/P right fem-pop bypass surgery with complaints of worsening claudication to the present status of rest claudication and limb threatening

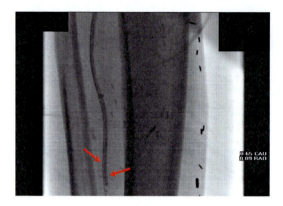

Fig. 27. 2.0×120 mm VascuTRAK 2. Note 2 Wires (*arrows*).

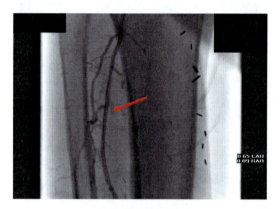

Fig. 28. Excellent final results (*arrow*).

ischemia. An initial CTA was performed to plan the procedure and also to evaluate the access site. The CTA revealed high grade stenosis of proximal anastomotic segment of the right fem-pop bypass graft. (Fig. 29)

Hardware Used: 7 F 42 cm contralateral cross-over sheath, 300 cm length Choice PT-extra support wire, Silverhawk Atherectomy device.

Procedure in detail: Initial angiogram was performed through the sheath parked in the right external iliac artery, which confirmed the CTA findings, also note sluggish flow in the profunda femoris artery (the most important source of collaterals in the lower extremities) (Fig. 30). After anticoagulation with bivalirudin, a 300-cm length Choice PT extra support wire was advanced into the right fem-pop bypass graft. The Silverhawk atherectomy device was tracked to the proximal edge of the lesion site and atherectomy was performed with four quadrant cuts (Fig. 31), large amount of fibrocalcific atheromatous debris was excised from the lesion site (Fig. 32). Final angiogram revealed excellent result with no residual disease and hence no further adjunctive therapy was needed (Fig. 33). Patient had quick resolution of his symptoms. This endovascular procedure has helped the patient avoid surgical endarterectomy and its associated morbidity and mortality in this patient with poor cardiopulmonary reserve.

Critical Limb Ischemia 65

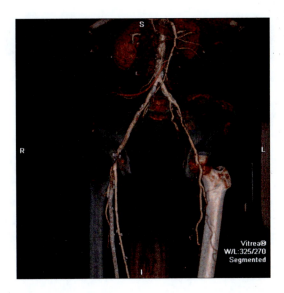

Fig. 29. High grade disease at the proximal anastomosis of fem-pop bypass graft.

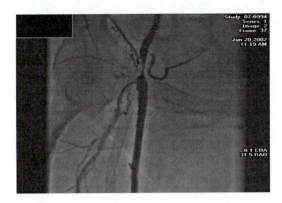

Fig. 30. Angiographic correlation of the peripheral CTA, revealing the "Graft Marker" at proximal anastomosis.

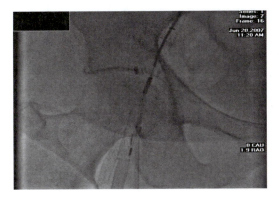

Fig. 31. Silverhawk atherectomy device performing multiquadrant atherectomy at proximal anastomosis.

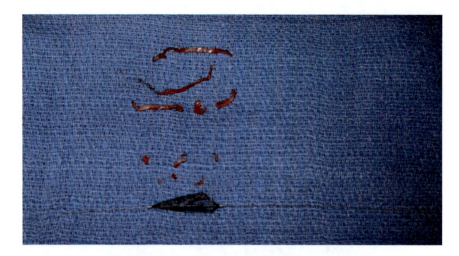

Fig. 32. Debris collected in the distal protection filter postatherectomy.

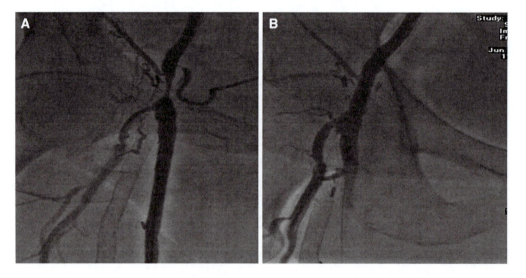

Fig. 33. Pre (**A**) and post (**B**) angiograms following Silverhawk atherectomy.

Case 4

History: 67-year-old Hispanic female patient with history of ESRD on hemodialysis, hypertension, diabetes mellitus referred by podiatrist for vascular evaluation and management for nonhealing ulcer on the dorsum of the foot (Fig. 34). An angiogram performed in the lab revealed occluded tibio-peroneal trunk with faint collateralization at the level of the ankle. The anterior tibial artery in the proximal segment was noted to have 99% fibrocalcific lesion (Fig. 35).

Hardware Used: 7 F 90 cm contralateral cross-over sheath, 300 cm length Choice PT-extra support wire, 130 cm length quick-cross catheter, CSI orbital atherectomy 2 mm orbit, Balloon expandable 5×40 mm stent.

Procedure in detail: The initial set-up angiogram was performed via the 7 F sheath parked in the popliteal artery. The high grade proximal anterior tibial artery lesion was

Critical Limb Ischemia

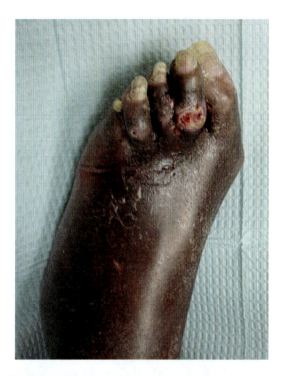

Fig. 34. Ischemic nonhealing ulcer on the dorsal foot.

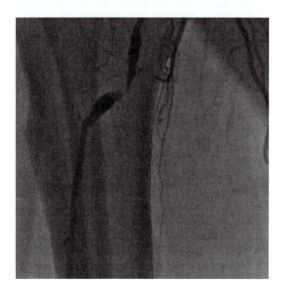

Fig. 35. Single vessel run-off with high grade lesion at the bend in anterior tibial artery.

initially crossed with Choice PT extra support wire. Then a 0.035-in. Quick cross catheter was tracked over the wire into the distal anterior tibial artery and then this wire was exchanged with VIPER wire (dedicated 0.018 wire to be used with CSI device). Orbital atherectomy was performed with 2-mm solid crown with escalating RPMs of low,

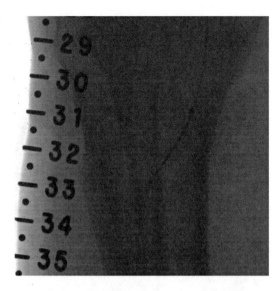

Fig. 36. Orbital atherectomy of the anterior tibial artery.

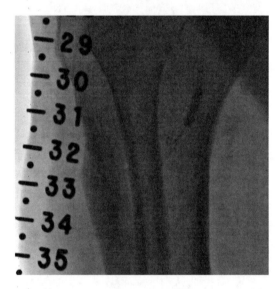

Fig. 37. Postatherectomy angioplasty performed with Focal Force angioplasty utilizing Vascutrak Balloon.

medium, and high (Fig. 36). There was a significant resolution of the lesion to 30%, since this was a limb salvage case with the last remaining vessel, a 5×40 mm balloon expandable stent was deployed (Fig. 37) with excellent angiographic results (Fig. 38). This patient went on to heal the ischemic ulcer on the dorsum of the foot. This is a good example of true limb salvage done the endovascular way.

Case 5

History: 77-year-old Asian female patient with past history of diabetes mellitus, hypertension, coronary artery disease, S/P CABG 5 years ago referred by her vascular

Critical Limb Ischemia

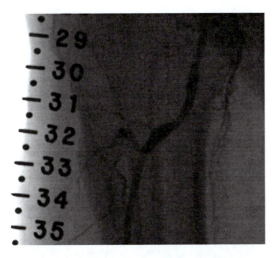

Fig. 38. Final result following balloon angioplasty.

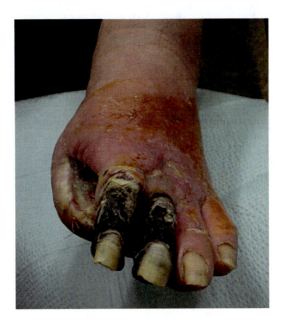

Fig. 39. Gangrene of the left foot toes. Also note auto-amputation of the great toe.

surgeon for PAD evaluation and management. She was seen by another physician in the last week and was recommended amputation of her right foot (Fig. 39). An angiogram was performed which revealed total occlusion of the bilateral tibial arteries, patent peroneal artery (Fig. 40).

Hardware Used: 7 F 90 cm contralateral cross-over sheath, 300 cm length Miracle Bro 6 gm and Choice PT-extra support wire, 130 cm length quick-cross catheter, 2.5×150 mm Vascutrak balloon.

Procedure in detail: The initial setup angiogram was performed using a 7-F sheath. The totally occluded PTA was attempted to cross with Choice PT wire using

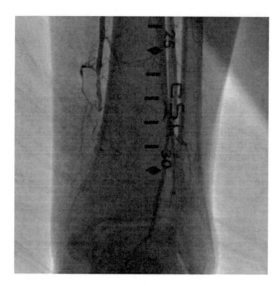

Fig. 40. Total occlusion of distal anterior tibial artery in a patient with nonhealing ulcer in the angiosomal distribution on the dorsal foot.

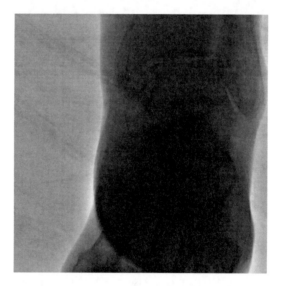

Fig. 41. Successful wire traversal of the anterior tibial artery.

0.014 Quick Cross support catheter, but the occlusion could not be crossed despite all prudent attempts. Hence a Miracle Bro 6 gm wire was used and after a brief manipulation, the wire crossed into the distal true lumen, now the wire was exchanged back to Choice PT (Fig. 41). Following which balloon angioplasty was performed with 2.5 × 150 mm balloon for about 3 min (Fig. 42). There was an excellent angiographic result (Fig. 43)

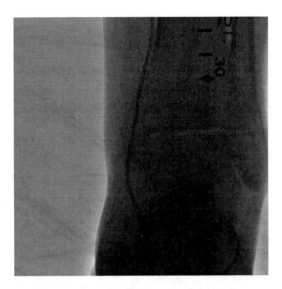

Fig. 42. Balloon angioplasty following wire traversal into the distal true lumen.

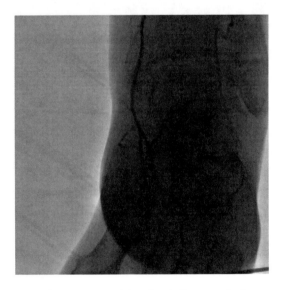

Fig. 43. Final result following balloon angioplasty.

Case 6

History: 69-year-old Hispanic female patient with past history of HTN, and diabetes mellitus and PAD with fem-tibial bypass, referred by her podiatrist for PAD evaluation and management. She had been complaining of lifestyle limiting rest claudication which was progressive for the last 8 months. Initial work-up also included a PV-CTA (Fig. 44). An angiogram was performed which revealed total occlusion of the TP-trunk. (Fig. 45)

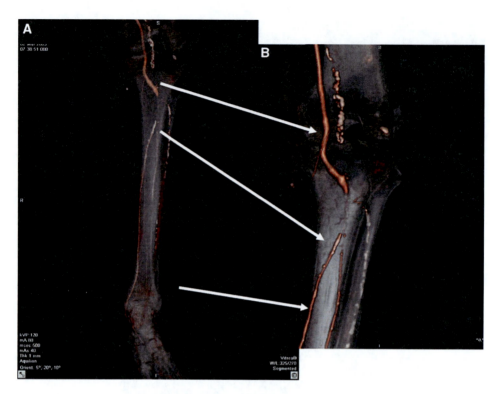

Fig. 44. (**A, B**) Failing bypass graft. Note patent distal runoff target; this was not seen on angiography (*arrows*).

(Note: Distal filling of the TP-trunk as visualized on PV-CTA delayed imaging, which was not otherwise visualized on diagnostic angiogram. This technology has greatly enhanced peripheral vascular imaging and for planning and guiding the interventions.)

Hardware Used: 7 F 90 cm contralateral cross-over sheath, 300 cm length Miracle Bro 12 gm and Choice PT-extra support wire, 130 cm length quick-cross catheter, 3.0×60 mm Cryoplasty balloon.

Procedure in detail: The initial setup angiogram was performed using a 7-F sheath. The totally occluded PTA was attempted to cross with Choice PT wire using 0.014 Quick Cross support catheter, but the occlusion could not be crossed. Hence a Miracle Bro 12 gm wire was used and after a brief manipulation the wire crossed into the distal true lumen, now the wire was exchanged back to Choice PT. Following which balloon angioplasty was performed with 3.0×60 mm Cryoplasty balloon (Fig. 46). Excellent angiographic result was obtained (Fig. 47)

Case 7

History: 46-year-old African male patient with history of HTN, dyslipidemia, polycystic kidney disease, now on HD for the last 7 years with rest claudication. PV-CTA revealed occluded tibial vessels with high grade segmental peroneal artery lesions which was heavily calcified (Figs. 48 and 49). In view of multiple comorbidities and high-risk candidate for surgical bypass, endovascular approach was recommended.

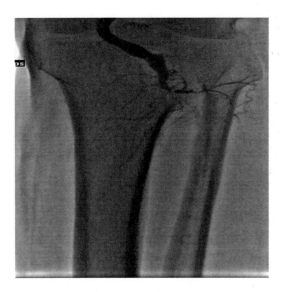

Fig. 45. Total occlusion of the TP trunk in a patient with CLI.

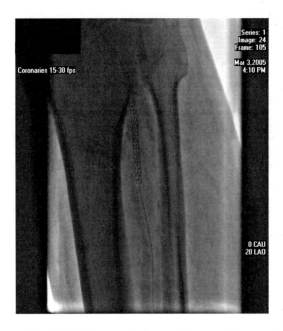

Fig. 46. Balloon angioplasty with cryoballoon.

Hardware Used: 7 F 90 cm contralateral cross-over sheath, 300 cm length Choice PT-extra support wire, 130 cm length quick-cross catheter, 0.018" Viper wire and 2 mm Orbital atherectomy burr.

Procedure in detail: The initial setup angiogram was performed using a 7-F sheath. The diffusely diseased peroneal artery was successfully traversed using Choice PT wire, which was then exchanged to 0.018" viper wire and orbital atherectomy was performed using 2-mm burr (Fig. 50) with progressive increase in the speed of spinning. Following

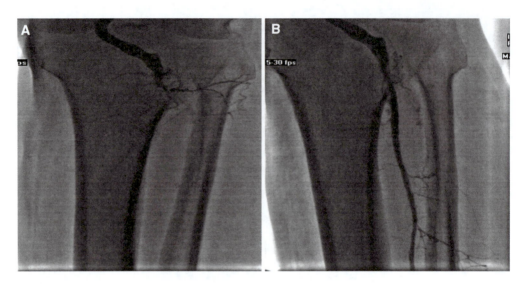

Fig. 47. Final angioplasty result following cryoplasty balloon angioplasty. (**A**) Pre; (**B**) Post.

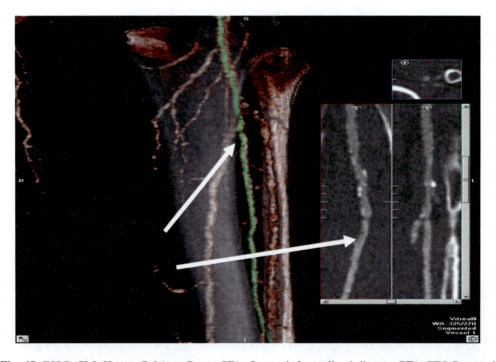

Fig. 48. ESRD CLI, Heavy *Calcium*, Patent SFA, Severe infrapopliteal disease. PTA CTO Peroneal 90% Stenosis (*arrows*).

Critical Limb Ischemia

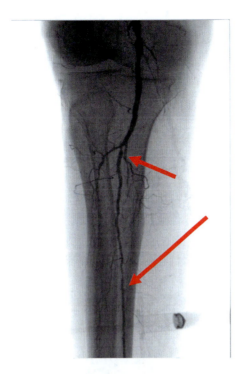

Fig. 49. Peroneal 90% and 95% stenosis (*arrows*).

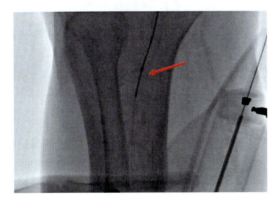

Fig. 50. CSI orbital atherectomy device (*arrow*).

two passes, excellent stand-alone angiographic result was obtained (Figs. 51 and 52) and this patient had almost immediate resolution of symptoms.

FUTURE PERSPECTIVES AND CONCLUSIONS

Endovascular interventions are minimally invasive techniques with a high technical success rate which help in alleviating symptoms, minimizing tissue loss, promoting wound healing, and avoiding amputation. However, at the present time there is no consensus on the best use of endovascular modality in most patients. There has been a paradigm shift in treating patients with CLI by endovascular techniques in recent years with encouraging results.

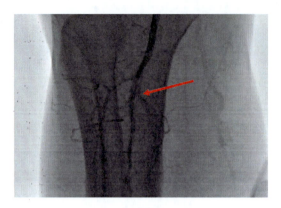

Fig. 51. Excellent proximal peroneal results (*arrow*).

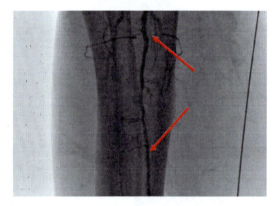

Fig. 52. Excellent distal peroneal results (*arrows*).

Since the publication of BASIL trial, we need no more debate that endovascular interventions should be considered the primary approach in this group of patients. Unfortunately due to the lack of the randomized data, no systematic guidelines can be written at this time. CLI imposes a major economic burden on health and social care resources. Patients presenting with CLI and getting treated only represent a minute proportion, the true dimensions of which are not yet completely defined. Every effort possible should be geared at these patients to salvage the threatened foot. Clinical examinations and vascular laboratory examinations remain the mainstay for the diagnosis of CLI. Both CTA and MRA performed with state-of-the-art technique can provide information to confirm diagnosis, to identify the level of arterial obstruction, and to plan an interventional procedure.

Endovascular treatment of CLI requires the physician to be very proficient with crossing and reconstruction of CTOs. Numerous techniques and devices are required to maximize the acute success. Future technology that combines image guidance and ablative devices may improve the ability to cross all CTOs. If untreated, CLI carries a high risk of limb loss, mortality, and morbidity. Excellent limb-salvage rates are now being achieved with a variety of endovascular therapies. As the armamentarium used is evolving and expanding including newer ablative atherectomy devices and, specialized guidewires for crossing chronic total occlusions, specialty balloon catheters, balloon-expandable and self-expanding covered and noncovered stents, drug-eluting balloons and drug-eluting stents, (though there is no randomized data), endovascular revascularization can restore straight line-flow in one or more of the tibial arteries which should translate into saving a limb, improving quality of life, and possibly decreasing the mortality.

REFERENCES

1. Norgren L, Hiatt WR, Dormandy JA, et al. Inter-society consensus for the management of peripheral arterial disease (TASC II). *J Vasc Surg.* 2007;45(supplS):S5.
2. TASC. Management of peripheral arterial disease (PAD). Trans-Atlantic inter-society consensus (TASC). *J Vasc Surg.* 2000;31(suppl1):S1–S287.
3. US Department of Health and Human Services. National Center for Health Statistics. National Hospital Discharge Survey: Annual Summary with Detailed Diagnosis and Procedure Data. Data from the National Hospital Discharge Survey. Series 13. 1983–2000.
4. Singh S, Evans L, Datta D, et al. The costs of managing lower limb ischemia. *Eur J Vasc Endovasc Surg.* 1996;12:359–362.
5. Ferraresi R, Centola M, Ferlini M, et al. Long-term outcomes after angioplasty of isolated, below-the-knee arteries in diabetic patients with critical limb ischemia. *Eur J Vasc Endovasc Surg.* 2009;:1–7.
6. Fisher RK, Harris PL. Epidemiological and economic considerations in the critically ischemic limb. In: Branchereau A, Jacobs M, eds. *Critical Limb Ischemia.* Armonk, NY: Futura Publishing Company, Inc.; 1999:19–25.
7. Adam DJ, Beard JD, Cleveland T, et al. BASIL trial participants. Bypass versus angioplasty in severe ischemia of the leg (BASIL): multicentre, randomized controlled trial. *Lancet.*2005;336:1925–1934.
8. Beschorner U, Sixt S, Schwarzwälder U, et al. Recanalization of the chronic occlusions of the superficial femoral artery using the Outback Rentry catheter: A single center experience. *Cath Cardiovasc Intervent.* 2009;74:934–938.
9. *J Vasc Surg.* 2009;50:54–60.
10. Bolia A, Brennan J, Bell PR. Recanalization of femoro-popliteal occlusions: improving success rate by subintimal recanalization. *Clin Radiol.* 1989;40:325.
11. Lazaris AM, Tsiamis AC, Fishwick G, et al. Clinical outcome of primary infrainguinal subintimal angioplasty in diabetic patients with critical lower limb ischemia. *J Endovasc Ther.* 2004;11:447–453.
12. Lazaris AM, Sala C, Tsiamis AC, et al. Factors affecting patency of subintimal infrainguinal angioplasty in patients with critical lower limb ischemia. *Euro J Vasc Endovasc Surg.* 2006;32:668–674.
13. Scott EC, Biuckians A, Light RE, et al. Subintimal Angioplasty for the treatment of claudication and critical limb ischemia: 3 year results. *J Vasc Surg.* 2007;46:959–964.
14. Patlola RR, Hebert C, et al. traversing peripheral chronic total occlusions with the COSSER device: the real world experience of 2050 CTOs (RESPECT trial): TCT 2010, Washington DC.
15. Mossop PJ, Amukotuwa SA, Whitbourn RJ. Controlled blunt microdissection for percutaneous recanalization of lower limb arterial chronic total occlusions: a single center experience. *Catheter Cardiovasc Interv.* 2006;68(2):304–310.
16. Weisinger B, Steinkamp H, Konig C, et al. Technical report and preliminary clinical data of a novel catheter for luminal reentry after subintimal dissection. *Invest Radiol.* 2205;40(11):725–728.
17. Hausegger KA, Georgieva B, Portugaller H, et al. The Outback catheter: a new device for true lumen reentry after dissection during recanalization of arterial occlusions. *Cardioavasc Intervent Radiol.* 2004;27(1):26–30.
18. Balmer H, Mahler F, Do D, et al. Balloon angioplasty in chronic critical limb ischemiaÑFactors affecting clinical and angiographic outcome. *J Endovasc Ther.* 2002;9:403–410.
19. Spinosa JD, Leung DA, Matsumoto AH, et al. Percutaneous intentional extraluminal recanalization in patients with chronic critical limb ischemia. *Radiology.* 2004;232:499–507.

20. Ansel GM, Sample NS, Botti CF, et al. Cutting balloon angioplasty of the popliteal and infrapopliteal vessels for symptomatic limb ischemia. *Cathet Cardiovasc Interv.* 2004;61:1–4.
21. Das TS, McNamara T, Gray B, et al. Primary cryoplasty therapy provides durable support for limb salvage in critical limb ischemia patients with infrapopliteal lesions: 12- month follow-up results from the BTK Chill Trial. *J Endovasc Ther.* 2009;16(suppl 2):
22. Patlola R, Hebert C, Allie D. Orbital atherectomy in treatment of peripheral arterial occlusive disease below the knee: a large single-center experience. Abstract presented at Transcatheter Cardiovascular Therapeutics, September 21–26, 2009; San Francisco, CA.
23. Safian RD, Niazi K, Runyon JP, et al. Orbital atherectomy for infrapopliteal disease: device concept and outcome data for the OASIS trial. *Cathet Cardiovasc Interv.* 2009;73:406–412
24. Ramaiah V, Gammon R, Kiesz S, et al. Midterm outcomes from the TALON registry: treating peripherals with Silverhawk: outcomes collection. *J Endovasc Ther.* 2006;13:592–602
25. McKinsey JF, Goldstein L, Khan HU, et al. Novel treatment of patients with lower extremity ischemia: use of percutaneous atherectomy in 579 lesions. *Ann Surg.* 2008;248:519–528.
26. Laird JR, Zeller T, Gray BH, et al. Limb salvage following laser-assisted angioplasty for critical limb ischemia: results of the LACI multicenter trial. *J Endovasc Ther.* 2006;13:1–11.
27. Feiring AJ. Preventing leg amputations in critical limb ischemia with below-the-knee drug-eluting stents: the PARADISE (Preventing Amputations Using Drug Eluting Stents) trial. *JACC.* 2010;55:1580–1589.
28. Rastan A, Schwarzwälder U, Noory E, et al. Primary use of sirolimus-eluting stents in the infrapopliteal arteries. *J Endovasc Ther.* 2010;17:480–487.
29. Rocha-Singh K. Interim results from the VIVA I: Xcell Trial. *Endovasc Today.* 2009:3:57–59.
30. Dosluoglu HH, O'Brien MS, Lukan J, et al. Does preferential use of endovascular interventions by vascular surgeons improve limb salvage, control for symptoms, and survival of patients with critical limb ischemia. *Am J Surg.* 2006;192(5):572–576.
31. Haider SN, Kavanagh EG, Forlee M, et al. Two-year outcome with preferential use of infrainguinal angioplasty for critical ischemia. *J Vasc Surg.* 2006;43(3):504–512.
32. Nasr MK, McCarthy RJ, Hardman J, et al. The increasing role of percutaneous transluminal angioplasty in the primary management of critical limb ischemia. *Eur J Vasc Endovasc Surg.* 2002;23(5):398-403.
33. Bosiers M, Cagiannos C, Deloose K, et al. The use of angiosculpt scoring balloon for infrapopliteal lesions in patients with critical limb ischemia: one year outcome. *Vascular.* 2009;17(1):29–35.
34. Robert Lookstein. Outcomes with drug-eluting stents for Infrapopliteal disease in the critical limb. TCT Conference, 2010, Washington DC.
35. McKinsey JF, Goldstein L, Khan HU, et al. Novel treatment of patients with lower extremity ischemia: use of percutaneous atherectomy in 579 lesions. *Ann Surg.* 2008;248:519–528.

4 Renal and Mesenteric Intervention

Ramy A. Badawi, MD,
and Christopher J. White, MD

CONTENTS

RENAL ARTERY INTERVENTION
MESENTERIC ARTERY INTERVENTION
REFERENCES

RENAL ARTERY INTERVENTION

Introduction

In 1934, Henry Goldblatt simulated occlusive renal vascular disease by clamping renal arteries in a canine model and inducing a hypertensive response which resolved with clamp removal *(1)*. Subsequent research into the pathophysiology of renal artery stenosis (RAS) has led to the elucidation of the renin–angiotensin–aldosterone system, which underlies our current understanding of how renal vascular disease results in renal ischemia, uncontrolled hypertension, and impaired renal function.

Renal Artery Stenosis: Prevalence and Natural History

Renal vascular disease is the most common cause of secondary hypertension accounting for approximately 5% of cases *(2)*. Atherosclerotic renal artery stenosis (ARAS) accounts for the majority of renal vascular disease and has a prevalence of almost 7% in a cohort of 834 Medicare patients *(3)*. The prevalence of ARAS increases to 25–35% in selected subsets including those with suspected coronary artery disease *(4–9)* and peripheral arterial disease (Table 1) *(10–12)*. Other causes of renal artery disease include fibromuscular dysplasia (Fig. 1), renal artery aneurysms, and more esoteric conditions such as Takayasu's arteritis, William's syndrome, neurofibromatosis, arteriovenous malformations or fistulas, atheroemboli, thromboemboli, trauma (e.g., lithotripsy, direct injury, surgery), past abdominal radiation therapy, or rarely retroperitoneal fibrosis *(13)*.

ARAS is a progressive disease *(14)* and the presence of RAS is an independent predictor of death *(15)*. Progression of lesion severity is related to increasing RAS severity.

From: *Peripheral and Cerebrovascular Intervention*, Contemporary Cardiology
Edited by: D. L. Bhatt, DOI 10.1007/978-1-60327-965-9_4
© Springer Science+Business Media, LLC 2012

Table 1
Prevalence of "Incidental" Renal Artery Stenosis at the Time
of Cardiac Catheterization

Study	N	RAS (%)	RAS >50%	Bilateral (%)
Crowley et al. (17)	14,152	11.4	6.3	21
Harding et al. (5)	1,302	30	15	36
Jean et al. (6)	196	29	18	NR
Vetrovec et al. (4)	116	NR	23	29
Conlon et al. (15)	3,987	34	9.1	17
Rihal et al. (7)	297	34	19	4
Weber-Mzell et al. (8)	177	25	11	8

RAS renal artery stenosis; NR not reported.

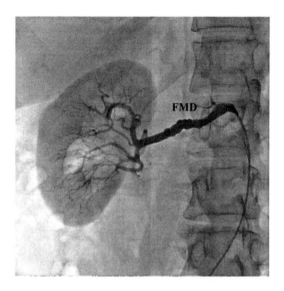

Fig. 1. Renal artery fibromuscular dysplasia. Angiography of right renal artery showing "stacked coin" appearance typical of fibromuscular dysplasia (FMD).

In a randomized trial of best medical therapy vs. angioplasty, 16% of the medically treated group progressed to complete renal artery occlusion within 1 year (16). Progression of RAS results in loss of renal function (17) accounting for up to 15% of new hemodialysis patients over 50 years old (18–20). Furthermore, RAS and ensuing renal failure are not slowed by adequate control of hypertension (21).

Indications for Screening for RAS

In patients who are deemed candidates for possible revascularization, current guidelines recommend screening diagnostic studies for RAS in patients who develop hypertension before the age of 30 or after the age of 55 years; patients with accelerated, resistant, or malignant hypertension; patients with new azotemia or worsening renal function after initiation of an angiotensin-converting enzyme (ACE) inhibitor or angiotensin receptor

Table 2
Clinical Presentations Warranting Renal Artery Stenosis (RAS) Screening

Onset of hypertension ≤30 or ≥55 years (Class I, LOE B)
Malignant, accelerated, or resistant hypertension (Class I, LOE C)
New azotemia or worsening renal function after administration of an ACE-I or ARB agent (Class I, LOE B)
Unexplained size discrepancy of ≥1.5 cm between kidneys or atrophic kidney (Class I, LOE B)
Unexplained renal dysfunction (Class IIa, LOE B)
Sudden, unexplained (flash) pulmonary edema (cardiac disturbance syndrome) (Class I, LOE B)
Multivessel (≥2) coronary artery disease (Class IIb, LOE B)
Peripheral arterial disease (abdominal aortic aneurysm or ABI <0.9) (Class IIb, LOE B)
Unexplained congestive heart failure (Class IIb, LOE C)
Refractory angina (Class IIb, LOE C)

Class I, IIa, IIb refers to ACC/AHA Clinical Practice Guideline Class Recommendations; LOE A, B, C refers to Level of Evidence as described in the ACC/AHA Clinical Practice Guidelines; ACE-I indicates angiotensin-converting enzyme inhibitors; *ARB* angiotensin-receptor blocker; *ABI* ankle brachial index.

blocker; patients with sudden (flash), unexplained pulmonary edema (cardiac destabilization syndrome); or patients with unexplained kidney atrophy or size discrepancy between kidneys >1.5 cm. Screening is also recommended in patients with unexplained renal failure starting renal replacement therapy, patients undergoing arteriography for multivessel coronary artery disease or peripheral arterial disease, or patients with unexplained congestive heart failure or refractory angina (Table 2) *(13, 22)*.

Screening Methods for RAS

Screening for RAS should be conducted noninvasively whenever feasible with Doppler ultrasound (Duplex) imaging, magnetic resonance angiography (MRA), or computed tomographic angiography (CTA). Duplex imaging is the most cost-effective of these modalities; however, it is technician dependent and thus most accurate and reliable in high-volume, experienced laboratories. Current CTA systems have superior spatial resolution compared with MRA but are associated with the use of ionizing radiation and iodinated contrast agents. MRA is of limited utility in patients with ferromagnetic implants (i.e., pacemaker–defibrillators) and is contraindicated in patients with renal failure *(23, 24)*. Radionuclide angiography, captopril scintigraphy, and plasma renin measurements are not useful screening tests. Invasive angiography is a screening tool in patients undergoing angiography for evaluation of multivessel coronary artery or peripheral artery disease *(13)*.

Diagnosis and Selection for RAS Revascularization

Once identified, the decision to proceed with revascularization requires a high clinical suspicion that the RAS is related to the patient's clinical symptoms. Characterization of the RAS on anatomic, hemodynamic, and physiologic grounds permits a better assessment of the lesion severity and its clinical significance.

- Anatomic characterization: this includes 1. measurement of kidney size (pole to pole, with a discrepancy of >1.5 cm between either kidney being a significant difference) and

2. RAS imaging by invasive angiography or intravascular ultrasound (IVUS). An angiographic stenosis of ≥70% (by visual estimation) is deemed to be significant. Moderate stenoses 50–69% (by visual estimation) are deemed to be significant if there is an accompanying translesional pressure gradient of ≥20 mmHg or a mean gradient of ≥10 mmHg as measured with a nonobstructive transcatheter (≤4 Fr) technique or a pressure wire.

- Physiological/functional characterization: this includes evaluation of renal fractional flow reserve (FFR) where a renal FFR <0.8 was found to predict improvement in blood pressure control after renal stenting with a sensitivity of 88% *(25, 26)*; translesional pressure gradient measurements where the ratio of distal pressure (Pd) to aortic pressure (Pa) was predictive for an increase in plasma renin concentration if the Pd/Pa ratio <0.90 *(27)*; renal frame count (RFC, analogous to thrombolysis in myocardial infarction, TIMI, frame count) where higher RFCs correlate with poorer renal perfusion *(28)*; renal radionuclide perfusion scans, selective renal vein renin and creatinine clearance determinations, and measurements of certain biomarkers such as brain natriuretic peptide (BNP) *(29)* all of which have shown promise in selecting patients who might benefit from renal revascularization *(22)*. Resistance index, an indicator of parenchymal renal disease obtained on duplex scanning for nephrosclerosis, is not a reliable predictor of improvement after renal revascularization *(30)*.

Evaluation of outcome usually involves a combination of assessing symptomatic improvement (e.g., improvement in blood pressure, angina frequency, or heart failure severity) and functional improvement as measured directly (improved kidney function) or indirectly (e.g., improved translesional pressures, FFR, RFC, creatinine clearance, or biomarkers).

Treatment Options and Clinical Outcomes for RAS

Three randomized studies (DRASTIC *(16)*, EMMA *(31)*, Scottish & Newcastle group *(32)*), a meta analysis *(33)*, and one cohort controlled study *(34)* have demonstrated the merits of percutaneous renal transluminal angioplasty (PRTA) for blood pressure control compared with medical (antihypertensive) therapy. Balloon angioplasty with stent (PRTAS) has been shown to be superior to PRTA in two trials (Fig. 2) *(35, 36)*. This data is supported by two meta-analyses showing a much higher procedural

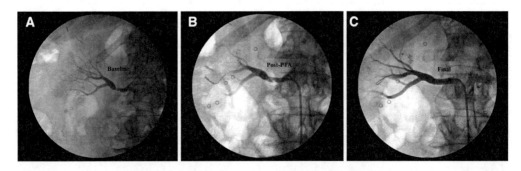

Fig. 2. Renal artery stenosis angioplasty and stenting. Serial angiograms of right renal artery stenosis before (**A**) and after balloon (**B**) angioplasty and subsequent stenting (**C**) due to suboptimal PTA result.

success rate (96–98% vs. 77%) in conjunction with a much lower restenosis rate in PRTAS (14%) as compared with PRTA (26%) *(37, 38)*. Two ongoing randomized clinical trials, Cardiovascular Outcomes in Renal Atherosclerotic Lesions (CORAL) and Angioplasty and Stent for Renal Artery Lesions (ASTRAL) seek to compare medical therapy to renal artery stenting and may provide further data on the value of PTRAS in renal revascularization *(39–41)*.

Renal Artery Intervention

TECHNICAL ASPECTS

Access

Common femoral arterial access with a 6-Fr sheath is the most common arterial access; however, if the renal artery is oriented in a caudal direction, radial or brachial artery access should be considered.

Sheath and Guide Selection

For tortuous iliac disease, consideration should be given to using a 25–45-cm sheath to lend control and support to the guiding catheter. We prefer to use a gently angulated guiding catheter such as a hockey stick or renal double curve from the femoral approach. From the upper extremity, a multipurpose shaped guiding catheter is usually the best fit. Caution regarding length from the radial artery access should be noted, in that often 110–125-cm guiding catheters are necessary.

Sheath/Guide Engagement

Direct engagement of the lesion using the guide catheter risks aortic trauma and renal artery complications such as abrupt vessel closure, dissection, and renal atheroembolism. Indirect engagement of the renal ostium has the advantage of a more controlled access and can be undertaken in one of two ways. The first involves telescoping the 6 Fr guide catheter over a 4 Fr diagnostic catheter (internal mammary shape) once the renal artery has been selected with the atraumatic diagnostic catheter. The interventional guidewire of choice (0.014 or 0.018 in.) is advanced across the lesion through the 4 Fr diagnostic catheter. In this scenario, the guide catheter is advanced over the atraumatic 4 Fr diagnostic catheter that has already engaged the renal ostium. The diagnostic catheter is then removed once the guide is coaxial with the renal ostium, leaving the guidewire in place. The second technique involves advancing the guide catheter from the femoral artery over an 0.035-in. J-wire placed into the thoracic aorta. The guide is advanced until it is in close proximity of the renal artery ostium without engaging it and then advancing a second 0.014-in. guidewire directly into the renal artery before removal of the 0.035-in. wire. This allows atraumatic engagement of the renal ostium and has been termed the "no touch" technique.

Interventional Guidewires

0.014 Inch wires are favored because most stent platforms, pressure wires, and distal protection devices conform to the 0.014-in. specification and 0.014-in. guidewires are less likely to cause trauma than 0.035-in. Hydrophilic wires should be avoided, if possible, as they are associated with a higher risk of renal vascular perforation.

PERCUTANEOUS MODALITIES

Percutaneous Renal Transluminal Angioplasty

Balloon angioplasty is used for predilation and sizing of the renal artery prior to stent placement (PRTAS). In general, confirming the expandability of the lesion with balloon predilation is recommended. In the setting of renal FMD, PRTA remains the treatment of choice.

Percutaneous Renal Transluminal Angioplasty Stent

Stent placement is the treatment of choice for atherosclerotic RAS, particularly in aorto-ostial lesions. Self-expanding stents lack precision and are difficult to place at the ostium of the renal artery, so balloon expandable stents are favored and sized 1:1 with the reference vessel diameter. Care needs to be taken, not to size the stents with the poststenotic dilated segment. The stent should be placed approximately 1 mm into the aorta to ensure complete coverage of the renal artery ostium. The stent balloon is inflated to its nominal diameter. If necessary, the ostium of the balloon can be "flared" with a high pressure inflation. The operator needs to be vigilant for inadequate stent expansion, and if this is identified, the stent should be further dilated under higher inflation pressures with larger balloons. This is an advantage of balloon predilation, as it avoids deployment of stents into undilatable lesions. Under-expanded stents result in a higher incidence of restenosis and target vessel revascularization.

Intravascular Ultrasound

IVUS permits quantitative cross-sectional evaluation of lesion morphology. Postintervention IVUS imaging also permits evaluation of stent apposition and expansion and lesion coverage. At present, there is no evidence that the use of IVUS results in improved clinical outcomes, but selective use, to answer specific questions, seems warranted.

ADJUNCTIVE THERAPIES

Antiplatelet Therapy

Premedication with aspirin (81–325 mg), at least 1 day prior to the intervention and long-term aspirin following intervention is the standard of care. There are no data supporting the use of additional oral antiplatelet agents such as clopidogrel or ticlopidine in renal artery revascularization and such use is at the discretion of the operator. The risk of subacute renal stent thrombosis is much less than in smaller coronary arteries. A recent study demonstrated that GpIIb/IIIa platelet inhibitors used in conjunction with an emboli protection device during renal artery revascularization can help preserve renal function though the arm of the study which used GpIIb/IIIa inhibitors without embolic protection did not show an improvement in renal function *(42)*. Further studies are needed to clarify the role of GpIIb/IIIa inhibitors in renal revascularization.

Anticoagulation Therapy

The use of unfractionated heparin to achieve an activated clotting time (ACT) >250 s during the procedure is the standard of care. There is no evidence that alternative anticoagulants such as low molecular weight heparins or bivalirudin offer any additional benefit to renovascular intervention.

Emboli Protection Devices (EPD)

There are no emboli protection devices (EPD) approved for use in the renal circulation. The aorto-ostial nature of most renal artery stenoses makes proximal occlusion devices difficult to use and distal occlusion balloons and filters the most likely devices to be used for renal protection. Given the bulky nature of the aorto-ostial plaque, the use of EPDs is attractive. However, use of EPD increases the complexity of the case and the risk of potential complications. Studies have shown that distal occlusion balloon (PercuSurge Guardwire, Medtronic, Minneapolis, MN) and guidewire-based distal filter (Angioguard, Cordis, Miami, FL) devices can be safely and effectively used in renal artery intervention *(43, 44)*. In these small series, angiographic success with stent placement was not impaired by the use of an EPD, debris was present in the majority of cases and renal function was preserved at follow up. The recent study by Cooper et al. suggests a renal function benefit with EPD only in the setting of adjunctive intravenous GpIIb/IIIa inhibition but the clinical use of EPD in renal artery revascularization requires further study *(42)*.

COMPLICATIONS

Vascular access complications are the most common complication in renal artery intervention. They include access site bleeding and hematoma (1.5–5%), access site vessel injury (1–2%), retroperitoneal hematoma (<1%), pseudoaneurysm (0.5–1%), and arteriovenous fistula and nerve injury (<1%) *(37, 38, 45)*.

1. Renal artery dissection can occur during catheter engagement or during stenting. Bailout stenting is required to correct the problem.
2. Atheroembolic and thromboembolic complications are best prevented by use of EPDs, possibly in conjunction with GpIIb/IIIa inhibitors.
3. Renal hematoma secondary to guidewire-induced renal vessel perforation is seen as extravasation of contrast into the parenchyma. Renal perforation may present as flank or abdominal pain with or without hemodynamic compromise. Depending on the severity of the bleeding, percutaneous renal vessel embolization, off-label use of a covered stent or surgical intervention may be required.
4. Stent thrombosis can occur and is often a consequence of impaired antegrade flow through the stent.
5. Contrast-related complications including contrast-induced nephropathy and contrast reactions may occur.

POSTINTERVENTION CARE AND FOLLOW UP

Blood pressure medications are held the morning of the procedure and titrated after the procedure. Patients are monitored overnight to adjust their medications after renal artery revascularization and to observe for procedural complications or hypotension following normalization of renal perfusion after intervention. Patients are discharged on lifelong aspirin therapy (81–325 mg daily) and optionally with 1 month of clopidogrel (75 mg daily) or ticlopidine (250 mg bid).

Follow-up evaluation at 1, 3, 6, and 12 months with renal artery duplex ultrasound to evaluate the baseline outcome, and determine blood pressure control, renal function, renal stent patency (with duplex), and treat cardiovascular disease and risk factors.

Restenosis

Renal artery stenting is associated with a restenosis rate of 10–20% and its treatment is still under study (46, 47). Defined as ≥50% in-stent cross-sectional diameter stenosis, it is more common in smaller vessels (less than 4.5 mm), in diabetics, in women, in long or calcified lesions, and in the setting of inadequate stent sizing, expansion, or placement (48). The need for the up-titration or addition of further antihypertensive medications, rising serum creatinine (>50% of baseline), or recurring angina or heart failure should all prompt evaluation for in-stent restenosis (ISR). ISR may also be identified by duplex ultrasound scanning and criteria include a postprocedure in-stent velocity (>100 cm/s) and peak systolic velocity renal/aortic >3.5 (49). Renal angiography with evaluation of pressure gradients is the gold standard for evaluation of ISR. ISR is deemed significant if there is a ≥70% diameter stenosis or a ≥50% stenosis in the setting of a translesional systolic pressure gradient of 20 mmHg or mean gradient of 10 mmHg.

Multiple approaches to the treatment of renal ISR have been reported including balloon angioplasty (46), repeat stenting (36), cutting balloon (50), and brachytherapy (51). Repeat stent placement appears to be superior to angioplasty alone for renal ISR but comparative controlled data is lacking (47). The use of drug-eluting stents has been reported (52) and if they had a similar impact on the reduction of renal ISR that they have had in coronary ISR this would be the treatment of choice (53). Currently, there are no drug-eluting stents approved for renal artery stenting.

Future Directions

The current procedure success rate for renal intervention in experienced hands is greater than 98%. The two major avenues for improvement in this technique are a reduction in restenosis and avoiding atheroembolic renal parenchymal injury during stent placement. Drug-eluting stents hold the greatest promise to reduce restenosis (54). The GREAT trial, a prospective, nonrandomized and un-blinded trial, demonstrated less ISR and target lesion revascularization out to 2 years but did not achieve statistical significance.

EPDs capture debris in the majority of PRTA(S) cases (65–100% in two series) (43, 44).

These observations support the need to protect the renal parenchyma from atheroembolism particularly in patients with abnormal renal function at baseline. However, to date only one trial has been published looking at the impact of EPDs on renal function after renal intervention and it has demonstrated benefit of EPDs only when used concomitantly with glycoprotein IIb/IIIa receptor antagonist antiplatelet therapy (42). Other approaches to improve primary patency and reduce restenosis are also under study including the use of covered stents (55) and novel aorto-ostial devices (56).

MESENTERIC ARTERY INTERVENTION

Incidence, Prevalence, Natural History

Mesenteric ischemia occurs as a consequence of compromise to the vascular supply of the small or large intestine. It can be either acute or chronic. Acute mesenteric ischemia (AMI) is the result of acute occlusion of a major visceral artery either secondary to embolization from a cardiac or aortic source or secondary to thrombus formation subsequent to atherosclerotic plaque rupture, in a manner akin to coronary plaque rupture. AMI most commonly involves the superior mesenteric artery and can occur in the setting of atrial fibrillation, iatrogenic disruption of atherosclerotic plaque, spontaneous or iatrogenic dissection, or systemic hypercoagulability *(57)*. AMI can also be nonocclusive, usually in the setting of a low flow state or shock *(58–63)* or exposure to vasoconstricting substances (e.g., cocaine, ergots, vasopressin, or norepinephrine) *(64, 65)* or following surgery in which collateral circulation has not been adequately re-established *(61, 66)*.

Chronic mesenteric ischemia (CMI) is uncommon accounting for less than 2% of all atheromatous revascularization procedures *(67)* and it is usually the consequence of atherosclerotic disease involving aorto-ostial stenosis of the celiac, superior mesenteric, and/or inferior mesenteric arteries often in the context of concomitant atherosclerotic disease of the aorta. Classical teaching suggests that CMI occurs when only one of three viscerals remains patent due to the rich collateral supply and the most commonly intervened on vessel is the superior mesenteric artery. Less commonly, CMI can have other etiologies including fibromuscular dysplasia (FMD), Buerger's disease, and aortic dissection.

Population-based studies of mesenteric artery stenosis using screening aortograms or abdominal ultrasound show a prevalence for significant stenosis (>50% diameter stenosis) between 8 and 17.5% with a strong predilection for the celiac artery and only 1.5% of patients having significant stenosis of more than one mesenteric artery. Only a minority of patients with multivessel mesenteric arterial stenoses will actually develop symptoms of CMI. Asymptomatic mesenteric artery stenosis is not associated with adverse cardiovascular events or death *(68, 69)* though there remains some controversy over this point *(70)*. The infrequent occurrence of CMI in clinical practice is ascribed to the redundancy of extensive mesenteric collaterals.

Acute Mesenteric Ischemia: Diagnosis and Treatment

Occlusive AMI should be suspected in a patient who develops abdominal pain that is out of proportion to physical findings. The discrepancy in symptoms and physical findings is due to the lag time of hours between developing peritoneal irritation and the full blown picture of an acute abdomen. The patient will usually have a history which provides a clue to the etiology of the occlusion be it cardiovascular (past atherosclerosis or arrhythmias) or iatrogenic (recent percutaneous or surgical intervention involving the aorta). Laboratory findings include leukocytosis and lactic acidosis. Though invasive angiography and duplex ultrasound can be used to identify acute occlusion of the mesenteric vessels, diagnostic imaging in the form of computed tomography is usually favored because it is most readily available and allows the evaluation for a wide spectrum of causes of acute abdominal pain. Intervention is usually surgical as this permits both revascularization and resection of necrotic bowel and the option for a "second look" operation at 24–48 h *(13)*. However, percutaneous intervention in select patients may be appropriate though patients may subsequently still require laparotomy *(13)*.

Nonocclusive AMI usually occurs in the setting of circulatory shock. Patients develop abdominal pain and/or distention and diagnosis is often delayed due to decreased levels of consciousness. The other category of patients who can develop non-occlusive AMI are those exposed to vasoactive substances such as ergot derivatives, cocaine, or amphetamines. There are no helpful clinical or laboratory findings to assist in the diagnosis of nonocclusive AMI. Invasive angiography is the preferred diagnostic modality as it provides information on mesenteric perfusion and arterial vasospasm *(60, 62, 64)*. In the setting of the latter it also allows for direct intra-arterial instillation of vasodilators *(59, 71)*. In the setting of circulatory shock treatment consists of treating the underlying physiologic insult and where needed laparotomy for resection of necrotic bowel *(13)*.

Chronic Mesenteric Ischemia

CMI is twice as common in women than men. The classic presentation is postprandial abdominal discomfort accompanied by a significant weight loss. Mesenteric ischemia, experienced as abdominal discomfort, is brought on by eating, leading patients to avoid food (food fear) and lose weight. Less typical presentations of ischemic gastropathy include: nausea, vomiting, diarrhea, constipation, ischemic colitis, and lower gastrointestinal bleeding. Such patients may have a history of systemic atherosclerosis and a history of past myocardial infarction, stroke, or claudication. The diagnosis may often be delayed as patients may be referred for a malignancy evaluation for weight loss. However, evidence of significant stenosis of two or more mesenteric vessels in conjunction with endoscopic findings of bowel ischemia should prompt the diagnosis *(72)*. CMI may occur in single mesenteric artery disease particularly after surgery if mesenteric collaterals have been disrupted.

Diagnostic Approach to Chronic Mesenteric Ischemia

CMI is a clinical diagnosis as there is no definitive diagnostic study. Clinical suspicion should be raised in any patient with functional bowel complaints associated with significant weight loss. This should prompt a work up for anatomic findings consistent with multivessel mesenteric arterial stenoses. Current noninvasive imaging using Doppler-ultrasound (Duplex) imaging, CTA, and/or MRA will delineate the mesenteric vasculature without the need for invasive angiography *(73–75)*.

Invasive angiography remains the gold standard for visualizing the mesenteric arterial tree. Visualization of the mesenteric vessels requires a lateral aortogram (Fig. 3). Anterior–posterior aortogram may reveal the arc of Riolan, an engorged collateral connecting the IMA to the SMA and indicative of proximal mesenteric artery disease. Critical stenosis ($\geq 70\%$) in symptomatic patients with weight loss should be considered for revascularization. Evaluation of borderline stenoses is hampered by the lack of an ischemic "stress" test.

Treatment of Chronic Mesenteric Ischemia

Historically, surgical revascularization has been the mainstay of treatment for CMI either by endarterectomy or bypass grafting with associated perioperative mortality and complications ranging from 8–12 to 33–47%, respectively *(76, 77)*. The highest incidence of adverse outcomes is in the elderly *(78)*.

Percutaneous transluminal angioplasty with or without stent (PTA(S)) circumvents the need for general anesthesia and results in lower mortality and morbidity (Table 3) *(67, 79–84)*.

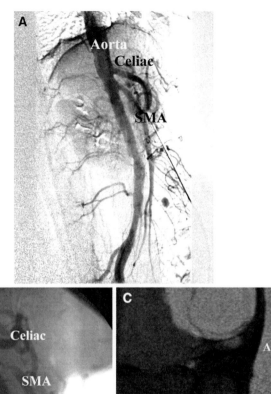

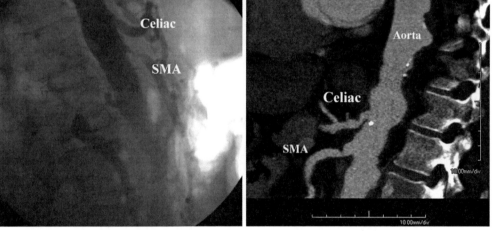

Fig. 3. Mesenteric aortogram. Serial lateral aortography showing an angiogram of a normal celiac artery and superior mesenteric artery (**A**), an angiogram of the superior mesenteric artery (SMA) stenosis (**B**) and a computed tomographic angiogram (CTA) of the celiac and superior mesenteric artery (SMA) stenosis (**C**).

The relative infrequency of this disease means there are no randomized trials comparing surgery to endovascular treatment for CMI. In the early 2000s, the Cleveland Clinic reported their surgical experience with an 8% perioperative mortality rate and a 33% perioperative morbidity *(77)*, which they found to be comparable to their endovascular mortality and morbidity (11 and 18% in 28 patients) *(83)*. Restenosis rates between the two groups were comparable ranging between 24 and 27% though symptom relief at follow up was sustained in 85% of surgically treated patients as opposed to 60% of endovascularly treated patients. Interestingly, when restenosis rates of patients treated with PTA alone as opposed to PTAS were compared there was a significant difference in patency (33% compared with 11.5%) *(83)*.

Table 3
Outcomes for Endovascular Revascularization in Chronic Mesenteric Ischemia

Authors	N	Technical success (%)	Clinical success (%)	Late clinical success (%)	Complication (%)	Mortality (30dy)	Restenosis (%)	Repeat PTA (%)	Mean follow up (≥2 years)
Maspes et al. (92)	23	87	87	78	9	0	17	17	91
Kasirajan et al. (83)	28	100	NA	60	18	11	18	68	68
Matsumoto et al. (79)	33	82	88	73	15	0	15	18	88
Sharafuddin et al. (86)	25	96	88	83	11	4	12	8	72
AbuRahma et al. (88)	22	95	95	50	0	0	32	23	82
van Wanroij, et al. (87)	27	93	81	67	11	0	22	NA	93
Landis et al. (81)	29	97	90	66	14	7	34	34	100[a]
Silva et al. (85)	59	97	85	79	3	0	29	29	88
Sarac et al. (84)[b]	65	NA	85	75	31	8	35	35	100[a]

Table includes all studies reporting more than 20 patients undergoing endovascular intervention for chronic mesenteric ischemia in the English literature.
N number of patients per study; *PTA* percutaneous transluminal angioplasty with or without stent. Clinical success indicates freedom from symptoms. Late clinical success indicates freedom from symptoms at follow up (1 year or more). NA indicates nonapplicable.

[a] These two studies had mean follow up of 1 year.
[b] 30% lesions reported in Sarac et al. were complete occlusions with a different technical success compared with stenotic lesions.

Almost a decade later, in the largest single series reported to date (65 patients), the Cleveland Clinic reported an unchanged perioperative mortality (8%) and morbidity (31%) with a similar rate of restenosis (35%) and a modest improvement in symptom relief (75%) *(84)*. In this series patients all had primary stenting. However, this experience for CMI is not representative of the other published contemporary series. In the second largest series published to date (59 patients), the Ochsner Clinic reported a high technical success rate (97%) with a considerably lower mortality (0%) and morbidity (3%) and comparable symptom relief rates at early (85%) and late (79%) follow up *(85)*. Patients in this series routinely underwent a primary stenting strategy.

Review of a number of other published case series with comparable numbers of patients undergoing endovascular revascularization for CMI shows similar clinical outcomes to the Ochsner's series with lower morbidity and mortality compared with traditional surgical series (Table 4.3) *(79, 81, 86–88)* suggesting that the Cleveland Clinic's experience may not be representative – perhaps due to patient and/or lesion selection, e.g., 30% of mesenteric artery lesions intervened upon were total occlusions (as opposed to 5–25% in previous series) *(81, 85)* lesions previously relegated to surgery, and 5% of patients required subsequent surgery for bowel ischemia or necrosis *(84)*.

In a recent review of the literature collating all endovascular series reporting more than 5 patients each, for a total of 328 patients, Kougias et al. concluded that endovascular mesenteric revascularization was associated with lower mortality and morbidity and shorter hospital stays than surgery but that open surgery still achieved better clinical outcomes (i.e., symptom relief) and slightly better patency rates *(67)*, findings echoed by a recent comparative series *(80)*. Further, it was noted that there was an increasing trend towards a strategy of primary stenting in endovascularly treated patients.

In conclusion, endovascular revascularization should be favored as the first choice for mesenteric revascularization, but is particularly important in elderly patients and those with comorbidities that make them high risk for surgery.

Mesenteric Artery Intervention

TECHNICAL ASPECTS

Vacular Access

Upper extremity (radial or brachial) access is favored due to the cephalad orientation of the celiac and superior mesenteric artery origins.

Sheath and Guide Selection

For tortuous iliac disease, consideration should be given to using a 25–45 cm sheath to lend control and support to the guiding catheter. From the upper extremity, multipurpose shaped guiding catheters work best. Caution regarding length from the radial artery access should be noted, in that often 110–125 cm guiding catheters are necessary. From the leg, angled catheters, such as renal double curves, hockey sticks, or internal mammary artery shaped catheters work best.

Sheath/Guide Engagement

From the femoral access, direct engagement of the lesion using a guide catheter risks complications such as vessel trauma, abrupt vessel closure, dissection, and atheroembolism. Indirect engagement of the diseased vessel has the advantage of a more controlled access and can be undertaken in one of two manners. The first involves telescoping the 6 Fr guide catheter over a 4 Fr diagnostic catheter once the vessel has been selectively engaged with a diagnostic catheter over a 0.035-in. J-wire. In this scenario, the guide catheter is advanced over the atraumatic 4 Fr diagnostic catheter that has already engaged the mesenteric artery ostium. The diagnostic catheter is removed once the guide is coaxial with the mesenteric ostium. The second technique involves advancing the guide catheter from the femoral artery, over a 0.035-in. wire placed into the thoracic aorta to close proximity of the mesenteric ostium without engaging it and then advancing a 0.014-in. guidewire into the mesenteric artery before removal of the 0.035-in. wire. This allows atraumatic engagement of the mesenteric artery ostium and has been termed the "no touch" technique.

Interventional Wires

0.014 Inch wires are favored because of the available stent platforms and because they are less likely to cause lesion trauma than 0.035-in. Hydrophilic wires are to be avoided as they are associated with a higher risk of perforation.

PERCUTANEOUS MODALITIES

Percutaneous Transluminal Angioplasty

Balloon angioplasty is used for predilation and sizing of the mesenteric artery prior to stent placement. Another benefit of balloon predilation is it gives the operator a sense of how much back-up support is needed to advance devices into the mesenteric artery.

Percutaneous Transluminal Angioplasty with Stent

Primary stent placement is favored in atherosclerotic mesenteric artery atherosclerosis, particularly in aorto-ostial lesions. Self-expanding stents lack precision and are difficult to place at the ostium of the mesenteric artery, so balloon expandable stents are favored and sized 1:1 with the reference vessel diameter. The stent should protrude slightly (approximately 1 mm) into the aorta to ensure complete coverage of the renal artery ostium. The stent balloon is inflated to its nominal diameter and then the balloon is withdrawn into the guide. If necessary, the ostium of the balloon can be "flared" with a high pressure inflation. The operator needs to be vigilant for inadequate stent expansion, and if this is identified, the stent should be further dilated under higher inflation pressures with larger balloons. This is an advantage of balloon predilation, as it avoids deployment of stents into undilatable lesions. Underexpanded stents result in a higher incidence of restenosis and target vessel revascularization.

ADJUNCTIVE THERAPIES

Antiplatelet Therapy

Premedication with aspirin (81–325 mg), at least 1 day prior to the intervention and long-term aspirin following intervention is the standard of care. There are no data supporting the use of additional oral antiplatelet agents such as clopidogrel or ticlopidine in mesenteric artery revascularization and such use is at the discretion of the operator. The risk of subacute mesenteric stent thrombosis is much less than in smaller coronary arteries and does not currently warrant adjunctive antiplatelet therapy.

Anticoagulation Therapy

The use of unfractionated heparin to achieve an activated clotting time (ACT) >250 s during the procedure is the standard of care. There is no evidence that alternative anticoagulants such as low molecular weight heparins or bivalirudin offer any additional benefit to mesenteric artery intervention at this time.

COMPLICATIONS

Vascular Access Complications

Vascular access complications are the most common complication in mesenteric artery intervention. They include access site bleeding, hematoma or thrombosis (3–15%), pseudoaneurysm (<1%), arteriovenous fistula (<1%), and nerve injury (<1%) *(67, 81, 84, 85)*.

Mesenteric Artery Dissection or Occlusion

Mesenteric artery dissection or occlusion is far less common and may occur during catheter engagement or stenting, requiring bail out stenting.

Bowel Ischemia

Bowel ischemia can occur as a result of unrecognized dissection or distal embolization and may require a repeat procedure.

Contrast-Related Complications

Contrast-related complications including contrast-induced nephropathy and contrast reactions are possible.

POSTINTERVENTION CARE

Patients are monitored overnight to observe for procedural complications. Patients are discharged on lifelong aspirin therapy (81–325 mg daily) and optionally with 1 month of clopidogrel (75 mg daily) or ticlopidine (250 mg bid).

Restenosis and Follow Up

Follow-up evaluation at 1, 3, 6, and 12 months with mesenteric artery duplex ultrasound to evaluate continued patency in conjunction with recurrence of symptoms along with modification of atherosclerotic disease risk factors is advisable. Doppler ultrasound (duplex) is the standard modality used by most centers *(67)* but the advent of CTA and MRA may provide alternative modalities for follow up in the future *(89, 90)*. Restenosis by duplex does not always correlate with recurrence of symptoms *(91)*.

REFERENCES

1. Goldblatt H, Lynch J, Hanzal RF, Summerville WW. Studies on experimental hypertension: I. The production of persistent elevation of systolic blood pressure by means of renal ischemia. *J Exp Med.* 1934;59(3):347–379.
2. Simon N, Franklin S, Bleifer K, Maxwell M. Clinical characteristics of renovascular hypertension. *JAMA.* 1972;220:1209–1218.
3. Hansen KJ, Edwards MS, Craven TE, et al. Prevalence of renovascular disease in the elderly: a population-based study. *J Vasc Surg.* 2002;36(3):443–451.
4. Vetrovec GW, Landwehr DM, Edwards VI. Incidence of renal artery stenosis in hypertensive patients undergoing coronary angiography. *J Interven Cardiol.* 1989;2(2):69–76.

5. Harding MB, Smith LR, Himmelstein SI, et al. Renal artery stenosis: prevalence and associated risk factors in patients undergoing routine cardiac catheterization. *J Am Soc Nephrol.* 1992;2:1608–1616.
6. Jean WJ, Al-Bitar I, Zwicke DL, Port SC, Schmidt DH, Bajwa TK. High incidence of renal artery stenosis in patients with coronary artery disease. *Cathet Cardiovasc Diagn.* 1994;32:8–10.
7. Rihal CS, Textor SC, Breen JF, et al. Incidental renal artery stenosis among a prospective cohort of hypertensive patients undergoing coronary angiography. *Mayo Clin Proc.* 2002;77:309–316.
8. Weber-Mzell D, Kotanko P, Schumacher M, Klein W, Skrabal F. Coronary anatomy predicts presence or absence of renal artery stenosis. A prospective study in patients undergoing cardiac catheterization for suspected coronary artery disease. *Eur Heart J.* 2002;23:1684–1691.
9. Aqel RA, Zoghbi GJ, Baldwin SA, et al. Prevalence of renal artery stenosis in high-risk veterans referred to cardiac catheterization. J Hypertens. 2003;21(6):1157–1162.
10. Schwartz CJ, White TA. Stenosis of renal artery: an unselected necropsy study. *Br Med J.* 1964;5422:1415–1421.
11. Olin J, Melia M, Young J, Graor R, Risius B. Prevalence of atherosclerosis renal artery stenosis in patients with atherosclerosis elsewhere. *Am J Med.* 1990;88:46 N–51 N.
12. Valentine R, Myers S, Miller G, Lopez M, Clagett G. Detection of unsuspected renal artery stenoses in patients with abdominal aortic aneurysms: refined indications for preoperative aortography. *Ann Vasc Surg.* 1993;7:220–224.
13. Hirsch AT, Haskal ZJ, Hertzer NR, et al. ACC/AHA 2005 practice guidelines for the management of patients with peripheral arterial disease (lower extremity, renal, mesenteric, and abdominal aortic): a collaborative report from the American Association for Vascular Surgery/Society for Vascular Surgery, Society for Cardiovascular Angiography and Interventions, Society for Vascular Medicine and Biology, Society of Interventional Radiology, and the ACC/AHA Task Force on Practice Guidelines (Writing Committee to Develop Guidelines for the Management of Patients With Peripheral Arterial Disease): endorsed by the American Association of Cardiovascular and Pulmonary Rehabilitation; National Heart, Lung, and Blood Institute; Society for Vascular Nursing; TransAtlantic Inter-Society Consensus; and Vascular Disease Foundation. *Circulation.* 2006;113(11):e463-e654.
14. Schreiber MJ, Pohl MA, Novick AC. The natural history of atherosclerotic and fibrous renal artery disease. *Urol Clin N Am.* 1984;11:383–392.
15. Conlon PJ, Little MA, Pieper K, Mark DB. Severity of renal vascular disease predicts mortality in patients undergoing coronary angiography. *Kidney Int.* 2001;60(4):1490–1497.
16. van Jaarsveld B, Krijnen P, Pieterman H, et al. The effect of balloon angioplasty on hypertension in atherosclerotic renal artery stenosis. *N Eng J Med.* 2000;342:1007–1014.
17. Crowley J, Santos R, Peter R, et al. Progression of renal artery stenosis in patients undergoing cardiac catheterization. *Am Heart J.* 1998;136:913–918.
18. Rimmer JM, Gennari FJ. Atherosclerotic renovascular disease and progressive renal failure. *Ann Intern Med.* 1993;118(9):712–719.
19. Scoble JE, Maher ER, Hamilton G, Dick R, Sweny P, Moorhead JF. Atherosclerotic renovascular disease causing renal impairment--a case for treatment. *Clin Nephrol.* 1989;31(3):119–122.
20. Mailloux LU, Napolitano B, Bellucci AG, Vernace M, Wilkes BM, Mossey RT. Renal vascular disease causing end-stage renal disease, incidence, clinical correlates, and outcomes: a 20-year clinical experience. *Am J Kidney Dis.* 1994;24(4):622–629.
21. Dean R, Kieffer R, Smith B, et al. Renovascular hypertension: anatomic and renal function changes during drug therapy. *Arch Surg.* 1981;116:1408–1415.
22. White CJ. Catheter-based therapy for atherosclerotic renal artery stenosis. *Circulation.* 2006;113(11):1464–1473.
23. Ledneva E, Karie S, Launay-Vacher V, Janus N, Deray G. Renal safety of gadolinium-based contrast media in patients with chronic renal insufficiency. *Radiology.* 2009;250(3):618–628.
24. ten Dam MA, Wetzels JF. Toxicity of contrast media: an update. *Neth J Med.* 2008;66(10):416–422.
25. Subramanian R, White CJ, Rosenfield K, et al. Renal fractional flow reserve: a hemodynamic evaluation of moderate renal artery stenoses. *Catheter Cardiovasc Interv.* 2005;64(4):480–486.
26. Mitchell J, Subramanian R, White C, et al. Predicting blood pressure improvement in hypertensive patients after renal artery stent placement. *Catheter Cardiovasc Interven.* 2007;69(5):685–689.
27. De Bruyne B, Manoharan G, Pijls NH, et al. Assessment of renal artery stenosis severity by pressure gradient measurements. *J Am Coll Cardiol.* 2006;48(9):1851–1855.

28. Mulumudi MS, White CJ. Renal frame count: a quantitative angiographic assessment of renal perfusion. *Catheter Cardiovasc Interv.* 2005;65(2):183–186.
29. Silva JA, Chan AW, White CJ, et al. Elevated brain natriuretic peptide predicts blood pressure response after stent revascularization in patients with renal artery stenosis. *Circulation.* 2005;111(3):328–333.
30. Zeller T, Muller C, Frank U, et al. Stent angioplasty of severe atherosclerotic ostial renal artery stenosis in patients with diabetes mellitus and nephrosclerosis. *Cathet Cardiovasc Intervent.* 2003;58:510–515.
31. Plouin PF, Chatellier G, Darne B, Raynaud A. Blood pressure outcome of angioplasty in atherosclerotic renal artery stenosis: a randomized trial. Essai Multicentrique Medicaments vs Angioplastie (EMMA) Study Group. *Hypertension.* 1998;31(3):823–9.
32. Webster J, Marshall F, Abdalla M, et al. Randomised comparison of percutaneous angioplasty vs continued medical therapy for hypertensive patients with atheromatous renal artery stenosis. Scottish and Newcastle Renal Artery Stenosis Collaborative Group. *J Hum Hypertens.* 1998;12(5):329–335.
33. Nordmann AJ, Woo K, Parkes R, Logan AG. Balloon angioplasty or medical therapy for hypertensive patients with atherosclerotic renal artery stenosis? A meta-analysis of randomized controlled trials. *Am J Med.* 2003;114(1):44–50.
34. Losito A, Errico R, Santirosi P, Lupattelli T, Scalera GB, Lupattelli L. Long-term follow-up of atherosclerotic renovascular disease. Beneficial effect of ACE inhibition. *Nephrol Dial Transplant.* 2005;20(8):1604–1609.
35. Dorros G, Prince C, Mathiak L. Stenting of a renal artery stenosis achieves better relief of the obstructive lesion than balloon angioplasty. *Cathet Cardiovasc Diagn.* 1993;29(3):191–198.
36. van de Ven PJ, Kaatee R, Beutler JJ, et al. Arterial stenting and balloon angioplasty in ostial atherosclerotic renovascular disease: a randomised trial. *Lancet.* 1999;353:282–286.
37. Isles CG, Robertson S, Hill D. Management of renovascular disease: a review of renal artery stenting in ten studies. *Quart J Med.* 1999;92:159–167.
38. Leertouwer TC, Gussenhoven EJ, Bosch JL, et al. Stent placement for renal arterial stenosis: where do we stand? A meta-analysis. *Radiology.* 2000;216(1):78–85.
39. Mistry S, Ives N, Harding J, et al. Angioplasty and STent for Renal Artery Lesions (ASTRAL trial): rationale, methods and results so far. *J Hum Hypertens.* 2007;21(7):511–515.
40. Dubel GJ, Murphy TP. The role of percutaneous revascularization for renal artery stenosis. *Vasc Med.* 2008;13(2):141–156.
41. Textor SC LL, McKusick M. The uncertain value of renal intervention: where are we now? *JAm Coll Cardiol Cardiovasc Interven.* 2009;2:175–182.
42. Cooper C, Haller S, Colyer W, et al. Embolic protection and platelet inhibition during renal artery stenting. *Circulation.* 2008 ;117:2752–2760.
43. Henry M, Klonaris C, Henry I, et al. Protected renal stenting with the PercuSurge GuardWire device: a pilot study. *J Endovasc Ther.* 2001;8(3):227–237.
44. Holden A, Hill A. Renal angioplasty and stenting with distal protection of the main renal artery in ischemic nephropathy: early experience. *J Vasc Surg.* 2003;38(5):962–968.
45. White CJ, Ramee SR, Collins TJ, Jenkins JS, Escobar A, Shaw D. Renal artery stent placement: utility in lesions difficult to treat with balloon angioplasty. *J Am Coll Cardiol.* 1997 Nov 15;30(6):1445–50.
46. Bax L, Mali WP, Van De Ven PJ, Beek FJ, Vos JA, Beutler JJ. Repeated intervention for in-stent restenosis of the renal arteries. *J Vasc Interv Radiol.* 2002;13(12):1219–1224.
47. N'Dandu ZM, Badawi RA, White CJ, et al. Optimal treatment of renal artery in-stent restenosis: repeat stent placement versus angioplasty alone. *Catheter Cardiovasc Interv.* 2008;71(5):701–705.
48. Lederman R, Mendelsohn F, Santos R, Phillips H, Stack R, Crowley J. Primary renal artery stenting: characteristics and outcomes after 363 procedure. *Am Heart J.* 2001;142:314–323.
49. Chi YW, White CJ, Thornton S, Milani RV. Ultrasound velocity criteria for renal in-stent restenosis. *J Vasc Surg.* 2009;50:119–123.
50. Munneke GJ, Engelke C, Morgan RA, Belli AM. Cutting balloon angioplasty for resistant renal artery in-stent restenosis. *J Vasc Interv Radiol.* 2002;13(3):327–331.
51. Jahraus CD, St Clair W, Gurley J, Meigooni AS. Endovascular brachytherapy for the treatment of renal artery in-stent restenosis using a beta-emitting source: a report of five patients. *South Med J.* 2003;96(11):1165–1168.

52. Zeller T, Sixt S, Rastan A, et al. Treatment of reoccurring instent restenosis following reintervention after stent-supported renal artery angioplasty. *Catheter Cardiovasc Interv.* 2007;70(2):296–300.
53. Zeller T, Rastan A, Rothenpieler U, Muller C. Restenosis after stenting of atherosclerotic renal artery stenosis: is there a rationale for the use of drug-eluting stents? *Catheter Cardiovasc Interv.* 2006;68(1):125–130.
54. Zahringer M, Pattynama PM, Talen A, Sapoval M. Drug-eluting stents in renal artery stenosis. *Eur Radiol.* 2008;18(4):678–682.
55. Yan BP, Kiernan TJ, Rosenfield K. Covered stent for the treatment of recurrent bilateral renal artery in-stent restenosis. *J Invasive Cardiol.* 2008;20(10):E288-E292.
56. Fischell TA, Malhotra S, Khan S. A new ostial stent positioning system (Ostial Pro) for the accurate placement of stents to treat aorto-ostial lesions. *Catheter Cardiovasc Interv.* 2008;71(3):353–357.
57. Wain RA, Hines G. Surgical management of mesenteric occlusive disease: a contemporary review of invasive and minimally invasive techniques. *Cardiol Rev.* 2008;16(2):69–75.
58. Ottinger LW, Austen WG. A study of 136 patients with mesenteric infarction. *Surg Gynecol Obstet.* 1967;124(2):251–261.
59. Boley SJ, Sprayregan S, Siegelman SS, Veith FJ. Initial results from an aggressive roentgenological and surgical approach to acute mesenteric ischemia. *Surgery.* 1977;82(6):848–855.
60. Kawauchi M, Tada Y, Asano K, Sudo K. Angiographic demonstration of mesenteric arterial changes in postcoarctectomy syndrome. *Surgery.* 1985;98(3):602–604.
61. Gewertz BL, Zarins CK. Postoperative vasospasm after antegrade mesenteric revascularization: a report of three cases. *J Vasc Surg.* 1991;14(3):382–385.
62. Siegelman SS, Sprayregen S, Boley SJ. Angiographic diagnosis of mesenteric arterial vasoconstriction. *Radiology.* 1974;112(3):533–542.
63. Ende N. Infarction of the bowel in cardiac failure. *N Engl J Med.* 1958;258(18):879–881.
64. Nalbandian H, Sheth N, Dietrich R, Georgiou J. Intestinal ischemia caused by cocaine ingestion: report of two cases. *Surgery.* 1985;97(3):374–376.
65. Greene FL, Ariyan S, Stansel HC Jr. Mesenteric and peripheral vascular ischemia secondary to ergotism. *Surgery.* 1977;81(2):176–179.
66. Cheatham JE Jr, Williams GR, Thompson WM, Luckstead EF, Razook JD, Elkins RC. Coarctation: a review of 80 children and adolescents. *Am J Surg.* 1979;138(6):889–893.
67. Kougias P, El Sayed HF, Zhou W, Lin PH. Management of chronic mesenteric ischemia. The role of endovascular therapy. *J Endovasc Ther.* 2007;14(3):395–405.
68. Thomas JH, Blake K, Pierce GE, Hermreck AS, Seigel E. The clinical course of asymptomatic mesenteric arterial stenosis. *J Vasc Surg.* 1998;27(5):840–844.
69. Wilson DB, Mostafavi K, Craven TE, Ayerdi J, Edwards MS, Hansen KJ. Clinical course of mesenteric artery stenosis in elderly Americans. *Arch Intern Med.* 2006;166(19):2095–2100.
70. Sreenarasimhaiah J. Chronic mesenteric ischemia. *Best Pract Res Clin Gastroenterol.* 2005;19(2):283–295.
71. Merhoff GC, Porter JM. Ergot intoxication: historical review and description of unusual clinical manifestations. *Ann Surg.* 1974;180(5):773–779.
72. Matsumoto AH, Tegtmeyer CJ, Fitzcharles EK, et al. Percutaneous transluminal angioplasty of visceral arterial stenoses: results and long-term clinical follow-up. *J Vasc Interv Radiol.* 1995;6(2):165–174.
73. Bowersox JC, Zwolak RM, Walsh DB, et al. Duplex ultrasonography in the diagnosis of celiac and mesenteric artery occlusive disease. *J Vasc Surg.* 1991;14(6):780–786; discussion 6–8.
74. Zwolak RM, Fillinger MF, Walsh DB, et al. Mesenteric and celiac duplex scanning: a validation study. *J Vasc Surg.* 1998;27(6):1078–1087; discussion 88.
75. Chow LC, Chan FP, Li KC. A comprehensive approach to MR imaging of mesenteric ischemia. *Abdom Imaging.* 2002;27(5):507–516.
76. Cunningham CG, Reilly LM, Rapp JH, Schneider PA, Stoney RJ. Chronic visceral ischemia. Three decades of progress. *Ann Surg.* 1991;214(3):276–287; discussion 87–88.
77. Mateo RB, O'Hara PJ, Hertzer NR, Mascha EJ, Beven EG, Krajewski LP. Elective surgical treatment of symptomatic chronic mesenteric occlusive disease: early results and late outcomes. *J Vasc Surg.* 1999;29(5):821–831; discussion 32.

78. Park WM, Cherry KJ Jr, Chua HK, et al. Current results of open revascularization for chronic mesenteric ischemia: a standard for comparison. *J Vasc Surg.* 2002;35(5):853–9.
79. Matsumoto AH, Angle JF, Spinosa DJ, et al. Percutaneous transluminal angioplasty and stenting in the treatment of chronic mesenteric ischemia: results and longterm followup. *J Am Coll Surg.* 2002;194(1Suppl):S22-S31.
80. Sivamurthy N, Rhodes JM, Lee D, Waldman DL, Green RM, Davies MG. Endovascular versus open mesenteric revascularization: immediate benefits do not equate with short-term functional outcomes. *J Am Coll Surg.* 2006;202(6):859–867.
81. Landis MS, Rajan DK, Simons ME, Hayeems EB, Kachura JR, Sniderman KW. Percutaneous management of chronic mesenteric ischemia: outcomes after intervention. J *Vasc Interv Radiol.* 2005;16(10):1319–1325.
82. Hallisey MJ, Deschaine J, Illescas FF, et al. Angioplasty for the treatment of visceral ischemia. *J Vasc Interv Radiol.* 1995;6(5):785–791.
83. Kasirajan K, O'Hara PJ, Gray BH, et al. Chronic mesenteric ischemia: open surgery versus percutaneous angioplasty and stenting. *J Vasc Surg.* 2001;33(1):63–71.
84. Sarac TP, Altinel O, Kashyap V, et al. Endovascular treatment of stenotic and occluded visceral arteries for chronic mesenteric ischemia. *J Vasc Surg.* 2008;47(3):485–491.
85. Silva JA, White CJ, Collins TJ, et al. Endovascular therapy for chronic mesenteric ischemia. *J Am Coll Cardiol.* 2006;47(5):944–950.
86. Sharafuddin MJ, Olson CH, Sun S, Kresowik TF, Corson JD. Endovascular treatment of celiac and mesenteric arteries stenoses: applications and results. *J Vasc Surg.* 2003;38(4):692–698.
87. van Wanroij JL, van Petersen AS, Huisman AB, et al. Endovascular treatment of chronic splanchnic syndrome. *Eur J Vasc Endovasc Surg.* 2004;28(2):193–200.
88. AbuRahma AF, Stone PA, Bates MC, Welch CA. Angioplasty/stenting of the superior mesenteric artery and celiac trunk: early and late outcomes. *J Endovasc Ther.* Dec;10(6):1046–1053.
89. Shih MC, Hagspiel KD. CTA and MRA in mesenteric ischemia: part 1, role in diagnosis and differential diagnosis. *AJR Am J Roentgenol.* 2007;188(2):452–461.
90. Shih MC, Angle JF, Leung DA, et al. CTA and MRA in mesenteric ischemia: part 2, normal findings and complications after surgical and endovascular treatment. *AJR Am J Roentgenol.* 2007;188(2):462–471.
91. Fenwick JL, Wright IA, Buckenham TM. Endovascular repair of chronic mesenteric occlusive disease: the role of duplex surveillance. *ANZ J Surg.* 2007;77(1–2):60–63.
92. Maspes F, MazzettidiPietralata G, Gandini R, et al. Percutaneous transluminal angioplasty in the treatment of chronic mesenteric ischemia: results and 3 years of follow-up in 23 patients. *Abdom Imaging.* 1998;23(4):358–363.

5 Subclavian and Upper Extremity Interventions

Khung Keong Yeo, MBBS, and John R. Laird, MD

CONTENTS
- ANATOMY
- CERVICAL RIB AND THORACIC OUTLET SYNDROME
- ETIOLOGY
- DIAGNOSIS
- NONINVASIVE TESTING
- INDICATIONS FOR INTERVENTION
- SURGICAL ALTERNATIVES
- ANGIOGRAPHIC EVALUATION
- TECHNICAL SUCCESS AND COMPLICATIONS
- ANTIPLATELET AND ANTICOAGULANT THERAPY
- FEMORAL APPROACH
- RETROGRADE BRACHIAL/RADIAL APPROACH
- COMPLICATIONS
- CASE EXAMPLES
- CONCLUSION
- REFERENCES

ANATOMY

An appreciation of the aortic arch anatomy is important for the interventionalist performing subclavian and upper extremity endovascular therapies. In the most common aortic arch configuration, the aortic arch gives rise to, from proximal to distal, the innominate, left common carotid and then left subclavian artery (Fig. 1). There are important anatomic variations of the aortic arch and great arch vessels *(1)*. These include: (1) "bovine" arch in which the left common carotid artery arises from the innominate artery (15–22%) (Fig. 2); (2) common ostium of the innominate and left carotid artery; (3) left vertebral artery arises from the arch between the left carotid and

From: *Peripheral and Cerebrovascular Intervention*, Contemporary Cardiology
Edited by: D. L. Bhatt, DOI 10.1007/978-1-60327-965-9_5
© Springer Science+Business Media, LLC 2012

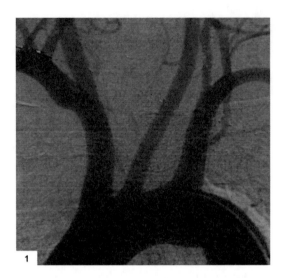

Fig. 1. This shows a normal configuration aortic arch with the innominate, left common carotid and left subclavian arteries arising from the aortic arch, proximal to distal.

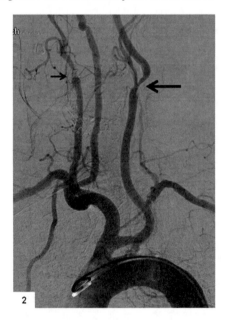

Fig. 2. This shows a "bovine" arch configuration with the left common carotid arising from the innominate artery. There is diffuse disease of the left subclavian artery. This patient has an occluded right internal carotid artery (*small arrow*) and moderate stenosis of the left internal carotid artery (*big arrow*). Access to the left internal carotid artery, if required, is likely to be difficult if approached from the femoral artery.

subclavian arteries; (4) right aortic arch; (5) arteria lusoria in which the right subclavian artery arises distal to the left subclavian artery and loops around behind the esophagus to the right arm. In addition, other, rarer variants have been reported.

The proximal subclavian artery diameter varies significantly in size and can range from 6 to 10 mm, tapering to 5–7 mm in the mid segment. The right subclavian artery arises from the innominate artery, which is the first major branch of the aortic arch. The left subclavian artery arises from the aortic arch as the third and most distal branch. Each subclavian artery in turn continues as the axillary artery after crossing the lateral margin of the first rib, and then as the brachial artery in the upper arm. The brachial artery then divides into the radial and ulnar arteries in the cubital fossa which supply the forearm and hand (Fig. 3).

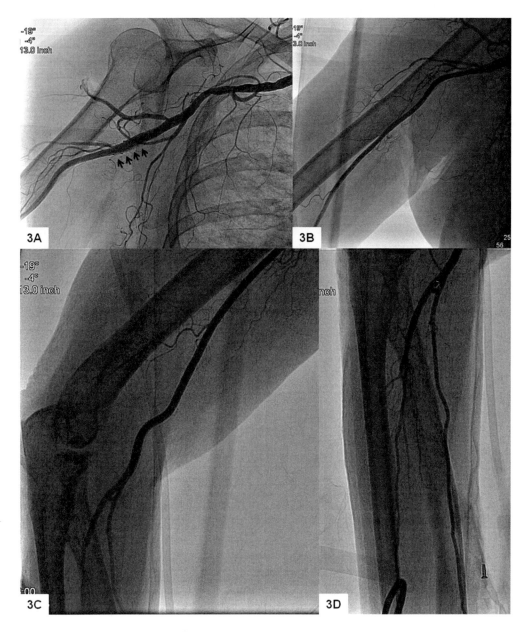

Fig. 3. (**A**) Shows the right subclavian artery continuing as the axillary artery. There are numerous collaterals noted (the patient had just undergone successful revascularization: a stent may be seen (*small arrows*). (**B**) Shows the axillary artery continuing as the brachial artery. (**C, D**) Show the brachial artery bifurcating into the radial and ulnar arteries.

The subclavian artery in its proximal (intrathoracic segment) gives rise to the vertebral artery, the thyrocervical trunk, and the internal mammary artery (IMA). After crossing the anterior scalene muscle, the subclavian artery gives rise to the costocervical trunk which gives rise to the superior intercostal artery and supplies part of the cervical spinal cord. The vertebral artery and IMA play an important role in percutaneous revascularization procedures because of their proximal location and the potential for devastating consequences should they be compromised.

CERVICAL RIB AND THORACIC OUTLET SYNDROME

The thoracic outlet syndrome is caused by either a taut congenital band from the first rib to the tip of an elongated C7 transverse process or to a rudimentary cervical rib. This structure can cause neuropathy or functional stenosis of the subclavian artery or vein. The most common vascular manifestation of thoracic outlet syndrome is venous obstruction which can lead to subclavian vein thrombosis (effort thrombosis). Impairment of arterial flow has also been reported, and repetitive injury can lead to the development of subclavian artery aneurysm. Surgical treatment with resection of the cervical rib and decompression is the definitive treatment of thoracic outlet syndrome.

ETIOLOGY

The most common underling etiology of subclavian stenosis is atherosclerosis and this most often affects the ostium or proximal part of the subclavian artery. Other disease processes can also result in subclavian or arch vessel stenosis or compromise. These include Takayasu's arteritis, fibromuscular dysplasia, giant cell arteritis, radiation arteriopathy, chronic dissection, and thoracic outlet syndrome. In Takayasu's arteritis and giant cell arteritis, lesions develop during the acute phase of the illness, and during this acute inflammatory phase, treatment consists primarily of anti-inflammatory agents such as glucocorticosteroids and immunosuppressants. Angioplasty and/or stenting are not recommended at this time because of a greater risk of complications (vessel rupture, pseudoaneurysm formation) and a high likelihood of early restenosis. During the chronic "burnt-out" phase of the disease, after irreversible stenosis has occurred, angioplasty and stenting can be performed if clinically indicated.

DIAGNOSIS

Most patients with subclavian artery stenosis or occlusion are asymptomatic. The diagnosis of subclavian stenosis should be suspected in patients with asymmetry between right and left arm blood pressure measurements. Typically, a pressure differential of ≥ 15 mmHg is considered significant (2, 3). On occasion, subclavian stenosis/occlusion is identified when a unilateral limb pulse is felt to be weaker than the contralateral side.

Upper extremity claudication may occur and is often described as arm fatigue, discomfort, weakness, or numbness with exertion. Other less common presentations include embolization to the digits (blue finger syndrome) or rarely, arm muscle atrophy. The subclavian steal syndrome is an important presenting manifestation in patients with severe proximal subclavian stenosis or occlusion. When severe proximal subclavian stenosis is present, the ipsilateral vertebral artery provides arterial blood flow to the upper extremity by "stealing" blood away from the posterior circulation of the brain via the contralateral vertebral artery and the basilar artery. This retrograde vertebral artery flow into the subclavian artery maintains circulation to the affected upper extremity but may result in neurologic symptoms due to vertebro-basilar ischemia (e.g., dizziness, vertigo, ataxia, nystagmus, syncope).

A similar phenomenon, coronary–subclavian steal, can be present in patients with a history of coronary artery bypass surgery (CABG)with use of the IMA as a conduit (usually to the left anterior descending coronary artery). When severe stenosis of the subclavian artery is present, upper extremity exercise provokes "stealing" of blood from the coronary artery resulting in myocardial ischemia and anginal symptoms.

NONINVASIVE TESTING

Noninvasive testing modalities to evaluate subclavian and upper extremity occlusive disease include duplex ultrasound, or CT *(4–6)* or MR angiography *(7, 8)*. Pressure decrements and abnormal Doppler and pulse volume recording waveforms may also allow for identification of the stenotic level. In the absence of contraindications, CT angiography is a useful diagnostic test because of the excellent image quality that can now be obtained with multi-detector CT technology, relative patient comfort and precise determination of anatomic relations of the diseased segments to the origins of the vertebral artery and IMA. Heavy calcification may complicate interpretation stenosis severity. MR angiography is similarly useful for establishing the anatomy of subclavian stenosis. In addition, it can also be used to demonstrate physiology such as the presence of subclavian steal or coronary steal phenomenon *(9–11)*.

Duplex ultrasound provides a useful, cheap, and noninvasive method of evaluating subclavian stenosis. Although the ostia of subclavian arteries can be difficult to visualize, the rest of the subclavian artery is easily imaged on ultrasound. In addition, retrograde flow in the vertebral artery is easily identified and suggests the presence of a hemodynamically significant subclavian artery stenosis or occlusion. Ultrasound duplex can directly visualize the stenotic artery and measure velocities; and color Doppler can demonstrate the presence of poststenotic turbulence. While definitive criteria have not been established, it is generally accepted that a doubling of peak systolic velocities suggest a ≥50% stenosis. Ultrasound can also visualize the presence of aneurysms which may be a source of emboli.

Natural history studies of atherosclerotic subclavian artery stenosis indicate a relatively benign course. Symptoms, when present, will often remain stable or may actually improve over time. Ackerman et al. reported a natural history study of subclavian stenosis (>50%) and occlusions (proximal to vertebral artery) in 67 patients with ultrasound correlation. Of these patients, all subsequent neurologic signs and symptoms occurring after diagnosis were transient. Only 15% of initially asymptomatic patients had vertebro-basilar transient ischemic attacks over a 2-year follow-up period. Using ultrasound follow-up of patients with stenoses, 17% had progression of disease. Due to the extensive collateral network which helps maintain perfusion to the upper extremity, many patients will remain asymptomatic despite progression to total occlusion of the subclavian artery. Stroke is a rare complication of subclavian artery disease. Flow reversal in the ipsilateral vertebral artery is generally thought to be protective *(12)*.

Given the favorable prognosis associated with this condition, subclavian artery intervention should generally be reserved for only those patients with symptoms. There may be certain circumstances (as outlined below); however, when preemptive intervention or treatment of an asymptomatic subclavian artery stenosis/occlusion may be warranted.

INDICATIONS FOR INTERVENTION

Claudication

In patients with lifestyle-limiting claudication, especially of the dominant arm, revascularization may provide symptomatic relief.

Bilateral Severe Stenosis

In patients with severe bilateral subclavian artery stenosis, reliable measurement of blood pressure is not possible as the measured upper extremity blood pressure will be significantly lower than the true systemic central aortic pressure. Many of these patients will have coexistent peripheral arterial disease that will also render measurements of leg/ankle pressures unreliable. In these situations, revascularization of one or both upper extremities will allow for accurate measurement of the blood pressure. The importance of reducing the risk of stroke and other end-organ complications of untreated hypertension cannot be understated.

Anticipated Use of the Internal Mammary Artery As a Coronary Bypass Conduit

In patients with severe coronary artery disease requiring CABG, the left (and less often, the right) IMA is used as an arterial conduit, most often to the left anterior descending coronary artery. If there is preexisting stenosis of the subclavian artery, flow into the left IMA graft may be compromised, leading to premature failure of the graft. Decisions regarding use of an alternative conduit or free IMA graft will depend upon the clinical scenario, but in some cases, treatment of the subclavian stenosis before the CABG may be indicated.

Coronary–Subclavian Steal

In patients who had prior CABG utilizing the IMA, development of proximal subclavian stenosis can result in a coronary–subclavian steal syndrome. This occurs due to inadequate flow through the proximal subclavian stenosis. As a result, the upper extremity "steals" blood from the IMA, which in turn draws blood from the coronary artery. This results in functional myocardial ischemia when the upper extremity is exercised (Fig. 4A–D). Treatment of the subclavian artery lesion is indicated to restore normal antegrade flow in the IMA graft for relief of myocardial ischemia symptoms and to preserve patency of the graft.

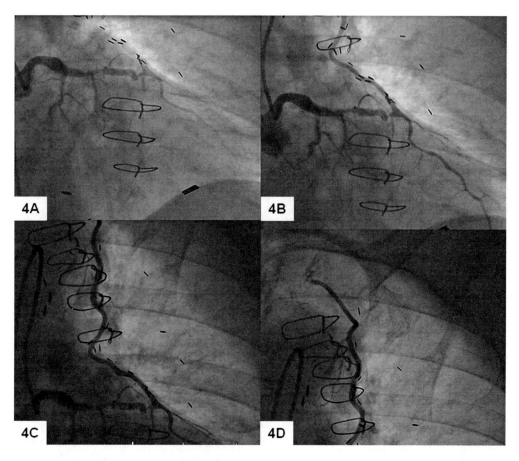

Fig. 4. (A–D) Demonstrate the typical angiographic features of coronary–subclavian steal during left coronary angiography. This patient was found to have total occlusion of the left subclavian artery. (**A**) Shows the native left anterior descending artery (LAD) filling first, followed by filling of the IMA graft all the way back to the subclavian artery (**B–D**).

Subclavian Steal Syndrome

Similar to coronary steal, proximal subclavian stenosis can result in insufficient arterial flow to the upper extremity. With exercise of the upper extremity, blood is drawn retrograde from the vertebral artery to the subclavian artery distal to the stenosis The classical subclavian steal syndrome involves posterior circulation symptoms such as dizziness, vertigo, ataxia, diplopia, and syncope (Figs. 5 and 6). Intervention is indicated for relief of subclavian steal symptoms.

Other, less common indications for subclavian artery intervention include preservation of flow into an axillary femoral bypass graft or an upper extremity dialysis graft or AV fistula. Treatment of a subclavian artery stenosis or occlusion may be necessary if embolization to the hand has occurred. A subclavian artery aneurysm may also be a source for emboli and may require treatment with surgery or covered stent technology. An ulcerated plaque in the subclavian artery may on occasion be the source of atheroemboli that threaten the hand even in the absence of hemodynamically significant stenosis.

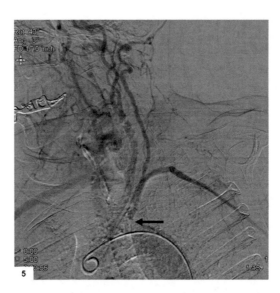

Fig. 5. This figure shows an arch aortogram with occlusion at the ostium of the left subclavian (*arrow*) artery and delayed filling of the left subclavian artery via retrograde flow down the left vertebral artery.

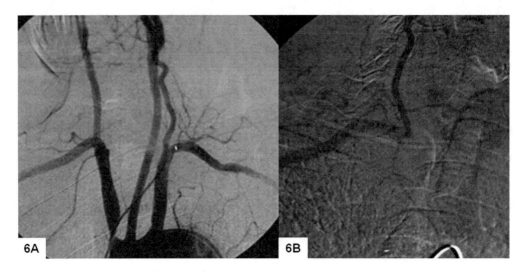

Fig. 6. (**A**) Shows severe proximal stenosis of the innominate artery. (**B**) Demonstrates delayed filling of the right subclavian artery via retrograde flow down the right vertebral artery.

SURGICAL ALTERNATIVES

The main surgical alternatives for proximal stenosis or occlusion of the subclavian artery are: carotid–subclavian bypass and subclavian to carotid artery transposition *(13–16)*. In carotid–subclavian bypass, both venous conduits and synthetic grafts have been used. Subclavian to carotid artery transposition has been reported to have the better long-term patency of the two operations. Less common surgical approaches include subclavian/innominate artery endarterectomy, aorta to subclavian bypass, and subclavian–subclavian artery bypass. A detailed discussion on the technical aspects of these procedures is beyond the scope of this chapter.

ANGIOGRAPHIC EVALUATION

It is advisable to begin the procedure with an arch aortogram in a 30–45° left anterior oblique projection in order to best delineate the aortic arch anatomy. This allows for visualization of the ostia and course of the great arch vessels, identification of arch vessel variants, assessment of the degree of atherosclerosis and calcification in the arch and evaluation of the aortic arch type (Types 1–3). The latter will provide useful information for catheter selection and will help predict difficulties with intubation of the subclavian artery or the other arch vessels. In the left anterior oblique projection, there is often overlap of the proximal right subclavian and right common carotid arteries. If disease of the proximal right subclavian artery is suspected, a 30° right anterior oblique projection will allow for appropriate visualization of the right carotid/subclavian bifurcation. When treating subclavian stenosis, the indication for intervention must be borne in mind. In cases of subclavian or coronary–subclavian steal, the ostia of the vertebral and IMA are critically important and will influence the interventional strategy. Whenever possible, stenting across the vertebral artery or IMA graft should be avoided. A right anterior oblique projection is often helpful to visualize the origin of the IMA graft to allow for precise positioning of the distal edge of the stent proximal to IMA origin.

TECHNICAL SUCCESS AND COMPLICATIONS

Reported success rates for subclavian artery intervention range from 84 to 98% *(17–20)*. Sullivan et al. reported a success rate of 93.9% in 66 subclavian interventions *(19)*, while Bates et al. reported technical success in 97% of 91 patients. Sixt et al. reported a technical success rate of 97% in 108 lesions treated in 107 patients over a 10-year period *(21)*. Technical success rates were 100% when treating subclavian stenosis and 87% when treating chronic total occlusion. The 1-year primary patency rate of the 97 patients eligible for follow-up was 88%; 79% for balloon angioplasty alone and 89% for stenting.

ANTIPLATELET AND ANTICOAGULANT THERAPY

There are limited data specific to subclavian artery interventions. Most data are extended from generalized studies involving different peripheral arteries, or carotid artery studies or coronary artery interventions. While the stakes are lower than for carotid or coronary artery interventions, the principles behind antiplatelet therapy use remain the same. Aspirin 81–325 mg daily should be given at least 3 days before the procedure, and continued indefinitely. Clopidogrel 75 mg daily should be given 5–7 days before the procedure, or a loading dose can be given at least 2 h before the procedure. Clopidogrel should be continued for at least 30 days after the intervention. Ticlopidine may be used if patients are intolerant or allergic to clopidogrel, although careful monitoring of blood counts is required. The use of prasugrel during peripheral arterial interventions has not yet been studied.

A total of 50–75 units/kg of heparin should be given to maintain an activated clotting time of 250–300 s. The use of low molecular weight heparin has not been well studied in peripheral arterial interventions. Bivalirudin is a reasonable alternative to heparin. The use of bivalirudin has not been formally examined in a randomized controlled trial in peripheral arterial interventions; however, retrospective studies have demonstrated efficacy and safety compared to unfractionated heparin *(22–24)*.

FEMORAL APPROACH

When approaching the subclavian artery from a femoral approach, the most important consideration is the arch anatomy and extent of disease in the aortic arch. In a severe, type III aortic arch, access to either subclavian artery can be challenging. This is made worse by the presence of a chronic total occlusion of the subclavian artery where adequate guide/sheath back-up support may be difficult or impossible. In the setting of proximal or "flush" occlusion of the subclavian or innominate artery, a retrograde (brachial or radial artery) approach may be necessary. The choice between a guide and a guide-sheath is largely determined by the arch anatomy and desire to minimize the size of the arterial puncture. A guiding catheter may allow easier access to the subclavian artery in patients with difficult arch anatomy. An 8–9-Fr guiding catheter will be necessary to accommodate the equipment usually required for subclavian interventions and thus will require a larger sheath in the femoral artery. On the other hand, use of a guide-sheath such as a Shuttle sheath (Cook, Bloomington, IN), will allow for a smaller arterial puncture (usually 6–7 Fr).

In Type 1 or Type II arch anatomy, a Judkins Right 4, Hockey stick or IMA catheter will usually be sufficient to engage the proximal left subclavian artery and perform diagnostic angiography. Numerous other cerebral catheters can also be used for this purpose. If intervention is to be performed, the diagnostic catheter can then be exchanged out for a 90 cm long guide-sheath for the intervention. In patients where there is a significant arch tortuosity or a Type III arch anatomy, a reverse curve catheter such as the Simmons or Vitek catheter (Cook Medical, Bloomington, IN) will more easily engage the innominate or left subclavian artery. The Vitek catheter is positioned just distal to the subclavian artery and then carefully advanced to engage the most distal arch vessel first. In order to engage the more proximal arch vessels, the catheter is then pushed forward until it prolapses out of the first artery it had engaged. Upon engaging the ostium of the target arch vessel, the Vitek catheter is then pulled back cautiously to 'seat' itself into the artery.

Telescoping Access Technique

An alternative method of advancing a guide sheath into the subclavian artery in patients with difficult arch anatomy is to telescope a diagnostic catheter such as a Vitek or Simmons catheter within the guide-sheath. The diagnostic catheter can be used to engage the subclavian or innominate artery. A 0.035 in. angled hydrophilic guidewire (Terumo, Somerset, NJ) can then be advanced across the stenosis into the distal subclavian artery. The diagnostic catheter is then advanced over the hydrophilic guidewire into the subclavian artery and the hydrophilic guidewire is exchanged for a more supportive guidewire. Finally, the guide-sheath can be advanced into the origin of the subclavian artery using the diagnostic catheter and wire as a rail. The intervention can then be performed over this supportive guidewire. Use of an extra stiff support wire helps provide a stable platform during delivery and positioning of the stent delivery system. In situations where the initial 5 Fr catheter does not cross the lesion or prolapses out of the subclavian artery, a 4 or 5 Fr hydrophilic catheter may be used to traverse the lesion. A stable platform for stent delivery is crucial for precise positioning in order to avoid the ostia of the IMA and vertebral artery.

If a lesion is heavily calcified with severe stenosis or a chronic total occlusion is present, a 0.035 in. guidewire or catheter may not easily traverse the lesion. In these circumstances, a 0.014 or 0.018 in. system may be utilized. 0.014 in. coronary CTO guidewires or hydrophilic tip guidewires can be very useful in these situations. 0.014 in. coronary balloons may be necessary to predilate the lesion before larger catheters and balloons will cross. 0.018 in. guidewires may be similarly used.

Stent

Bare metal stents are most often chosen for this location, although covered stents may be necessary to treat complications following subclavian intervention or to treat subclavian artery aneurysms or pseudoaneurysms. In general, balloon expandable stents are preferred for the treatment of proximal or ostial subclavian lesions because they can be more precisely positioned and deployed. A 0.035 in. balloon expandable stent platform will provide greater resistance to elastic recoil and is well suited for lesions in this location. For ostial lesions, the stent will need to be extended approximately 1 mm into the aorta to ensure complete ostial coverage. For lesions that extend close to the origin of the vertebral artery or IMA, balloon expandable stents allow for precise positioning just proximal to these important branches. Distal to the vertebral or IMA, a self-expanding nitinol stent is preferred because the artery is subject to compression and flexion forces in this location. There are no Food and Drug Administration approved stents with a subclavian artery indication; therefore, stents are used in an off-label manner in this location.

RETROGRADE BRACHIAL/RADIAL APPROACH

In cases of chronic total occlusion or severe stenosis near the origin of the subclavian artery, a femoral approach may be technically challenging due to inability to obtain adequate guide catheter or sheath back-up support. This is particularly true if there is proximal or "flush" occlusion with little or no proximal subclavian artery "stump." In such situations, a retrograde approach may be considered. Access via the brachial or radial arteries are both acceptable although brachial access may be preferred if larger sheath/guide size is required. Alternatively, after crossing the lesion with standard CTO techniques, the wire may be snared in the aorta and externalized via the femoral artery, to allow for delivery of the stent platform through a larger femoral artery sheath (Fig. 7A–C).

In the setting of severe subclavian artery stenosis or occlusion, the brachial pulse may be weak or absent. Ultrasound guided puncture of the brachial artery with a micropuncture kit is preferred in this situation and may minimize the potential for access site complications. Another challenge associated with the retrograde approach is adequate

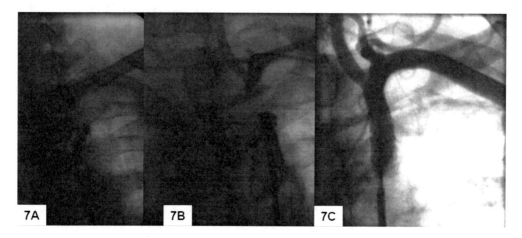

Fig. 7. This series of panels demonstrates the use of a retrograde approach in a patient with proximal left subclavian artery occlusion. (**A**) Shows the proximal stump of the occlusion. (**B**) Shows simultaneous contrast injection in the proximal stump and in the distal stump via a retrograde catheter. (**C**) Shows the final angiographic result.

visualization of the ostium of the subclavian artery when injecting contrast against the flow of blood. Care must be taken to adequately visualize the "true" ostium prior to stent deployment.

COMPLICATIONS

Complications that can occur with subclavian artery interventions can be life and limb threatening. These include aortic dissection, stroke, subclavian artery rupture/perforation, distal embolization, and upper extremity ischemia. However, available data from published case series suggest a low incidence of complications. In a series of 177 treated subclavian or innominate arteries (in 170 patients), technical success was achieved in 98.7% of treated arteries with no procedure-related deaths, 1 stroke (0.6%) and 1 TIA (0.6%) *(20)*. There were three flow-limiting dissections in this report, all of which were successfully treated with placement of a second stent. Arterial thrombosis occurred in one patient (0.6%). In another series of 108 interventions (107 patients) by Sixt et al., there were no major complications reported *(21)*. Bates et al. reported distal embolization successfully treated with thrombolysis in 2 of 91 treated patients (2.2%), brachial artery thrombosis related to access requiring embolectomy (1.1%), and reperfusion edema without compartment syndrome (1.1%) *(17)*.

Stroke Prevention

As previously described, flow reversal in the vertebral artery is protective during subclavian artery interventions and likely accounts for the low risk of stroke associated with these procedures. The routine use of distal embolic protection devices in the vertebral artery has not been studied, and is currently not recommended. Potential downsides to use of an embolic protection device include spasm or dissection of the vertebral artery, and entrapment of the device on the subclavian artery stent. If the subclavian stenosis is in close proximity to the ostium of the vertebral artery, and the ostium of the vertebral artery is diseased, placement of a guidewire into the vessel to maintain access while the subclavian artery is treated may be necessary. Rarely, rescue angioplasty of the vertebral artery may need to be performed. Because of the limited published literature on this scenario, treatment has to be individualized to the anatomy and clinical scenario.

CASE EXAMPLES

Case 1

A 74-year-old man with a history of coronary artery disease with prior multivessel coronary artery bypass surgery presented with progressive anginal symptoms. He had an abnormal nuclear stress test with myocardial ischemia in the anterior wall. Diagnostic cardiac catheterization was performed and showed severe native three-vessel coronary artery disease, with patent vein grafts to his right posterior-descending artery and obtuse marginal arteries. His left IMA was patent as well and inserted into the distal left anterior descending artery. However, he had severe proximal left subclavian artery stenosis, which was felt to be the cause of his ischemic symptoms. Percutaneous revascularization of the left subclavian artery was then performed.

A 0.035 guidewire was advanced up into the descending thoracic aorta and a 7-Fr, 90 cm long shuttle sheath was advanced to the descending thoracic aorta. Anticoagulation with intravenous heparin was given to achieve an activated clotting time of >250 s. The left subclavian artery was engaged with a 5-Fr Vitek catheter which confirmed subtotal occlusion of the left subclavian artery (Fig. 8A). Attempts were made to cross the subtotal occlusion with a variety of guidewires including a 0.014 in. PT Graphix wire (Boston Scientific, Natick, MA), 0.035 in. angled Terumo glide wire (Terumo, Somerset, NJ), and a 0.014 in. Confianza Pro wire (Abbott, Abbott Park, IL). Despite multiple attempts, the subtotal occlusions could not be successfully crossed. The 7-Fr shuttle sheath was removed and exchanged for an 8-Fr short sheath in the right common femoral artery. The left subclavian artery was then intubated with an 8-Fr JR4 guiding catheter. Attempts were made again to cross the subtotal occlusion, but were unsuccessful. The JR4 guiding catheter was subsequently exchanged for an 8-Fr left coronary bypass guiding catheter. The left subclavian artery was intubated, and the subtotal occlusion was crossed with a 0.018 Terumo gold-tipped guidewire (Terumo, Somerset, NJ). A microcatheter was advanced over this wire into the distal left subclavian artery. The wire was then exchanged for a 0.014 in. extra support wire. The left subclavian artery was dilated with a 4 mm diameter by 3 cm long balloon. The angiography demonstrated significant improvement, but with residual high-grade stenosis. The wire in the subclavian artery was then exchanged for a 0.035 in. Supracore wire (Abbott, Abbott Park, IL), and the 8-Fr guiding catheter was exchanged for a 7-Fr shuttle sheath. The left subclavian artery stenosis was then further dilated with a 6 mm diameter × 2 cm long balloon. This was followed by implantation of a 7 mm diameter × 24 mm long Genesis stent (Cordis, Bridgewater, NJ) (Fig. 8B). Subsequent angiography demonstrated an excellent angiographic result with no significant residual narrowing of the proximal left subclavian artery (Fig. 8C). There was normal antegrade flow down the left IMA bypass graft to the LAD, and normal antegrade flow into the left vertebral artery.

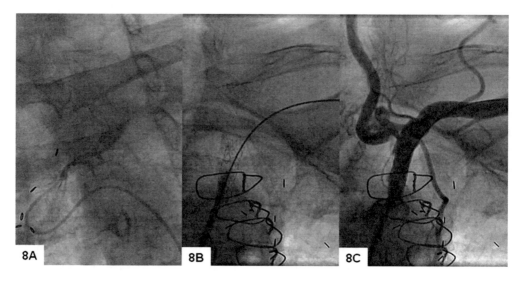

Fig. 8. (**A**) Shows subtotal occlusion of the left subclavian artery. It is engaged with a 5-Fr Vitek catheter. (**B**) Shows a wire across the occlusion with a stent deployed. (**C**) Demonstrates the location of the stent just proximal to the ostia of the IMA and vertebral artery.

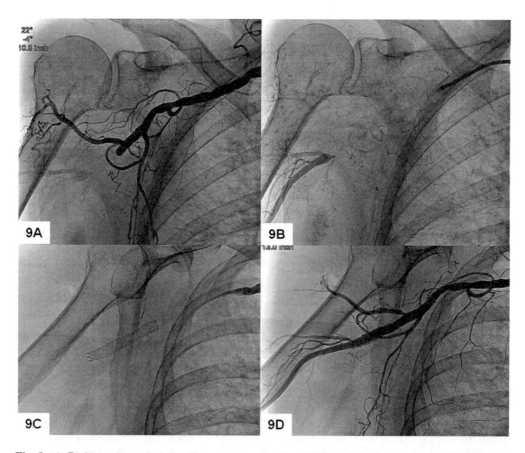

Fig. 9. (**A, B**) Show the occluded axillary artery and delayed filling via collaterals beyond the segment of occlusion. (**C**) Shows the stent within the axillary artery and (**D**) shows the final angiographic result.

Case 2

A 65-year-old woman with a history of coronary artery disease presented with lifestyle-limiting right arm claudication. Her right radial and brachial pulses were not palpable on physical examination. Duplex ultrasound showed peak velocities of 250 cm/s in the proximal subclavian artery. Because of her severe symptoms, angiography was performed. This showed the presence of mild stenosis in the innominate and proximal right subclavian artery. In addition, the right axillary artery had a short-segment occlusion with distal reconstitution (Fig. 9A, B).

Catheter-based intervention was performed. The innominate artery was engaged with a 5 Fr Vitek catheter and a 0.035 in. angled hydrophilic guidewire was advanced into the proximal axillary artery. The Vitek catheter was then used to exchange out the wire for a short-tipped 0.035 in. Amplatz super stiff wire. This was used to deliver and position a 6-Fr 90-cm Shuttle sheath at the subclavian artery. A 0.014 in. Confianza Pro wire, using a 5.0×20 mm over-the-wire balloon as support, was used to cross the occlusion. End-hole injection through the balloon confirmed entry into the distal true lumen. Balloon angioplasty was then performed followed by the deployment of an 8×40 mm SMART Control stent (Cordis, Bridgewater, NJ). Postdilation with a 6×30 balloon was performed. Final angiographic results were excellent showing no dissection, embolization, perforation, or residual stenosis (Fig. 9C, D). Postprocedure, the patient reported resolution of her right arm claudication. Physical examination showed normal right radial and brachial pulses.

CONCLUSION

In summary, subclavian and upper extremity arterial stenoses are usually benign and can be medically managed. However, revascularization may be necessary in specific occasions. Common indications include the following: (1) when significant symptoms such as claudication are present; (2) there is associated subclavian steal or coronary–subclavian steal syndrome; (3) the IMA is required as a conduit for coronary bypass surgery; and (4) there are bilateral severe subclavian artery stenoses and accurate blood pressure measurements are required. Important technical pointers include the use of a stable platform with supportive guidewire for accurate stent delivery. In the proximal and mid subclavian artery, balloon expandable stents are generally preferred for precise deployment, in order to avoid the IMA and the vertebral artery. When properly performed, subclavian and upper extremity interventions can be safely and effectively performed in the majority of cases.

REFERENCES

1. Natsis KI, Tsitouridis IA, Didagelos MV, Fillipidis AA, Vlasis KG, Tsikaras PD. Anatomical variations in the branches of the human aortic arch in 633 angiographies: clinical significance and literature review. *Surg Radiol Anat.* 2009;31:319–323.
2. English JA, Carell ES, Guidera SA, Tripp HF. Angiographic prevalence and clinical predictors of left subclavian stenosis in patients undergoing diagnostic cardiac catheterization. *Catheter Cardiovasc Interven.* 2001;54:8–11.
3. Osborn LA, Vernon SM, Reynolds B, Timm TC, Allen K. Screening for subclavian artery stenosis in patients who are candidates for coronary bypass surgery. *Catheter Cardiovasc Interven.* 2002;56:162–165.

4. Moussa F, Kumar P, Pen V. Cardiac CT scan for preoperative planning in a patient with bilateral subclavian stenosis needing coronary artery bypass. *J Card Surg.* 2009;24:196–197.
5. Peloschek P, Sailer J, Loewe C, Schillinger M, Lammer J. The role of multi-slice spiral CT angiography in patient management after endovascular therapy. *Cardiovasc Intervent Radiol.* 2006;29:756–761.
6. Remy-Jardin M, Remy J, Masson P, et al. Helical CT angiography of thoracic outlet syndrome: functional anatomy. *AJR Am J Roentgenol.* 2000;174:1667–1674.
7. Bitar R, Gladstone D, Sahlas D, Moody A. MR angiography of subclavian steal syndrome: pitfalls and solutions. *AJR Am J Roentgenol.* 2004;183:1840–1841.
8. Cosottini M, Zampa V, Petruzzi P, Ortori S, Cioni R, Bartolozzi C. Contrast-enhanced three-dimensional MR angiography in the assessment of subclavian artery diseases. *Eur Radiol.* 2000;10:1737–1744.
9. Patil S. Images in Medicine. Subclavian steal syndrome diagnosed by MR angiography. *Med Health RI.* 2001;84:173.
10. Sheehy N, MacNally S, Smith CS, Boyle G, Madhavan P, Meaney JF. Contrast-enhanced MR angiography of subclavian steal syndrome: value of the 2D time-of-flight "localizer" sign. *AJR Am J Roentgenol.* 2005;185:1069–1073.
11. Virmani R, Carroll TJ, Hung J, Hopkins J, Diniz L, Carr J. Diagnosis of subclavian steal syndrome using dynamic time-resolved magnetic resonance angiography: a technical note. *Magn Reson Imaging.* 2008;26:287–292.
12. Ringelstein EB, Zeumer H. Delayed reversal of vertebral artery blood flow following percutaneous transluminal angioplasty for subclavian steal syndrome. *Neuroradiology.* 1984;26:189–198.
13. Cohn LH, Fogarty TJ, Daily PO, Silverman JF, Shumway NE. Surgical treatment of atherosclerotic lesions of the subclavian artery. *Calif Med.* 1972;116:8–12.
14. Deriu GP, Milite D, Verlato F, et al. Surgical treatment of atherosclerotic lesions of subclavian artery: carotid-subclavian bypass versus subclavian-carotid transposition. *J Cardiovasc Surg.* 1998;39:729–734.
15. Gerety RL, Andrus CH, May AG, Rob CG, Green R, DeWeese JA. Surgical treatment of occlusive subclavian artery disease. *Circulation.* 1981;64:II228-II230.
16. Linni K, Ugurluoglu A, Mader N, Hitzl W, Magometschnigg H, Holzenbein TJ. Endovascular management versus surgery for proximal subclavian artery lesions. *Ann Vasc Surg.* 2008;22:769–775.
17. Bates MC, Broce M, Lavigne PS, Stone P. Subclavian artery stenting: factors influencing long-term outcome. *Catheter Cardiovasc Interven.* 2004;61:5–11.
18. Korner M, Baumgartner I, Do DD, Mahler F, Schroth G. PTA of the subclavian and innominate arteries: long-term results. *Vasa.* 1999;28:117–122.
19. Sullivan TM, Gray BH, Bacharach JM, et al. Angioplasty and primary stenting of the subclavian, innominate, and common carotid arteries in 83 patients. *J Vasc Surg.* 1998;28:1059–1065.
20. Patel SN, White CJ, Collins TJ, et al. Catheter-based treatment of the subclavian and innominate arteries. *Catheter Cardiovasc Interven.* 2008;71:963–968.
21. Sixt S, Rastan A, Schwarzwalder U, et al. Results after balloon angioplasty or stenting of atherosclerotic subclavian artery obstruction. *Catheter Cardiovasc Interven.* 2009;73:395–403.
22. Maclean AA, Pena CS, Katzen BT. Bivalirudin in peripheral interventions. *Tech Vasc en Radiol.* 2006;9:80–83.
23. Katzen BT, Ardid MI, MacLean AA, et al. Bivalirudin as an anticoagulation agent: safety and efficacy in peripheral interventions. *J Vasc Interven Radiol.* 2005;16:1183–1187; quiz 7.
24. Sheikh IR, Ahmed SH, Mori N, et al. Comparison of safety and efficacy of bivalirudin versus unfractionated heparin in percutaneous peripheral intervention: a single-center experience. *JACC Cardiovasc Interven.* 2009;2:871–876.

6 Carotid and Vertebral Intervention

Douglas E. Drachman, MD,
Nicholas J. Ruggiero II, MD,
and Kenneth Rosenfield, MD

CONTENTS

INTRODUCTION
CAROTID ENDARTERECTOMY
CAS: HISTORY AND TRIALS
INDICATIONS FOR CAS
CAS: TECHNICAL ASPECTS
VERTEBRAL ARTERY STENOSIS
ANATOMY OF THE VERTEBRAL ARTERY
THERAPY FOR VERTEBRAL ARTERY STENOSIS
ENDOVASCULAR TECHNIQUE FOR
    VERTEBRAL INTERVENTION
CONCLUSIONS AND FUTURE DIRECTIONS
REFERENCES

INTRODUCTION

Following cardiovascular disease and cancer, stroke represents the third most common cause of death in the United States, claiming 150,000 lives annually. Equally significant, stroke is the leading cause of disability. Approximately 795,000 individuals experience a new or recurrent stroke each year, of which 600,000 are first attacks, and 185,000 are recurrent *(1, 2)*. Nearly 20% of all strokes occur as the result of atherosclerotic disease in the carotid artery *(3)*. The prevalence of carotid stenosis in the United States is significant, afflicting 5–10% of those over the age of 65 with at least 50% stenosis, and 1% with greater than 80% stenosis *(4)*. The risk of stroke in individuals with known carotid atherosclerosis varies depending on the degree of stenosis and whether or not there have been previous symptoms associated with the lesion. Historically, clinical studies have shown that asymptomatic individuals with a >60%

From: *Peripheral and Cerebrovascular Intervention*, Contemporary Cardiology
Edited by: D. L. Bhatt, DOI 10.1007/978-1-60327-965-9_6
© Springer Science+Business Media, LLC 2012

carotid stenosis have a 2-year ipsilateral stroke rate of 5%; while symptomatic individuals with a >70% stenosis have a 2-year stroke rate as high as 26% *(5, 6)*.

In select patients, carotid revascularization may provide an opportunity to reduce the morbidity and mortality associated with severe atherosclerotic stenosis. Carotid endarterectomy (CEA), refined over the past five decades since its development, has long been held as the "gold standard" revascularization strategy. In more recent years, however, endovascular therapy – and in particular carotid artery stenting (CAS) – has evolved as an alternative, minimally invasive approach. Clinical trials designed to compare these techniques have engendered tremendous controversy. At present, data do not clearly indicate that "one size fits all," or that one revascularization modality is superior to the other in all patients and in all carotid atherosclerotic lesions. Rather, patient- and lesion-specific considerations must be taken into account when tailoring the approach to the individual. Through careful review of the data regarding medical therapy, surgical revascularization, and endovascular therapy for carotid stenosis, we may gain insight into the promise and pitfalls of each approach and may determine the best practice for our patients. In this chapter, we will also review the contemporary management of vertebral artery stenosis, with analogous focus on the data regarding medical, surgical, and endovascular approaches.

CAROTID ENDARTERECTOMY

CEA was first performed in the 1950s *(7)*. It was not until the 1980s–1990s, however, that randomized clinical trials demonstrated that CEA reduces stroke when compared with medical therapy in patients with severe carotid artery stenosis (Table 1). In broad terms, these early trials may be grouped based on their focus on patients with either symptomatic or asymptomatic or carotid stenosis. Such a distinction remains valuable in determining clinical practice, since patients with symptomatic disease are at higher risk of a subsequent stroke *(8)* and may have more to gain from revascularization, at least in the short term.

The North American Symptomatic Carotid Endarterectomy Trial (NASCET) examined 2,226 patients with symptomatic internal carotid artery stenosis randomized to medical therapy vs. endarterectomy. Patients in the trial had sustained either a transient ischemic attack or stroke within 4 months of enrollment, and were demonstrated to have a 30–99% stenosis of the internal carotid artery. For patients with a ≥70% stenosis, CEA reduced the risk of any ipsilateral stroke from 26 to 9% at 2 years ($P<0.001$) *(5)*.

Rothwell et al. performed a pooled analysis of 6,092 patients from three randomized trials of CEA vs. medical therapy in symptomatic patients: NASCET, ECST, and the Veterans Affairs Trial. In this analysis, there was a 7.1% incidence of stroke or death at 30 days after carotid endarterectomy. In patients with 50–69% carotid stenosis, the 5-year relative risk reduction of ipsilateral stroke following CEA was 28%; in those with 70–99% stenosis, the relative risk reduction was 48%. There was no benefit to CEA in patients with stenosis less than 50%. Additionally, for patients with near-total occlusion of the carotid artery ("string sign"), the benefit of CEA was also not detectable *(9, 10)*.

In the Asymptomatic Carotid Atherosclerosis Study (ACAS), 1,662 patients with asymptomatic 60–99% carotid stenosis were randomized to undergo surgery or receive

Table 1
Trials of Carotid Endarterectomy Versus Medical therapy for Carotid Artery Stenosis (17)

Trial	N	Stenosis	Follow-up (yrs)	Endpoint	Medical (%)	CEA (%)	P	RRR(%)	ARR	NNT(%)
Symptomatic										
ECST	3018	≥80%	3	Major stroke or death	26.5	14.9	<0.001	44	11.6	8.6
VA 309	189	>50%	1	Ipsilateral stroke or TIA or surgical death	19.4	7.7	0.011	60	11.7	8.5
NASCET	659	≥70%	2	Ipsilateral stroke	26	9	<0.001	65	17	5.9
NASCET	858	50–69%	5	Ipsilateral stroke	22.2	15.7	0.045	29	6.5	15.4
NASCET	1368	≤50%	5	Ipsilateral stroke	18.7	14.9	0.16	20	3.8	26.3
Asymptomatic										
ACAS	1662	>60%	5	Ipsilateral stroke or surgical death	11	5.1	0.004	54	5.9	16.9
ACST	3120	≥60%	5	Any stroke	11.8	6.4	<0.001	46	5.4	18.5
VA	444	≥60%	4	Ipsilateral stroke	9.4	4.7	<0.06	50	4.7	21.3

ACAS Asymptomatic Carotid Atherosclerotic Study (6); *ACST* Asymptomatic Carotid Surgery Trial (18); *ARR* Absolute Risk Reduction *CEA* Carotid Endarterectomy *ECST* European Carotid Surgery Trial (10), *NASCET* North American Symptomatic Carotid Endarterectomy Trial(5) *NNT* Number to Treat *RRR* Relative Risk Reduction *TIA* Transient Ischemic Attack *VA* Veterans Affairs.
Reproduced with permission of Kenneth Rosenfield MD, CathSAP 3 ACC/SCAI © 2008(17).

medical therapy. The study was conducted at 39 centers with a <3% stroke risk associated with CEA. At 5 years, the risk of stroke or death was 5.1% in patients who underwent CEA, and 11.3% in patients receiving medical therapy *(6)*.

When reviewing these seminal randomized trials comparing CEA to medical therapy in the 1980s and 1990s, it is critical to observe that the "medical therapy" arm often consisted of aspirin alone. Since then, our awareness of the importance of managing risk factors for primary and secondary stroke prevention has increased; correspondingly, medical therapy has improved. In the HOPE trial, ramipril was administered to patients at high cardiovascular risk and MACE events were evaluated in comparison to placebo. In patients who received ramipril, there was a statistically significant reduction in stroke (3.4 vs. 4.9%; relative risk, 0.68; $P<0.001$) *(11)*. In the SPARCL trial, high-dose atorvastatin reduced the risk of ischemic stroke by 12% *(12)*. In the JUPITER trial, the use of rosuvastatin in subjects with LDL <130 but with elevated CRP (≥ 2.0) reduced the risk of stroke by 48% compared with placebo *(13)*. Therefore, a reevaluation of the merits of CEA against the current "best medical therapy," particularly for the asymptomatic patient populations, is warranted.

The entry criteria for the early CEA studies were designed to select low-risk patients. As a result, the dramatic results may not be applicable to higher-risk groups. This is particularly true of elderly patients (>79 years), patients with concomitant cardiovascular disease, and patients with high-risk lesions such as restenosis after a prior CEA, radiation-induced stenosis, lesions following radical neck surgery or those with difficult surgical access. Features previously demonstrated to contribute to high surgical risk for CEA are outlined in Table 2.

Carotid atherosclerosis predominantly occurs at the carotid bifurcation, which is typically readily accessible for conventional surgical technique. Carotid disease that extends beyond the bifurcation or involves the origin or proximal aspect of the common carotid artery is not uncommon, and may be difficult to treat surgically, however. Surgical management of carotid stenosis at these proximal locations has historically required thoracotomy or subclavian–carotid bypass procedure. Similarly, stenosis that extends significantly distal to the bifurcation may also require a complex surgical

Table 2
High-risk Criteria for Carotid Endarterectomy (CEA) *(3)*

Anatomical criteria	*Medical comorbidities*
Lesion at C-2 or higher	Age ≥ 80 yrs
Lesion below clavicle	Class III/IV congestive heart failure
Prior radical neck surgery or radiation	Class III/IV angina pectoris
Contralateral carotid occlusion	Left main/≥ 2-vessel coronary disease
Prior ipsilateral CEA	Urgent (<30 days) heart surgery
Contralateral laryngeal nerve palsy	Left ventricular ejection fraction $\leq 30\%$
Tracheostoma	Recent (<30 days) myocardial infarction
	Severe chronic lung disease
	Severe renal disease

(Reprinted with permission of the American College of Cardiology.)

approach, potentially including disarticulation of the jaw in order to access otherwise "hard to reach" sites of distal disease.

Current recommendations for CEA are based primarily on the symptomatic status of the patient, the severity of stenosis, and the experience and historical outcomes of the surgeon. Current AHA guidelines recommend CEA in symptomatic patients with stenosis 50–99%, if the risk of perioperative stroke or death is <6%. For asymptomatic patients, AHA guidelines recommend CEA for stenosis 60–99%, if the risk of perioperative stroke or death is <3%. These guidelines may be influenced by other important clinical factors such as anticipated life expectancy, age, gender and presence of other comorbid medical conditions. The American Academy of Neurology recommends that eligible patients should be 40–75 years old and have a life expectancy of at least 5 years *(14, 15)*.

Surgical experience is also very important when anticipating risk of stroke with CEA. Wennberg et al. showed that morbidity of the procedure was inversely related to the volume of CEA performed. In low-volume hospitals, there was a 2.5% mortality whereas, in the NASCET hospitals, there was a 1.4% mortality *(16)*.

CEA is contraindicated when the predicted perioperative risk of stroke or death is >3% for asymptomatic patients, >6% for symptomatic patients, and >10% for repeat CEA *(14)*. Anatomic features and comorbid medical conditions that are associated with increased complications after CEA are listed in Table 2.

The complications most often described following CEA include: adverse cardiovascular events such as hypertension (20%), hypotension (5%), and myocardial infarction (1%); neurological events including stroke (2–6%), hyperperfusion syndrome, intracranial hemorrhage, seizures, cranial nerve injury (7%); wound infection (1%), hematoma (5%), injury to carotid artery (dissection, thrombosis, restenosis 5–10%), and death (1%) *(14)*.

CAS: HISTORY AND TRIALS

While CEA has long been held as the procedure of choice for the management of carotid artery disease, endovascular therapy now offers a minimally invasive alternative. By reviewing the contemporary literature comparing these techniques, we may gain insight into scenarios where one strategy may offer advantage over another. As with CEA trials, studies of carotid stenting have been designed based on symptomatic status. In addition, carotid stenting trials may involve patients deemed to be high- or conventional-risk for CEA, based on comorbid conditions or surgically unfeasible issues, as articulated in Table 2. The grid below the Table 3 represents a schema for considering carotid stenting trials.

The first balloon angioplasty for carotid artery stenosis was reported in 1980 *(19)*. The first embolic protection device (EPD) involving transient balloon occlusion of the distal internal carotid artery, with aspiration of vascular debris following intervention was introduced in the 1980s. Subsequently, the use of EPD – although never rigorously subjected to randomized-controlled investigation – has been found to reduce periprocedural CVA profoundly in carotid stenting procedures *(20)*. The first balloon-expandable stent was deployed in the carotid artery in 1989 *(21)*. Subsequent use of the Wallstent, and later use of self-expanding nitinol stents, has increased the success rate for

Table 3
Schematic Categorization of Carotid Stent Trials

Surgical risk	Symptomatic status	
	High risk Symptomatic	High risk Asymptomatic
	Low risk Symptomatic	Low risk Asymptomatic

endovascular therapy of carotid stenosis. The iterative development of better devices and procedural techniques has resulted in continued improvement in the outcomes of carotid endovascular therapy.

Still, carotid stenting remains one of the most controversial topics in cardiovascular medicine. The findings of several major clinical trials in the field have been inconsistent, and have contributed to the delay in widespread acceptance of this technique. In 2001, Roubin et al. published a 5-year single center follow-up of 528 consecutive patients undergoing carotid stenting. In this study, the authors reported a 98% procedural success rate, a 1.6% mortality rate, and a combined 30-day endpoint of death and stroke of 7.4% (22). While this single-center registry demonstrated the feasibility of the current carotid stenting technique, subsequent large, multicenter, randomized and controlled studies were needed.

The first randomized controlled trial was the Carotid and Vertebral Artery Transluminal Angioplasty Study (CAVATAS) trial. A total of 504 patients, with asymptomatic carotid stenosis greater than 90% were randomized to CEA ($n=253$) or carotid angioplasty ($n=251$). Stent insertion was performed in only 26% of patients; the rest were treated with balloon angioplasty alone. Embolic protection devices (EPD) were not widely available, and were not used in CAVATAS. Despite these significant limitations, the 30-day endpoint of disabling stroke or death showed no difference between the angioplasty arm (10%) or the surgical arm (9.9%, $P=0.9$). Long-term follow-up has shown no difference between the two groups. The authors therefore concluded that angioplasty and surgery were equivalent for safety and efficacy, although the angioplasty group experienced less procedural morbidity. Additionally, patients undergoing CEA were more likely to develop cranial nerve palsy (8.7 vs. 0%, $P<0.0001$) or a major hematoma in the neck (7 vs. 1%, $P<0.0015$), than those who underwent endovascular treatment (23).

The SAPPHIRE (Stenting and Angioplasty with Protection in Patients at High Risk for Endarterectomy) trial was the first randomized clinical trial to compare contemporary CAS technique including EPD and self-expanding nitinol stents against CEA in high surgical-risk patients (24). A total of 334 patients from 29 American centers were randomized. Entry criteria included asymptomatic carotid stenosis (>80% by ultrasound) or symptomatic stenosis (>50%), plus at least one feature putting the patient at higher risk for surgical endarterectomy. These features included age greater than 80 years, the presence of congestive heart failure, severe COPD, previous endarterectomy with restenosis, previous radiation therapy or radical neck surgery, or lesions distal or proximal to the usual cervical location (see Table 2). Patients were screened by a team including a vascular surgeon, an interventionalist, and a neurologist, all of whom had to agree that the patient was appropriate for revascularization and could undergo either procedure.

The primary endpoint of the SAPPHIRE trial included stroke, death, or myocardial infarction at 30 days, or ipsilateral stroke or death between 31 days and 1 year following the carotid revascularization procedure. The primary endpoint was reached in 12.2% of patients treated with stenting, and in 20.1% of those who underwent CEA ($P=0.004$ for noninferiority). The rate of cranial nerve palsy was 0% in CAS and 4.9% in CEA patients at 1 year ($P=0.004$). The rate of target vessel revascularization was 0.6% in CAS and 4.3% in CEA patients at 1 year ($P=0.04$) *(24)*. The results of the SAPPHIRE trial led to the Food and Drug Administration's approval of the carotid stenting procedure for patients at high surgical risk. At 3 years' follow-up, the prespecified secondary endpoint of 30-day stroke, death, or myocardial infarction or 31–1,080-day incidence of death or ipsilateral stroke was reached in 24.6% of those in the stenting group and 26.9% of those in the CEA group ($P=0.27$). The 3-year outcomes of the SAPPHIRE trial demonstrate, in rigorous fashion, the durability of stroke reduction following endovascular therapy for carotid stenosis in a surgical high-risk population *(25)*.

Two subsequent prospective multicenter trials, the Acculink for Revascularization of Carotids in High Risk Patient (ARCHeR) and the Registry Study to Evaluate the Neuroshield Bare-Wire Cerebral Protection System and X-Act Stent in patients at high risk for Carotid Endarterectomy (SECuRITY) have demonstrated equally impressive results with the combination of specifically designed carotid stents and embolic protection devices.

The ARCHeR trial evaluated patients considered to be high-risk surgical candidates who were treated with CAS with or without embolic protection. The trial is comprised of a series of three prospective, nonrandomized, multicenter studies at 48 sites in the United States, Europe, and Argentina, which enrolled 581 consecutive patients. The ARCHeR 1 trial evaluated the ACCULINK stent alone; the ARCHeR 2 trial included the stent and an embolic protection device (ACCUNET filter); and ARCHeR 3 evaluated updated catheter design for stent and embolic filter delivery, using rapid exchange systems. Taken collectively, the 30-day adverse event rate of the ARCHeR trials, including stroke, death, and myocardial infarction, was 8.3%; and, the 30-day major/fatal stroke rate was 1.5%. The primary composite endpoint of 30-day death/stroke/MI plus ipsilateral stroke at 1 year was 9.6%. Restenosis and the need for clinically driven target lesion revascularization were low, at 2.2 and 2.9% at 1 and 2 years, respectively *(26)*.

The utility of carotid stenting in standard-surgical-risk patients has recently come under fire. Three studies published in high impact journals concluded that CAS was inferior to CEA in standard-risk patients. Subsequent re-evaluation, and the identification of several methodological flaws, calls the conclusions drawn from these studies into question. The first study, the EVA-3S (Endarterectomy versus Angioplasty in Patients with Symptomatic Severe Carotid Stenosis) trial is a multicenter, randomized, noninferiority trial performed in 30 French institutions. In this study, 527 patients with symptomatic stenosis greater than 60% were enrolled. The study was stopped prematurely for reasons of safety and futility. The primary endpoints of any stroke or death at

30 days occurred in 9.6% after CAS and 3.9% after CEA. The 30-day incidence of severe disabling stroke or death was 3.4% after CAS and 1.5% after CEA. At 6 months the incidence of stroke or death was 11.7% for CAS and 6.1% for CEA. In light of these findings, the authors concluded that in patients with symptomatic carotid stenosis of 60% or greater, the rates of death and stroke at 1 and 6 months are lower with CEA than CAS (27). In the critique of this study, several procedural issues were identified with carotid stent technique which may have contributed to the lack of efficacy: lesions were not routinely predilated before stent implantation; distal embolic protection was seldom used; there was a high rate of stenting after prior CEA; and there was an unusually high rate of stent failure (13 patients, 5%) when compared with the experience in other, comparable clinical trials. Perhaps the most important factor identified was the exceptional inexperience of CAS operators enrolling in the trial, which allowed individuals with very little experience to stent randomized subjects. The low level of experience in the CAS arm was contrasted with a very high level in the surgeons performing CEA.

The SPACE trial (Stent-Supported Percutaneous Angioplasty of the Carotid Artery versus Endarterectomy) was designed to demonstrate equivalence or superiority of either CEA or CAS in symptomatic patients with carotid artery stenosis. In this study, 1,200 patients with symptomatic carotid-artery stenosis were randomly assigned within 180 days of transient ischemic attack or moderate stroke (modified Rankin scale score of ≤3) to undergo either carotid-artery stenting ($n=605$) or CEA ($n=595$). The primary endpoint was 30-day ipsilateral ischemic stroke or death. The noninferiority margin was defined as less than 2.5% on the basis of an expected event rate of 5%. Analyses were on an intention-to-treat basis. A total of 1,183 patients were included in the analysis. The rate of death or ipsilateral ischemic stroke from randomization to 30 days after the procedure was 6.84% with carotid-artery stenting and 6.34% with CEA (absolute difference 0.51, 90% CI −1.89–2.91%). The one-sided p value for noninferiority was 0.09 (28).

The SPACE trial therefore failed to prove noninferiority of carotid-artery stenting compared with CEA for the periprocedural complication rate. The authors concluded based on the short-term results of the trial that the use of CAS for the widespread treatment of carotid artery stenosis is not justified. After 2 years of follow-up, the rate of recurrent ipsilateral ischemic strokes reported was similar in both treatment groups. The incidence of recurrent carotid stenosis at 2 years, as defined by ultrasound, was significantly higher after CAS than CEA (28, 29). It cannot be excluded, however, that the degree of in-stent stenosis is slightly overestimated by conventional ultrasound criteria. In critique of this study: the study was stopped due to a lack of funding; the noninferiority endpoint was not reached due to decreased enrollment; and 73% of procedures did not utilize EPDs; yet the endpoints for CAS vs. CEA were still statistically close. Had the trial gone to completion, the endpoint of noninferiority may well have been met, but the trial as it stands is inconclusive. Interestingly, patients under the age of 68 had a statistically better outcome after CAS than after CEA, raising the possibility that one may be able to define subsets who do better with CAS, and others who do better with CEA.

In addition to EVA-3S and SPACE, the interim results of the International Carotid Stenting (ICSS) trial have recently been published, evaluating outcomes in standard-risk surgical patients with symptomatic carotid stenosis. In the randomized multicenter trial, 1,713 patients were randomized 1:1 to CAS or CEA. At the interim (120-day) analysis point, the composite endpoint of CVA/death/MI was reached in 8.5% of patients treated with CAS and 5.2% of patients who underwent CEA (HR 1.69, $P=0.006$). Although embolic protection was used more frequently in ICSS (72% of the 828 patients randomized to CAS) than in EVA-3S or SPACE, more than a quarter of patients were "unprotected," other methodological concerns persist as well. To participate in the study, investigators need only have performed 50 stenting procedures total, with ten being in the carotid artery. As a result, inexperience amongst the interventionalists – particularly relative to that of the surgeons performing CEA – may have biased the stent outcomes negatively. In two of the centers participating in the trial, 5 out of the 11 enrolled patients suffered disabling stroke or death after CAS (30).

In a meta-analysis of EVA-3S, SPACE, and ICSS, the outcomes of 3,433 patients with symptomatic carotid stenosis treated with CAS or CEA were analyzed on an intention-to-treat basis. Overall, the 120-day outcome of stroke/death was 8.9% in patients treated with CAS and 5.8% in those who underwent CEA (RR 1.53, $P=0.0006$). When the analysis was stratified based on patient age, a break-point at the age of 70 was identified. In patients under 70, the stroke/death rate for CAS was 5.8% and CEA was 5.7% (RR 1.00); but, for patients over 70, the rate of stroke/death following CAS was 12.0%, and for CEA was 5.9% (RR 2.04, $P=0.0053$) (31). Critics have pointed to the multiple methodological flaws in these trials, including lack of embolic protection, incomplete enrollment, and performance of CAS by operators with minimal prior experience. In addition, while patients were excluded from enrollment on the basis of nonqualification for CEA, little was known about reasons to exclude patients for nonsuitability for CAS.

The Carotid Revascularization Endarterectomy versus Stenting Trial (CREST) was recently published, and represents the largest multicenter randomized study of CAS vs. CEA to date. The study enrolled 2,502 patients, with both symptomatic (53%) and asymptomatic (47%) carotid stenosis, with a median follow-up of 2.5 years. This landmark trial was performed with careful adjudication of outcomes. Efforts were made to ensure at least a basic level of skill for the operators performing CAS and CEA. The trial showed equivalency between CAS and CEA in this population of conventional-risk patients. Specifically, the primary endpoint of periprocedural stroke/death/MI or ipsilateral stroke within 4 years after randomization was not significantly different between CAS (7.2%) and CEA (6.8%; HR 1.11, $P=0.51$). The rates of periprocedural ipsilateral CVA were higher in CAS (4.1%) than in CEA (2.3%; HR 1.79, $P=0.01$), although this was fueled by minor rather than major events. There was no difference in major stroke between the two cohorts. Conversely, periprocedural myocardial infarction occurred less commonly in CAS (1.1%) than in CEA (2.3%; HR 0.50, $P=0.03$). Cranial nerve palsy developed in 0.3% of those with CAS and in 4.7% of those who underwent CEA (32).

Of interest, subgroup analysis in the CREST trial identified a significant correlation between patient age and treatment efficacy. As was identified in the meta-analysis of EVA-3S, SPACE, and ICSS, the CREST study demonstrated more favorable outcomes in CAS – relative to CEA – for patients under 70 than for those older than 70 (31, 32). Conversely, patients over the age of 80 had more favorable outcomes with CEA. One must be cautious not to overinterpret these results, as 90% of the randomized patients were between the ages of 69 and 80. The difference in outcomes in patients above 80 was therefore "driven" by an extremely small number of events in a very small subset of patients.

Additionally, significant debate has evolved regarding the evaluation of periprocedural MI in recent studies of CAS vs. CEA. EVA-3S, SPACE, and ICSS examined patients for MI only when clinical signs or symptoms were evident to the investigator. SAPPHIRE and CREST mandated the measurement of CK and CK-MB postrevascularization. The criteria for MI in CREST were more stringent and required the presence of a clinical event or EKG changes accompanying the enzyme rise; events were adjudicated by a committee dedicated to evaluating for MI. The composite primary endpoints of SAPPHIRE and CREST include periprocedural MI, and are significantly driven by the proportionally higher measure this clinical event following CEA than CAS. Some trialists debate that a potentially clinically silent event, such as CK-MB elevation, has less impact on quality of life than does periprocedural stroke. A body of clinical literature, however, supports the concept that CK-MB elevation – even when not accompanied by clinically appreciable stigmata of coronary ischemia or infarction – may have significant implications on morbidity and mortality following vascular surgery *(33, 34)*. Preliminary analysis from the CREST trial, examining intermediate term mortality, would seem to support the negative implications of periprocedural MI.

While the initial response to publication of the European trials called the benefit of CAS into question, subsequent exposure of the major methodological concerns surrounding these trials have helped us understand both the risk and benefit of endovascular therapy. Studies such as the CREATE trial aided in this discussion. In this prospective, nonrandomized, multicenter registry, 419 patients who were felt to be at high risk for CEA were enrolled for CAS, using the Protégé self-expanding nitinol stent and the SPIDER embolic protection system. Technical success was achieved in 408 of 419 patients (97.4%). The primary endpoint of MACCE at 30 days after the index procedure was observed in 26 patients (6.2%), including death in 8 (1.9%), nonfatal stroke in 14 (3.3%) and nonfatal myocardial infarction in 4 (1%). The authors concluded that, in some patients with severe carotid artery stenosis and high-risk features, CAS is a reasonable alternative to CEA for revascularization *(35)*.

Additional, more contemporary premarket single arm studies enrolling high-surgical-risk patients, aimed at obtaining FDA approval for newer EPDs and stents, have demonstrated further reduction in events after CAS. For example, the PROTECT trial, utilizing the EmboPro device (Abbott Vascular Devices, Menlo Park, CA) had combined 30-day stroke, death and MI rate of 1.8%; the EPIC trial, utilizing a novel EPD comprised of a bundle of fibers, demonstrated a 30-day MAE rate of 3.0%. One of the more important advances has been the development of so-called "proximal protection devices," wherein antegrade flow to the distal carotid is either arrested or reversed during the procedure, then restored after placement of the stent and removal of the (potentially debris-laden) stagnant column of blood. The Empire Trial, utilizing flow reversal, and the ARMOUR Trial, with transient flow arrest, had 30-day MAE rates of 2.9 and 2.7%, respectively *(36)*. Importantly, using these flow arrest devices, the MAE rates in symptomatic patients were even lower than in asymptomatic individuals, suggesting (contrary to the belief promulgated by EVA-3S) that symptomatic patients can be treated effectively with CAS, when utilizing proper technique and equipment, and with skilled/experienced operators.

Further evidence supporting improved results with CAS over time comes from the postmarket surveillance (PMS) trials that have been mandated by FDA and CMS. Gray et al. published results from the Xact and CAPTURE PMS trials: amongst a cohort of 4,282 asymptomatic and 589 symptomatic nonoctogenarian patients, MAE was less than 3% and 6%, respectively *(37)*. This is the first demonstration of achieving – in high-surgical-risk patients – target MAE rates that were established by the AHA for conventional-risk patients.

In addition to CREST, the ACT-1 clinical trial will help to solidify our understanding of the role for carotid stenting in standard-surgical-risk patients. ACT-1 is a prospective, randomized, multicenter trial designed to demonstrate noninferiority of CAS vs. CEA in asymptomatic, normal-risk patients. Approximately 1,658 patients will be enrolled, with a 3:1 ratio of CAS to CEA. The primary endpoint is combined 30-day rate of stroke, MI, or death, plus ipsilateral stroke 31–365 days postprocedure.

INDICATIONS FOR CAS

Compared with CEA, CAS poses theoretic advantage in light of its minimally invasive nature. The SAPPHIRE trial showed a clinical advantage for carotid stenting in surgical high-risk patients (Table 2) with a symptomatic stenosis greater than 50% or an asymptomatic stenosis greater than 80% *(24)*. The results of the ongoing randomized trials will define the future role of CAS in standard-risk patients. It is also important to note that certain patients may be poor candidates for CAS; these contraindications are listed in Table 4.

The potential benefit of carotid stenting is less well established in older patients (>80 years), particularly in the context of asymptomatic stenosis. Additionally, small studies have suggested an increased risk of embolic events associated with endovascular carotid therapy in the elderly. Some octogenarian patients may indeed benefit from CAS (as has been the case in SAPPHIRE, other PMA trials, and the PMS trials). In one recently published

Table 4
Contraindications or Relative Contraindications to CAS *(3)*

Neurological
Major functional impairment
Significant cognitive impairment (poor cerebral "reserve")
Major stroke within 4 weeks
Anatomical
Inability to achieve safe vascular access
Severe tortuosity or friability of aortic arch
Severe tortuosity of CCA or ICA
Intracranial aneurysm or AVM requiring treatment
Heavy concentric lesion calcification
Visible thrombus in lesion
Total occlusion
Long subtotal (recanalized) occlusion (string sign)
Clinical
Short life expectancy (<5 years for asymptomatic patients)
Contraindication to aspirin and/or thienopyridines
Renal dysfunction precluding safe contrast medium administration

(Reprinted with permission of the American College of Cardiology.)

retrospective case series, CAS outcomes in 418 consecutive octogenarian patients from four high-volume centers demonstrated a 30-day stroke or death rate of 2.8% *(38)*. Accordingly, it has been postulated that the poorer outcomes of CAS in patients over 80 is less of a "class effect" than it is a case of poor case selection. All patients – regardless of age – must be carefully assessed as to their suitability for CAS before undertaking it. Much as surgeons over time have identified the characteristics that render a patient high risk for CEA, CAS operators are now increasingly aware of what constitutes "high risk for stenting," and are avoiding those patients. These characteristics may be more frequent in the very elderly, but many octogenarians remain reasonable CAS candidates.

CAS: TECHNICAL ASPECTS

The technical approach to carotid intervention must always take into account each patient's unique anatomic, clinical, and comorbid features. From the moment of obtaining arterial access, sensitivity to vessel disease state – particularly with respect to the status of the aortic arch – should be considered when advancing catheters to the carotid origin. The geometric relationship of the common carotid origin to the adjacent segment of the aorta has tremendous bearing on the ability to access the vessel with an interventional guiding sheath or catheter.

Types of aortic arches (per the definitions developed by Subby Myla, M.D. and described in Uflacker et al.) *(39)*.

Types of Aortic Arches

TYPE I ARCH (FIG. 1)

The arch vessels arise in a relatively horizontal plane from the top of aortic arch; specifically, the innominate artery's origin arises just beneath the tangent to the top of the aortic arch, at a distance that is less than the diameter of the innominate artery (Fig. 1).

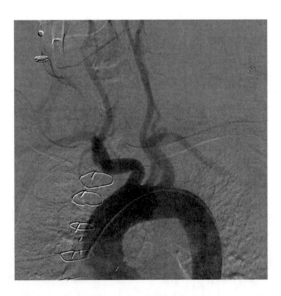

Fig. 1. Type I Arch.

Type II Arch (Fig. 2)

The arch vessels arise between the parallel planes delineated by the outer and inner curves of the arch (moderate angulation). The innominate artery arises beneath the tangent to the top of the aortic arch at a distance that is twice the diameter of the innominate artery (Fig. 2).

Type III Arch (Fig. 3)

The arch vessels arise proximal or caudal to the lesser curvature of the arch or off the ascending aorta (severe angulation). The vertical distance from the origin of the innominate artery to the top of the arch is three times the diameter of the innominate artery (see below).

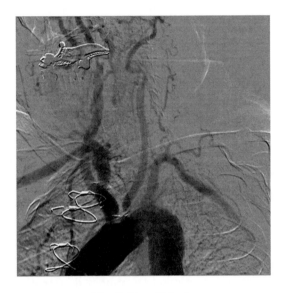

Fig. 2. Type II Arch.

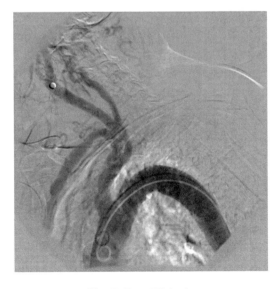

Fig. 3. Type III Arch.

In most cases, retrograde femoral arterial access provides a stable, straightforward platform from which to access either carotid artery. In some circumstances, particularly with severe angulation of the origin of the right common carotid artery from the ascending aorta (Type III aortic arch, described above), or in cases where the left common carotid artery originates from the innominate artery ("bovine arch" configuration), right brachial or radial access may be considered.

When possible, a straight 6-French sheath (90 cm, with lubricious coating) should be considered, since this platform optimizes usable internal diameter, while maintaining relatively small external diameter, and consequent arteriotomy. It also provides excellent support for stent advancement and enables one to minimize manipulation once in the common carotid artery. In cases with more significant angulation of common carotid origin or proximal vessel, a coronary guiding catheter (typically 8 F) placed at the Common Carotid origin may also be considered. In either case, it is often advantageous to engage the common carotid artery first with a 5-French diagnostic catheter, advance a relatively atraumatic wire into the common or external carotid artery, transitioning as needed for a more supportive wire, then advancing the interventional sheath or guide over the diagnostic catheter (or appropriate sheath dilator) to engage the common carotid artery securely. When using an interventional sheath or multipurpose guiding catheter, the tip is usually positioned in the distal CCA but using a more aggressive guiding catheter shape, the tip of the guide is usually positioned in the proximal (intrathoracic) segment of the CCA. Careful attention to the placement of the tip of guiding catheter or interventional sheath will help prevent spasm, thrombosis, or dissection of the common carotid artery.

Throughout the procedure, meticulous attention should be paid to catheter flushing and backbleeding (particularly after advancement of bulky stent-delivery platforms) so as to eliminate the possibility of injecting any air that may become entrained in the system, and to minimize the risk of air embolization. Additionally, the activated clotting (ACT) time should be maintained at 250–300 s to minimize the chance of developing catheter or wire-associated thrombus. Unfractionated heparin and the direct thrombin inhibitor bivalirudin are presently most commonly used for this purpose.

Prior to embarking on the interventional procedure, formal intracerebral angiography should be performed. At least a two-vessel angiogram involving both carotid arteries and their intracranial territories should be examined carefully. In some cases, four-vessel investigation involving both vertebral arteries may provide additional anatomic and clinically relevant data upon which to base the procedural approach. Following the intervention, intracranial angiograms should also be performed, and compared carefully with the baseline assessment to assure that embolization, intracranial hemorrhage, or other vascular disruption have not occurred.

Once the interventional sheath or guide is positioned, the ensuing steps include: wire access (typically with embolic protection device), balloon angioplasty predilatation, stent deployment, and stent postdilatation. In cases of severe stenosis, complex eccentric plaque, or critical angulation in the diseased carotid segment, the use of a 0.014" "buddy wire" may facilitate advancement and deployment of the EPD. In rare cases, gentle and undersized (2.0 mm) predilatation of the lesion may be required in order to permit passage of the EPD; understandably, predilatation in the absence of a deployed EPD may engender increased risk of ipsilateral stroke, and should be avoided when possible.

Once the EPD is deployed, balloon angioplasty serves to predilate the carotid stenosis and permit easier passage and positioning of the stent. Additionally, predilatation may be used to gauge whether a lesion is highly recalcitrant in nature. Lesions that are circumferentially calcified or that demonstrate highly recalcitrant (i.e., "nondilatable") nature during predilatation should not be treated with stenting, since profoundly constrained or underexpanded stent segments may be prone to thrombosis or restenosis. In general principle, balloon dilatation should consider:

1. The target lesion should be subjected to as little mechanical injury as possible, to minimize the risk of plaque embolization,
2. Undersized angioplasty balloons (3–4 mm in diameter and 15–40 mm in length; a balloon:ICA ratio of 0.5–0.6) are selected for predilatation of the vessel to allow passage of the stent delivery system,
3. Undersized postdilatation angioplasty balloons are then selected to expand the stent.

Stent Choice

Balloon expandable stents are generally used for intrathoracic lesions at the origin of the CCA. However, over 90% of stenoses involve the cervical portion of the distal CCA or proximal ICA; and self-expanding stents are preferable to balloon-expandable stents because of superior conformability and resistance to stent deformation during neck movement or extrinsic compression. Nitinol self-expanding stents are preferred by most operators over stainless steel stents because of better conformability, less stent foreshortening during expansion, and more predictable positioning during deployment. Many nitinol stents are available in tapered designs to conform to the tapered transition from the larger CCA (8–10 mm in diameter) to the smaller ICA (5–7 mm in diameter), although there are no data to suggest that tapered stents result in better outcomes compared with nontapered designs. Stent lengths (most commonly 30–40 mm) are usually chosen to achieve complete lesion coverage (proximal and distal margins of the stent land in nondiseased segments) from the distal CCA to the proximal ICA (see Fig. 4).

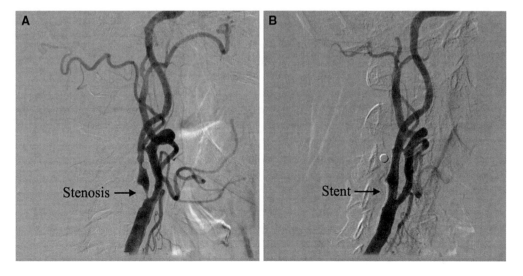

Fig. 4. Carotid stenosis before (**A**) and after (**B**) stenting.

Complications

Manipulation and stimulation of the carotid baroreceptors may be provoked during balloon angioplasty and stent deployment, and may lead to hypotension and/or bradycardia. Treatment may involve a combination of fluid resuscitation, atropine, and alpha-adrenergic agents. Temporary transvenous RV pacing is rarely needed, but should be made readily available. Postprocedure hypertension (systolic >180 mmHg) must be avoided to minimize the risk of "hyperperfusion syndrome" and cerebral hemorrhage which carries a very high mortality rate, particularly in elderly patients with previous near-occlusion of the carotid artery and under-perfused cerebral hemisphere.

Neuroprotection

The risk of embolic stroke has been a major limitation of early endovascular therapy. The majority of neurological complications are due to intracerebral embolism from plaque fragments or thrombus during the endovascular procedure. At some level, embolic risk exists irrespective of patient-, lesion-, or technique-specific factors. The focus of current treatment strategies has shifted from neurological rescue (with intra-arterial fibrinolytic agents and/or catheter-directed techniques) to neurological protection using embolic protection devices (EPD) to capture and remove embolic debris that were generated during the procedure.

In broad terms, there are two types of EPDs: proximal EPDs and distal EPDs. Proximal EPDs rely on transient occlusion of the CCA proximal to the stenosis and the ECA, resulting in stagnant or reversed flow in the ICA. Proximal EPDs have the theoretical advantage of providing embolic protection before the lesion is crossed with a guidewire. After intervention is completed, aspiration of blood from the carotid bifurcation removes any debris, followed by removal of the proximal EPD. Proximal EPDs must maintain a tight seal and static column of blood. Even transient restoration of flow during the interventional procedure may allow cerebral embolization.

Distal EPDs require first crossing the lesion with a guidewire, followed by deployment of the EPD distal to the target lesion. There are many designs of distal EPDs in the form of either a filter or occlusive balloon. After intervention is completed, the filter is captured and removed along with embolic debris in the filter. Large-scale studies of proximal EPDs and comparative studies of various distal EPDs have not been performed. Although all distal EPDs appear to be able to capture and remove embolic debris, no device has been shown to completely prevent distal embolization.

Although there are no randomized studies comparing CAS with and without EPDs, the majority of published series have shown a large reduction (at least 60%) in neurological complications rate with these devices and few or no major strokes in most of these studies *(40)*. The use of EPDs should be routine and mandatory when technically feasible in all cases of CAS.

VERTEBRAL ARTERY STENOSIS

The clinical importance and standards for management of vertebral artery stenosis are less well-characterized than those for carotid stenosis. In large part, vertebrobasilar insufficiency (VBI) is underappreciated, because the symptoms may be quite nonspecific. Typical symptoms of VBI include dizziness, ataxia, diplopia, hemiparesis, and bilateral lower extremity weakness and numbness *(41–43)*. Primarily afflicting the elderly, these symptoms of VBI may have a broad differential diagnosis. While duplex ultrasonography may be readily available and inexpensive, the sensitivity to diagnose vertebral artery stenosis is unreliable. MRA, CTA, and invasive angiography have higher yield and accuracy, and should be considered when vertebral stenosis is suspected.

The primary etiology of clinical events in the posterior circulation is embolization, accounting for 40% of clinical events. Emboli may arise from the heart (typically thrombotic in nature), from the aorta (typically atheromatous), or from proximal portions of the vertebral arteries themselves (athero/thrombotic). Posterior circulation hypoperfusion – due to a combination of large vessel stenosis and transient dips in perfusion pressure – is the second most common cause of posterior circulation events, accounting for 32% of VBI. Atherosclerosis is the most common etiology of vertebral artery stenosis, and primarily involves the vessel origin. Other, less common causes of vertebral artery stenosis include: arterial dissection, fibromuscular dysplasia, migraine, and vasculitides *(41, 43)*.

ANATOMY OF THE VERTEBRAL ARTERY

Although anatomic variants do exist, the vertebral artery most commonly originates from the proximal portion of the subclavian artery. Of the anatomic variants, the most common (in 5% of patients) involves a separate origin for the left vertebral artery from the aorta, between the left common carotid and left subclavian arteries' origins.

The vertebral artery's course may be divided into four regions (see Fig. 5):

V1 – The section of the artery which extends from its origin (typically off of the subclavian artery) to the point where it enters the transverse foramina of the vertebra, usually at C5 or C6.
V2 – The section in which the vertebral artery travels through the intervertebral foramina, to the point where it emerges behind the atlas (C2).
V3 – The section where the vertebral artery passes extracranially from C2 into the base of the skull via the foramen magnum.
V4 – The intracranial portion of the vessel, where it penetrates into the dura and arachnoid mater of the brain at the skull base, and merges with the contralateral vertebral artery to form the basilar artery.

The left vertebral artery is more often the larger of the two; and in such cases is considered the "dominant" vessel. In cases of unilateral vertebral stenosis, it is more common to identify symptoms when the dominant vessel is involved *(44)*.

THERAPY FOR VERTEBRAL ARTERY STENOSIS

There remains considerable debate regarding the management of stenosis of the extracranial vertebral artery (ECVA). Historically, surgical treatment of vertebral stenosis has resulted in dismal outcomes, with morbidity and mortality of 20% *(45, 46)*. Surgical strategies include: transection of the vertebral artery distal to the stenosis with re-implantation of the vessel to the ipsilateral carotid or subclavian artery; vertebral endarterectomy; and vein patch angioplasty. In the context of poor surgical outcomes,

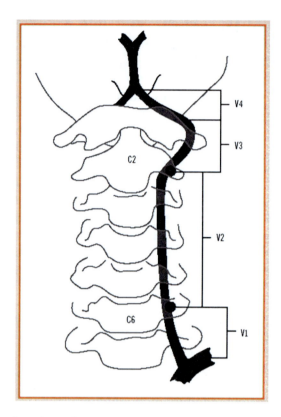

Fig. 5. The four anatomic regions of the vertebral artery *(44)* (Reprinted with permission of Oxford University Press).

therapy of vertebral stenosis has historically been relegated to medical management. When symptoms of vertebrobasilar insufficiency persist despite medical management, however, the risk of CVA or death at 1 year is 5–11%. Additionally, if vertebral stenosis contributes to TIA, the likelihood of a CVA at 5 years is 30% *(47, 48)*.

Endovascular strategies may offer a unique, effective, and minimally invasive approach to the treatment of patients with symptomatic ECVA atherosclerotic disease. The first angioplasty for vertebrobasilar stenosis was performed by Sundt in 1980 *(49)*. Since then, several medical centers have developed decades of experience, and a high degree of proficiency in the endovascular treatment of ECVA stenosis; but the data justifying this therapeutic approach are limited, consisting primarily of small single-center registries (Table 5).

In a recently published single-center registry, Jenkins et al. describe the experience at Ochsner clinic in treating 105 consecutive patients with symptomatic vertebral artery stenosis between 1995 and 2006. They achieved technical success in endovascular treatment of the stenoses in 100% of the patients, with only one stroke in the vertebrobasilar system less than 30 days after the intervention, and no in-hospital stroke/death. Additionally, there was one patient death <30 days postprocedure, due to MI. At a median follow-up of 29.1 months, 71.4% of the patients were alive. Target vessel revascularization was required in 13.1% of patients at the median follow-up time of 29.1 months. No embolic protection devices were used in the study *(48)*.

Table 5
Registries of Vertebral Artery Stenting

Author	N	Technical success	Procedural complications	Improvement in symptoms	Mean follow-up (m)	Late stroke	Restenosis
Mukherjee et al. (50)	12	100%	None	12/12	6.4	0	1/12
Malek et al. (51)	13	100%	1 TIA	11/13	20.7	0	N/A
Jenkins et al. (52)	32	100%	1 TIA	31/32	10.6	0	1/32
Chastain et al. (53)	50	98%	None	48/50	25	1	5/50

With permission from Mukherjee and Rosenfield (43).

Endovascular revascularization of ECVA stenosis is generally reserved for patients who are symptomatic, and who have not responded to or are intolerant of medical therapy. Endovascular treatment of asymptomatic individuals remains hotly debated. In evaluating asymptomatic patients with high-grade vertebral stenosis, a comprehensive assessment by both a neurologist and an interventionalist should be obtained, and a decision by committee should be made. Factors which should be considered are (1) severity of stenosis; (2) morphologic considerations of the stenosis noted at angiography (ulceration, thrombus, friability, or other predictors of high risk for embolic events); (3) adequacy of collateral flow; and (4) patient age and comorbidity (43).

ENDOVASCULAR TECHNIQUE FOR VERTEBRAL INTERVENTION

As with all endovascular procedures, arterial access for vertebral intervention represents a critical element of the technique. Most commonly, arterial access is obtained retrograde in the common femoral artery. In patients with severe bilateral aortoiliac disease, an ipsilateral brachial or radial artery approach may be an effective alternative. A brachial or radial approach may also be advantageous in patients with severe stenosis or tortuosity of the proximal subclavian arteries or a Type III aortic arch. If arterial access is obtained via the arm, care must be taken to administer 3000–5000 U of unfractionated heparin after sheath insertion to minimize the risk of thrombosis. If radial access is used, intra-arterial nitroglycerin and/or verapamil should also be administered via the sheath to minimize vessel spasm.

Diagnostic aortic arch angiography should be performed before selective cannulation of the vertebral arteries is undertaken. Using 30–45 degrees of LAO projection, aortography permits delineation of the aortic arch configuration, including the sites of origin of the arch vessels. Typical arch anatomy with separate ostia of the brachiocephalic, left common carotid and left subclavian arteries is noted in >70% of patients. A shared origin of the brachiocephalic trunk and left common carotid artery is seen in 15% of cases, while a bovine arch (left common carotid artery arising from the brachiocephalic trunk) is noted in 8–10% of cases. With increasing patient age, chronic hypertension, and atherosclerotic vascular degeneration, the ascending portion of the arch tends to sag deeper into the thoracic cavity, drawing the great vessels with it, distorting the angle and origins of the great vessels. Given the potential variability in arch configuration – and the marked impact that anomalous configurations have on procedural technique – arch aortography represents an important step in planning one's interventional approach in each patient *(43)*.

Selective angiography should be performed with catheter shapes that minimize the need for manipulation in the arch and great vessels, in order to reduce the risk of atheroembolism. Most vertebral arteries may be selectively engaged with a Right Judkins number 4 catheter (JR4). In patients with an angulated or tortuous aortic arch, a Vitek, Headhunter, or Simmons catheter may be utilized. Since the liberation of even very small cerebral emboli to the posterior circulation may have devastating clinical impact, gentle and meticulous technique is imperative. Nonselective vertebral angiography with the catheter tip near the origin of the vertebral artery may also reduce complications. This is especially true if there is severe stenosis in the proximal portion or origin of the vessel, i.e., in the V1 segment. Inflating a blood pressure cuff on the ipsilateral arm during nonselective vertebral angiography may help to improve visualization of the vertebral artery, by reducing the ability for contrast to runoff to the ipsilateral arm.

The origins of the vertebral arteries are best visualized in the contralateral oblique projection, although minor variations in angulation may be required. The remainder of the V1 as well as the V2 and V3 segments are visualized using the postero-anterior (PA) and lateral views. Alternatively, a single ipsilateral oblique view may suffice. The intracranial posterior circulation is best visualized in a steep (approximately 40 degrees) AP cranial view (Townes view), and in a cross-table lateral projection.

Anticipating vertebral intervention, patients should be pretreated with aspirin 325 mg daily and clopidogrel 300–600 mg load followed by 75 mg daily, started at least 2 days prior to the procedure. Unfractionated heparin – weight based at 60 u/kg IV bolus – should be used to achieve a target activated clotting time (ACT) greater than 250 s. Bivalirudin may be used in patients who have a history of heparin-induced thorombocytopenia (HIT), or at the discretion of the operator. The use of glycoprotein IIb/IIIa inhibitors during vertebral artery intervention is not well defined and therefore is not recommended.

The procedure may be performed using either a long sheath or a guiding catheter. If brachial or radial access is selected, a 6-French sheath (35 or 55 cm long) may be preferred over a guide, since sheath use maximizes the outer to inner diameter ratio, minimizing the arteriotomy size in the arm vessel, while maximizing the allowable lumen caliber for delivery of peripheral balloons and stents. A long (80 cm) 6-French sheath may be used with retrograde femoral arterial access. If a guiding catheter is selected, either an 8-French – or possibly a 7-French – system should be utilized to provide adequate support and a large enough lumen for stent passage.

The telescoping technique, described previously for carotid intervention, may also be employed effectively for vertebral intervention. With this technique, a long 125 cm diagnostic catheter (e.g., JR4) is telescoped through the guide and is used to engage the ostium of the subclavian/innominate artery. A wire (Wholey or stiff-angled glidewire) is then advanced into the axillary artery, and the diagnostic catheter is advanced into the distal portion of the subclavian artery. The guide is then advanced over the wire/catheter system into the proximal subclavian artery, near the origin of the vertebral artery. The guide is then advanced to the origin of the vertebral artery without intubating it. The same technique may also be used to manipulate a long sheath into proximity of the vertebral artery origin for subsequent intervention.

A 0.014" exchange length wire is then placed across the lesion in the vertebral artery. Hydrophilic wires should be avoided if possible, but are sometimes necessary to traverse extremely tortuous vascular segments. If a hydrophilic wire is used to cross a lesion, it should subsequently be exchanged over a balloon catheter to a nonhydrophilic wire to minimize the chance of distal wire migration. In tortuous vessels there is a high propensity for the development of wire bias (pleating of the vessel, or pseudostenosis) which may not only compromise flow, but may encourage consideration of balloon dilatation at a site without a clinically relevant flow-limiting stenosis.

The typical diameter of the proximal vertebral artery is 3–6 mm. Predilatation with a balloon allows for the passage of subsequent equipment and also permits estimation of the vessel diameter and length of the lesion. In order to minimize the chance of causing arterial dissection, a balloon that is two-thirds of the vessel diameter should be selected for the initial dilatation of the vertebral stenosis. A stent is then placed, sized to match the lumen diameter of the portion of vessel treated (typically 3.5–6 mm). The type of stent selected for vertebral intervention has been a matter of debate; if the lesion does not lie in a tortuous segment of the vessel, a balloon-expandable peripheral stent – inherently more rigid and with greater radial strength – may be preferred. Conversely, in lesions which lie in tortuous segments of a vessel, or where extrinsic compressive forces may be an issue, the superior conformability of a self-expanding stent may be preferred. At the conclusion of stent deployment, an angiogram should be performed in multiple projections to assure that the lesion is adequately dilated and covered, particularly in cases involving the very origin of the vertebral artery. It is often necessary to allow 1–2 mm of the stent protruding proximally from the lesion into the subclavian artery, in order to assure that the vessel's origin is entirely covered and is adequately buttressed by the stent. The degree of stent protrusion may often appear somewhat asymmetric due to the angle between the vertebral takeoff and the subclavian artery.

Lesions that do not involve the origin of the vertebral artery occur less frequently, but are usually more straightforward to treat from a technical standpoint. In such cases, the type of stent selected may be critical; in general, balloon-expandable stents should be selected for lesions in the extracranial (V1 and) V2 segments, and self-expanding stents for lesions in the V3 segments (*see* Fig. 6).

Distal embolic protection devices are not commonly used in vertebral artery intervention. It is often technically difficult to advance embolic protection devices into the vertebral artery, since severe disease may often be present at the very origin of the vessel, since the proximal segment of the vessel may be highly angulated, and since passage of the device – given these technical constraints – may engender more risk than potential benefit. Moreover, successful use of embolic protection may be contingent upon finding a suitable "landing zone" in the V2 segment for device deployment; and, contralateral vertebral artery patency may be required for certain embolic protection devices which may temporarily interrupt antegrade flow in the vessel when deployed.

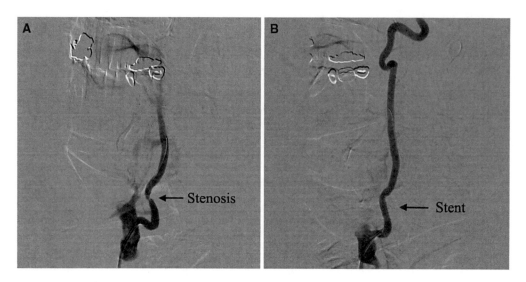

Fig. 6. Right vertebral artery proximal stenosis before (**A**) and after (**B**) stenting.

Given these technical considerations, most operators reserve the use of embolic protection devices for vertebral intervention where lesion morphology carries high-risk features for embolization: bulky plaque, complex or "hazy" appearance, friable substrate.

Major complications, occurring in 1% of vertebral intervention, include transient ischemic attack or stroke from atheromatous embolization to the posterior circulation.

Vertebral dissection and vasospasm have also been reported. Other complications include those related to vascular access: hematoma, pseudoaneurysm, and arteriovenous fistula *(43)*.

Following vertebral intervention, patients should be observed in the hospital overnight, permitting frequent neurologic evaluations. Blood pressure should be meticulously controlled to prevent hypertension, which may precipitate reperfusion hemorrhage, or hypotension, which may cause cerebral hypoperfusion. Optimal blood pressure parameters are 110–130 mmHg/70–85 mmHg. Patients should receive daily aspirin indefinitely, and clopidogrel 75 mg daily for 1–12 months. Long-term follow-up should include serial clinical assessments screening for recurrent VBI symptoms, noninvasive imaging as clinically warranted, and global focus on secondary risk factor modification.

CONCLUSIONS AND FUTURE DIRECTIONS

Ever since the relationship was identified between cerebrovascular atherosclerosis and stroke, there has been a need to identify the optimal strategy for patient management. Over the past several decades, the terrain involved in this assessment has changed dramatically, as medical therapy has improved, surgical and anesthetic technique has advanced, and minimally invasive options, such as endovascular therapy, have entered the domain.

The landscape remains a hotly contested one. The management of patients with cerebrovascular disease now exists in a delta which includes physicians from diverse backgrounds, including internal medicine, vascular surgery, vascular medicine, cardiology, neurology, interventional radiology, neurosurgery, and neurointerventional radiology, to name a few. Additionally, the patients who manifest cerebrovascular disease whether symptomatic or asymptomatic often have risk for vascular events and the attendant comorbidity, in other vascular territories. As a result, it is difficult to establish consensus about which physician should treat which patient with which strategy, in a manner that takes all of these variables into account. Moreover, the decision as to who is best qualified to make such a determination remains a very politically charged issue.

The treatment modalities for carotid disease themselves are in a state of evolution. While insight from large-scale, randomized, prospective, multicenter clinical trials informs some of our day-to-day clinical decisions, those trials have certain limitations and do not necessarily apply to all patients. Furthermore, as the landscape changes, time and resources are required to develop the evidence base to support an altered therapeutic approach. Through continued investigation, we may understand the ways in which optimal medical therapies may reduce future cerebrovascular events in our patients; we may reflect on the long and well-established history that demonstrates the role for surgical revascularization in select patients; and, we may acknowledge that endovascular carotid therapy may represent an advantageous and less-invasive alternative to surgery – one which will be preferred in certain patients and clinical scenarios. As interventional technique continues to improve and future clinical investigation is completed, it is anticipated that the role of carotid stenting as a mainstay of therapy will continue to expand. Ultimately, amongst patients in whom revascularization is appropriate, it is likely that there will be a cohort identified in whom CEA will be clearly preferable, a cohort in whom CAS will be clearly preferable, and then a group in whom either therapy would be suitable and reasonable. For the latter group of patients, individualization of therapy based on patient and physician preference and careful assessment of relative benefits and liabilities of each modality will be essential.

While it is unlikely that we will ever identify a "one size fits all" strategy to approach patients with cerebrovascular disease, we may hope that – through continued multidisciplinary investigation – we may establish a collaborative mechanism by which each patient may be evaluated, and may receive the most advanced and appropriately tailored strategy to suit their specific clinical profile.

REFERENCES

1. Lloyd-Jones D, Adams RJ, Brown TM, et al. Heart disease and stroke statistics--2010 update: a report from the American Heart Association. *Circulation*. 2010;121(7):e46–e215.
2. Lloyd-Jones D, Adams RJ, Carnethon M, et al. Heart Disease and Stroke Statistics—2009 Update; A Report From the American Heart Association Statistics Committee and Stroke Statistics Subcommittee. *Circulation*. 2009;119: e21–e181.
3. Bates ER, Babb JD, Casey DE Jr, et al. ACCF/SCAI/SVMB/SIR/ASITN 2007 clinical expert consensus document on carotid stenting: a report of the American College of Cardiology Foundation Task Force on Clinical Expert Consensus Documents (ACCF/SCAI/SVMB/SIR/ASITN Clinical Expert Consensus Document Committee on Carotid Stenting). *J Am Coll Cardiol*. 2007;49:126–170.
4. Goldstein LB, Adams R, Alberts MJ, et al. Primary prevention of ischemic stroke: a guideline from the American Heart Association/American Stroke Association Stroke Council: cosponsored by the Atherosclerotic Peripheral Vascular Disease Interdisciplinary Working Group; Cardiovascular Nursing Council; Clinical Cardiology Council; Nutrition, Physical Activity, and Metabolism Council; and the

Quality of Care and Outcomes Research Interdisciplinary Working Group. *Circulation*. 2006;113:e873–e923.
5. North American Symptomatic Carotid Endarterectomy Trial Collaborators. Beneficial effect of carotid endarterectomy in symptomatic patients with high-grade carotid stenosis. *N Engl J Med*. 1991;325:445–453.
6. Endarterectomy for asymptomatic carotid artery stenosis. Executive Committee for the Asymptomatic Carotid Atherosclerosis Study. *JAMA*. 1995;273:1421–1428.
7. Debakey ME, Crawford ES, Cooley DA, Morris GC Jr, Garret HE, Fields WS. Cerebral arterial insufficiency: one to 11-year results following arterial reconstructive operation. *Ann Surg*. 1965;161:921–945.
8. Thacker EL, Wiggins KL, Rice KM, et al. Short-term and long-term risk of incident ischemic stroke after transient ischemic attack. *Stroke*. 2010;41(2):239–243.
9. Rothwell PM, Eliasziw M, Gutnikov SA, et al. Analysis of pooled data from the randomised controlled trials of endarterectomy for symptomatic carotid stenosis. *Lancet*. 2003;361:107–116.
10. European Carotid Surgery Trialists' Collaborative Group. Randomised trial of endarterectomy for recently symptomatic carotid stenosis: final results of the MRC European Carotid Surgery Trial (ECST). *Lancet*. 1998;351:1379–1387.
11. Yusuf S, Sleight P, Pogue J, Bosch J, Davies R, Dagenais G. Effects of an angiotensin-converting-enzyme inhibitor, ramipril, on cardiovascular events in high-risk patients. The Heart Outcomes Prevention Evaluation Study Investigators. *N Engl J Med*. 2000;342:145–153.
12. Amarenco P, Bogousslavsky J, Callahan A 3 rd, et al. High-dose atorvastatin after stroke or transient ischemic attack. *N Engl J Med*. 2006;355:549–559.
13. Everett BM, Glynn RJ, MacFadyen JG, Ridker PM. Rosuvastatin in the prevention of stroke among men and women with elevated levels of C-reactive protein: justification for the use of statins in prevention: an intervention trial evaluating rosuvastatin (JUPITER). *Circulation*;121:143–150.
14. Sacco RL, Adams R, Albers G, et al. Guidelines for prevention of stroke in patients with ischemic stroke or transient ischemic attack: a statement for healthcare professionals from the American Heart Association/American Stroke Association Council on Stroke: co-sponsored by the Council on Cardiovascular Radiology and Intervention: the American Academy of Neurology affirms the value of this guideline. *Stroke*. 2006;37:577–617.
15. Biller J, Feinberg WM, Castaldo JE, et al. Guidelines for carotid endarterectomy: a statement for healthcare professionals from a special writing group of the Stroke Council, American Heart Association. *Stroke*. 1998;29:554–562.
16. Wennberg DE, Lucas FL, Birkmeyer JD, Bredenberg CE, Fisher ES. Variation in carotid endarterectomy mortality in the Medicare population: trial hospitals, volume, and patient characteristics. *JAMA*. 1998;279:1278–1281.
17. Rosenfield K. Carotid and Cerebrovascular Disease. In *Cath SAP 3*, ed. Moliterno DJ, section editor Mukherjee D. Washington DC: American College of Cardiology Foundation; 2008: 1012–1019.
18. Halliday A, Mansfield A, Marro J, et al. Prevention of disabling and fatal strokes by successful carotid endarterectomy in patients without recent neurological symptoms: randomised controlled trial. *Lancet*. 2004;363:1491–1502.
19. Kerber CW, Cromwell LD, Loehden OL. Catheter dilatation of proximal carotid stenosis during distal bifurcation endarterectomy. *AJNR Am J Neuroradiol*. 1980;1:348–349.
20. Garg N, Karagiorgos N, Pisimisis GT, et al. Cerebral protection devices reduce periprocedural strokes during carotid angioplasty and stenting: a systematic review of the current literature. *J Endovasc Ther*. 2009;16:412–427.
21. Chaturvedi S, Bruno A, Feasby T, et al. Carotid endarterectomy—an evidence-based review: report of the Therapeutics and Technology Assessment Subcommittee of the American Academy of Neurology. *Neurology*. 2005;65:794–801.
22. Roubin GS, New G, Iyer SS, et al. Immediate and late clinical outcomes of carotid artery stenting in patients with symptomatic and asymptomatic carotid artery stenosis: a 5-year prospective analysis. *Circulation*. 2001;103:532–537.
23. Endovascular versus surgical treatment in patients with carotid stenosis in the Carotid and Vertebral Artery Transluminal Angioplasty Study (CAVATAS): a randomised trial. *Lancet*. 2001;357: 1729–1737.

24. Yadav JS, Wholey MH, Kuntz RE, et al. Protected carotid-artery stenting versus endarterectomy in high-risk patients. *N Engl J Med.* 2004;351:1493–1501.
25. Gurm HS, Yadav JS, Fayad P, et al. Long-term results of carotid stenting versus endarterectomy in high-risk patients. *N Engl J Med.* 2008;358:1572–1579.
26. Gray WA, Hopkins LN, Yadav S, et al. Protected carotid stenting in high-surgical-risk patients: the ARCHeR results. *J Vasc Surg.* 2006;44:258–268.
27. Mas JL, Chatellier G, Beyssen B, et al. Endarterectomy versus stenting in patients with symptomatic severe carotid stenosis. *N Engl J Med.* 2006;355:1660–1671.
28. Ringleb PA, Allenberg J, Bruckmann H, et al. 30 day results from the SPACE trial of stent-protected angioplasty versus carotid endarterectomy in symptomatic patients: a randomised non-inferiority trial. *Lancet.* 2006;368:1239–1247.
29. Eckstein HH, Ringleb P, Allenberg JR, et al. Results of the Stent-Protected Angioplasty versus Carotid Endarterectomy (SPACE) study to treat symptomatic stenoses at 2 years: a multinational, prospective, randomised trial. *Lancet Neurol.* 2008;7:893–902.
30. Ederle J, Dobson J, Featherstone RL, et al. Carotid artery stenting compared with endarterectomy in patients with symptomatic carotid stenosis (International Carotid Stenting Study): an interim analysis of a randomised controlled trial. *Lancet.* 2010;375:985–997.
31. Bonati LH, Dobson J, Algra A, et al. Short-term outcome after stenting versus endarterectomy for symptomatic carotid stenosis: a preplanned meta-analysis of individual patient data. *Lancet.* 2010;376:1062–1073.
32. Brott TG, Hobson RW 2nd, Howard G, et al. Stenting versus endarterectomy for treatment of carotid-artery stenosis. *N Engl J Med.* 2010;363:11–23.
33. Landesberg G, Shatz V, Akopnik I, et al. Association of cardiac troponin, CK-MB, and postoperative myocardial ischemia with long-term survival after major vascular surgery. *J Am Coll Cardiol.* 2003;42:1547–1554.
34. Kertai MD, Boersma E, Klein J, Van Urk H, Bax JJ, Poldermans D. Long-term prognostic value of asymptomatic cardiac troponin T elevations in patients after major vascular surgery. *Eur J Vasc Endovasc Surg.* 2004;28:59–66.
35. Safian RD, Bresnahan JF, Jaff MR, et al. Protected carotid stenting in high-risk patients with severe carotid artery stenosis. *J Am Coll Cardiol.* 2006;47:2384–2389.
36. Ansel GM, Hopkins LN, Jaff MR, et al. Safety and effectiveness of the INVATEC MO.MA proximal cerebral protection device during carotid artery stenting: results from the ARMOUR pivotal trial. *Catheter Cardiovasc Interv.* 2010;76:1–8.
37. Gray WA, Chaturvedi S, Verta P. Thirty-day outcomes for carotid artery stenting in 6320 patients from 2 prospective, multicenter, high-surgical-risk registries. *Circ Cardiovasc Interv.* 2009;2:159–166.
38. Grant A, White C, Ansel G, Bacharach M, Metzger C, Velez C. Safety and efficacy of carotid stenting in the very elderly. *Catheter Cardiovasc Interv.* 2010;75:651–655.
39. Uflacker R. *Atlas of Vascular Anatomy: An Angiographic Approach.* 2nd ed. Philadelphia: Lippincott Williams & Wilkins; 2007.
40. Atkins MD, Bush RL. Embolic protection devices for carotid artery stenting: have they made a significant difference in outcomes? *Semin Vasc Surg.* 2007;20:244–251.
41. Caplan LR, Wityk RJ, Glass TA, et al. New England Medical Center Posterior Circulation Registry. *Ann Neurol.* 2004;56:389–398.
42. Savitz SI, Caplan LR. Vertebrobasilar disease. *N Engl J Med.* 2005;352:2618–2626.
43. Mukherjee D, Rosenfield K. *Manual of Peripheral Vascular Interventions.* Philadelphia: Lippincott, Williams & Wilkins; 2005.
44. Cloud GC, Markus HS. Diagnosis and management of vertebral artery stenosis. *QJM.* 2003;96:27–54.
45. Imparato AM. Vertebral arterial reconstruction: a nineteen-year experience. *J Vasc Surg.* 1985;2:626–634.
46. Thevenet A, Ruotolo C. Surgical repair of vertebral artery stenoses. *J Cardiovasc Surg.* 1984;25:101–110.
47. Sivenius J, Riekkinen PJ, Smets P, Laakso M, Lowenthal A. The European Stroke Prevention Study (ESPS): results by arterial distribution. *Ann Neurol.* 1991;29:596–600.
48. Jenkins JS, Patel SN, White CJ, et al. Endovascular stenting for vertebral artery stenosis. *J Am Coll Cardiol*;55:538–542.
49. Sundt TM Jr, Smith HC, Campbell JK, Vlietstra RE, Cucchiara RF, Stanson AW. Transluminal angioplasty for basilar artery stenosis. *Mayo Clin Proc.* 1980;55:673–680.

50. Mukherjee D, Roffi M, Kapadia SR, et al. Percutaneous intervention for symptomatic vertebral artery stenosis using coronary stents. *J Invasive Cardiol.* 2001;13:363–366.
51. Malek AM, Higashida RT, Phatouros CC, et al. Treatment of posterior circulation ischemia with extracranial percutaneous balloon angioplasty and stent placement. *Stroke.* 1999;30:2073–2085.
52. Jenkins JS, White CJ, Ramee SR, et al. Vertebral artery stenting. *Catheter Cardiovasc Interv.* 2001;54:1–5.
53. Chastain HD 2nd, Campbell MS, Iyer S, et al. Extracranial vertebral artery stent placement: in-hospital and follow-up results. *J Neurosurg.* 1999;91:547–552.

7 Intracranial Intervention

Muhammad Shazam Hussain, MD, FRCP(C), and Rishi Gupta, MD

CONTENTS

INTRODUCTION TO CEREBROVASCULAR ANATOMY
ANGIOPLASTY AND STENTING FOR INTRACRANIAL
  ATHEROSCLEROTIC DISEASE (ICAD)
INDICATIONS FOR TREATMENT OF CEREBRAL ANEURYSMS
ACUTE STROKE INTERVENTIONS
REFERENCES

The indications and practice of intracranial endovascular interventions have expanded rapidly over the last decade, particularly for the treatment of hemorrhagic and ischemic cerebrovascular disease. Better understanding of the underlying pathophysiology of these conditions in combination with the use of advanced neuroimaging techniques, has led to improved diagnosis and identification of patients at risk. Sophisticated new device technology has improved the safety and efficacy of many intracranial interventions. These developments have changed a once nihilistic approach to cerebrovascular disease into one of expanding interventions to the benefit of many patients.

INTRODUCTION TO CEREBROVASCULAR ANATOMY

A thorough understanding of cerebrovascular anatomy is critical to perform safe and effective intracranial interventions. A detailed description of cerebrovascular anatomy and its variations is beyond the scope of this chapter, but many excellent sources are available *(1)*. A brief introduction will be reviewed here.

Following the carotid bifurcation, the internal carotid artery (ICA) is divided into seven segments (Fig. 1A, B). The cervical portion (C1) extends from the carotid bifurcation to the skull base. Here the petrous portion (C2) begins, and consists of a vertical and horizontal segment until it reaches the foramen lacerum, where a short lacerum

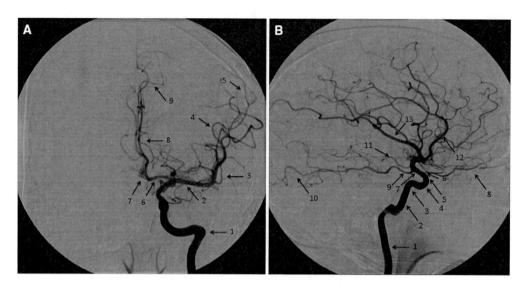

Fig. 1. (A) PA view of left internal carotid artery injection. *1* Left internal carotid artery. *2* M1 segment of the left middle cerebral artery (MCA). *3* M2 segment of the left MCA. *4* M3 segment of the left MCA. *5* M4 segment of the left MCA. *6* A1 segment of the left anterior cerebral artery (ACA). *7* Anterior communicating artery. *8* A2 segment of the left ACA. *9* A3 and A4 segments of the left ACA. **(B)** Lateral projection of left internal carotid artery injection. *1* Cervical (C1) segment of the left internal carotid artery (ICA). *2* Petrous (C2) segment of the left ICA. *3* 0 Lacerum (C3) segment of the left ICA. *4* Cavernous (C4) segment of the left ICA. *5* Clinoid (C5) segment of the left ICA. *6* Ophthalmic (C6) segment of the left ICA. *7* Communicating (C7) segment of the left ICA. *8* Left ophthalmic artery. *9* Left posterior communicating artery (PCOM). *10* Left posterior cerebral artery (filling via the left PCOM). *11* Left anterior choroidal artery. *12* Anterior cerebral artery. *13* Middle cerebral artery.

segment (C3) is present. The ICA then enters the cavernous sinus and is thus called the cavernous segment (C4) where it again has vertical and horizontal portions. The ICA then crosses the anterior clinoid process and is named the clinoid segment (C5). The ophthalmic segment (C6) and communicating segment (C7) then follow, named for the ophthalmic and posterior communicating (PCOM) artery origins which originate from these segments, respectively. The anterior choroidal artery, a major perforating artery, usually arises shortly after the PCOM artery, and supplies portions of the internal capsule and mesial temporal lobe.

The ICA then terminates into two major arteries (Fig. 1a, b). The middle cerebral artery (MCA) projects laterally and is responsible for the majority of the blood supply to the cerebral hemispheres. The MCA is also divided into segments. The M1 segment is the portion of the MCA from its origin to the Sylvian fissure. The M2 insular segments are those portions of the MCA that are within the Sylvian fissure, and the M3 opercular segments are those segments which overly the opercular areas. The MCA branches end in the M4 cortical branches. It is also useful to describe the MCA for its branches and the areas which they supply. The proximal segment (M1) gives rise to the lateral lenticulostriate arteries, which supply the deep areas of the cerebral hemisphere, including the internal capsule and basal ganglia. Shortly after this group, the anterior temporal artery arises, which supplies the anterior temporal pole. The MCA then typically bifurcates into a superior and inferior division. The superior division typically supplies the orbitofrontal and prefrontal arteries, as well as the arteries of the Rolandic area (pre-Rolandic, Rolandic, and post-Rolandic arteries). The inferior division typically supplies the posterior parietal artery, angular artery, temporo-occipital artery, and the temporal arteries.

The second terminal branch of the ICA is the anterior cerebral artery (ACA), which courses medially and supplies a significant portion of the mesial surface of the brain. The ACA is also divided into segments: the A1 segment from its origin to the anterior communicating (ACOM) artery, the A2 segment from the ACOM artery to the genu of the corpus callosum, and the distal A3 segments. From the A1 segment, the medial lenticulostriate arteries arise, the most major of which is the recurrent artery of Huebner, which supplies the anterior limb of the internal capsule, head of the caudate and portions of the anterior lentiform nucleus. The cortical branches of the ACA arise from the A2 segment and are as follows: orbitofrontal artery, frontopolar artery, pericallosal artery, and callosomarginal artery.

The vertebral arteries (Fig. 2A, B) provide the majority of the blood supply to the brainstem and cerebellum. The portion of the vertebral artery from its origin from the subclavian artery to its entrance into the vertebral transverse foramina is called the V1 segment. The V2 segment is the portion of the vertebral artery within the transverse foramina. The V3 segment extends from the exiting point at the C1 vertebral body transverse foramina until the vertebral artery pierces the dura, where it becomes the V4

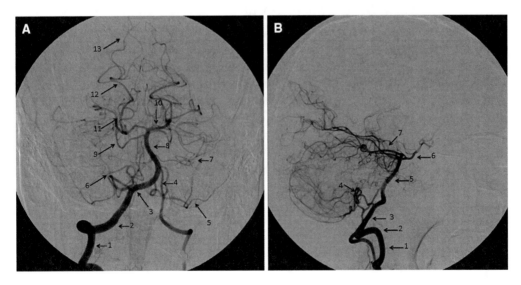

Fig. 2. (**A**) PA projection of a right vertebral artery injection. *1* V2 segment of the right vertebral artery. *2* V3 segment of the right vertebral artery. *3* V4 segment of the right vertebral artery. *4* V4 segment of the left vertebral artery (hypoplastic). *5* Left posterior inferior cerebellar artery (PICA). *6* Right PICA. *7* Left anterior inferior cerebellar artery (AICA). *8* Basilar artery. *9* Right superior cerebellar artery (SCA). *10* P1 segment of the left posterior cerebral artery (PCA). *11* P2 segment of the right PCA. *12* P3 segment of the right PCA. *13* P4 segment of the right PCA. (**B**) Lateral projection of a right vertebral artery injection. *1* V2 segment of the right vertebral artery. *2* V3 segment of the right vertebral artery. *3* V4 segment of the right vertebral artery. *4* Right PICA. *5* Basilar artery. *6* PCOM artery. *7* Posterior cerebral arteries.

segment. Typically, the V4 segment gives rise to two major branches, the anterior spinal artery and the posterior inferior cerebellar artery. The two vertebral arteries then join to form the basilar artery, which gives off the anterior inferior cerebellar artery, the superior cerebellar artery, as well as many perforating arteries to the brainstem. The basilar artery terminates in the posterior cerebral arteries (PCA). The PCA are also described in segments: the P1 segment of the PCA is the segment until its connection with the PCOM, the P2 segment from the PCOM to the dorsal midbrain, the P3 segment from the dorsal midbrain to the calcarine fissure, and the P4 segment describing the terminal branches. The PCA typically has two major branches: the medial branch, which gives rise to the parietooccipital artery and calcarine artery, and the lateral branch, which gives rise to the anterior, middle, and posterior inferior temporal arteries. Other important branches to note are the thalamoperforators, which mainly arise from the P1 and P2 segments *(2)*.

At the base of the brain, connections between these systems allow for collateral circulation. These connections are termed the Circle of Willis. The Circle of Willis is formed by the A1 segments of the ACA, connected by the ACOM, the P1 segments of the PCA, the supraclinoid ICA, which are connected to the PCAs by the PCOM. It is important to note, however, that only 40–60% of individuals have a complete Circle of Willis, as the remainder have hypoplastic or aplastic segments *(3, 4)*.

ANGIOPLASTY AND STENTING FOR INTRACRANIAL ATHEROSCLEROTIC DISEASE (ICAD)

Natural History and Medical Management of ICAD

Intracranial atherosclerotic disease (ICAD) likely accounts for 10–15% of all ischemic strokes, with increased incidence seen in Asian, Black, and Hispanic populations *(5)*. Stroke in this setting likely occurs due to two main mechanisms, which are not mutually exclusive: thrombus at the site of stenosis with distal embolization and hemodynamic flow reduction to areas which are unable to recruit adequate collateral flow. As with other atherosclerotic lesions, plaque rupture can initiate a cascade which results in thrombus formation at the site of the lesion, resulting in occlusion of the vessel and perforating arteries which may arise from the segment *(6)*. Emboli from the thrombus may go downstream and cause occlusion of distal vessels *(6)*. In addition, the lack of cerebral blood flow to the distal vessel may result in ischemia in watershed areas between major vessels, particularly when good collaterals are not present *(7)*.

Symptomatic ICAD carries a high risk of subsequent stroke. The best data to date comes from the Warfarin vs. Aspirin for Symptomatic Intracranial Disease (WASID) trial *(8)*. This randomized, double-blind controlled trial compared warfarin vs. aspirin for the management of ICAD in patients with 50–99% symptomatic stenosis. From this trial, 106 reached the endpoint of an ischemic stroke, 77 (73%) of which were in the territory of the stenotic artery *(8)*. The factors that were most predictive of stroke in the area of the stenotic artery included stenosis measuring 70–99%, time for qualifying event (<17 days), and female gender *(9)*. One of the strongest predictors was having stenosis 70–99%, with stroke rates of 18% at 1 year and 19% at 2 years (as compared to 6% at 1 year and 10% at 2 years for those with <70% stenosis) *(9, 10)*. Clearly, risk of stroke is greatest in the first year following the initial event, highlighting the need for urgent assessment and management. In the WASID trial, strokes in the area of the stenotic artery were mostly non-lacunar (70 out of 77; 91%) and can be quite disabling (34 out of 77; 44%) *(11)*.

The medical management of ICAD is similar to that of atherosclerosis in other arterial beds and is important regardless of whether intervention is undertaken or not. From the WASID trial, insight as to the use of antithrombotics was gained. No difference ischemic stroke was seen between the two groups (15% in the aspirin group and 13% in the warfarin group at 2 years) but a higher rate of hemorrhage was observed in the warfarin group (8.3 vs. 3.2% in the aspirin group). This has led to the general recommendation that aspirin should be preferred over warfarin for the management of this condition. It is also important to address other atherosclerotic risk factors including hypertension, hyperlipidemia, diabetes, smoking, diet, and sedentary lifestyle. In the WASID trial, very few patients were at blood pressure and LDL targets (50% of patients had systolic blood pressure >140, and 58% had LDL>100 mg/dL) *(12)*. Modification of vascular risk factors in stroke patients, including those with ICAD, has been shown to reduce subsequent stroke risk, making this an extremely important aspect of management.

Technical Approach and Potential Pitfalls of Endovascular Management of ICAD

Baseline angiography should be obtained to assess the degree of stenosis. Presently, the convention for measurement of ICAD is by the WASID method. The measurement is $1-(D_{min}-D_{prox}) \times 100$, where D_{min} is the minimal luminal diameter of the stenotic segment and D_{prox} is the normal vessel diameter proximal to the diseased segment *(13)*. It is also important to note the length of stenosis and whether the stenosis is concentric or eccentric, as these factors will be important for device sizing and may influence the risk of the procedure *(14)*. After baseline angiography, a guide catheter (typically 6F) is placed in the ICA or vertebral artery. Patients are given heparin to achieve an activated clotting time of 250 s for the procedure and the blood pressure is maintained higher on the autoregulation curve to allow for perfusion if the lesion is critical. A 2.3 Fr microcatheter over a 0.014″ microwire is then advanced across the stenosis using roadmap assistance. The microwire is removed and an exchange length (300 cm) 0.014″ microwire is advanced into the distal vessel. If utilizing a self-expanding stent, the microcatheter can then be removed and an angioplasty balloon advanced to the stenosis and inflated to nominal pressure. The balloon is typically sized to approximately 80% of the vessel diameter. After inflation, angiographic imaging should be performed to assess for dissection or rupture. The balloon can then be exchanged for the stent delivery system, which is placed across the stenosis and deployed. The sizing of a self-expanding stent is operator dependant, but in our experience we select a diameter 1.5× that of the native vessel to achieve increased radial force. Angiographic imaging is again performed. If the residual stenosis is sufficient (~>30%), repeat angioplasty may be considered. If done, care must be taken to keep the balloon within the stent as the stent tines of a self-expanding stent may make it difficult to traverse with a balloon. Final angiographic images can then be obtained, with care taken to assess for branch occlusions.

For balloon-mounted stent-delivery systems, the initial microcatheter can usually be exchanged for the stent-delivery system directly, with preceding angioplasty only required if the stenosis is too severe to allow for passage of a stent across the lesion.

Patients with ICAD often have very tortuous vascular anatomy, making access to the lesion challenging. By utilizing guide catheters to provide adequate proximal access and supportive exchange wires, most lesions can be traversed for angioplasty and stent deployment. In order to maximize support, the use of a long shuttle sheath (70 or 80 cm) placed in the common carotid artery allows for reduction of aorto-iliac tortuosity. Coaxially through the shuttle sheath, placement of a 6 Fr guide catheter (90–105 cm) placed near the petrous carotid artery can provide additional support. In patients with tortuous intracranial anatomy, a 5.2 Fr 115 cm length distal access catheter (Concentric Medical, Mountain View, CA) can be placed in the cavernous ICA thereby reducing the distance to the target lesion. Often times, the lesion can be traversed with a microwire without exchanging and monorail balloon and stent systems may be utilized over this wire. Vessel tortuosity may also be a consideration in the choice between balloon-mounted stent delivery systems as opposed to self-expanding stent delivery systems, as balloon-mounted stents are typically stiffer and more difficult to advance through tortuous anatomy.

Blood pressure management during endovascular management for ICAD is important. Patients are typically treated while under general anesthesia, which will lower blood pressure. Care must be taken to maintain higher mean arterial pressures until the stenosis has been opened by angioplasty, after which it is important to lower the blood pressure to lessen the risk of reperfusion injury *(15, 16)*.

Data for Angioplasty and Stenting of ICAD

As it was recognized that symptomatic, high-grade ICAD carries a great risk of subsequent stroke, attention was given to possible intracranial intervention to reduce this risk. Angioplasty and stenting for ICAD have gained attention, but due to high risk of procedural complications, have to be applied carefully in selected patients by properly trained interventionalists. Data is emerging on these techniques, and presently a large, randomized clinical trial underway to assess stenting against best medical management for the management of ICAD.

Angioplasty alone has been advocated by some groups as good luminal flow can be obtained with no permanent implant left in place, reducing the need for dual antiplatelet agents. Angioplasty has been reported in many retrospective studies to have reasonable success rates with periprocedural complication rates reported from 4 to 40% *(10, 17)*. Concerns about angioplasty alone including acute intimal dissection, vessel rupture, immediate recoil of the vessel, and poor post-procedure residual stenosis have limited its use among interventionalists. In a study by Marks et al., dissection of the treated vessel occurred in 11 of 36 treated patients; although none of these patients had clinical sequelae *(18)*. High restenosis rates of 24–40% have also been reported *(19)*. Prospective and randomized controlled studies are required to further assess this approach but may be reasonable in patients with small vessel diameters or if the anatomy precludes safe placement of a stent.

To reduce the risk of periprocedural dissection and immediate recoil of the vessel, stenting emerged as a potential therapeutic option. Initial retrospective trials also reported reasonable technical success rates with varied complication rates. The first major prospective non-randomized trial was the stenting of symptomatic atherosclerotic lesions in the vertebral or intracranial arteries (SSYLVIA) trial *(20)*, using a balloon-expanding bare metal stent. This stent was placed at total of 61 patients, 43 of whom had symptomatic ICAD. Technical success was seen in 95% of cases, with an overall complication rate of 7.2% at 30 days *(20)*. In a recent systematic review of stenting reports and trials for ICAD, technical success varied from 71 to 100% in the various studies, with complication rates were reported ranging from 0 to 50%, with a median of 7.7% *(21)*. Restenosis rates varied from 0 to 50% *(21)*.

Stent Designs and Types: Self-Expanding Versus Balloon-Mounted

Two main stent types exist for the treatment of ICAD: Self-expanding stents and balloon-mounted stents. At present, the only FDA-approved stent for the management of ICAD is the Wingspan (Boston Scientific, Fremont, CA) stent. This nitinol stent received approval in 2005 and has been used in a substantial number of interventions in the United States. Two concurrent registries were performed following approval of the device. The US Wingspan registry, funded by Boston Scientific, tracked patients in whom the device was placed in five US centers. Initially, periprocedural results were reported, with a technical success rate of 98.8%. The mean reported residual stenosis was 27.2 ± 16.7%. Five (6.1%) periprocedural complications were seen, four of which led to mortality *(22)*. Later, the group published their long-term results. Of the total of 129 lesions treated, 36 (27.9%) developed in-stent restenosis (ISR), defined as >50% stenosis by WASID method *(23)*. ISR was more frequently seen in younger patients and more frequently in the anterior circulation, with rates in the supraclinoid ICA reaching as high as 59% *(24)*. The NIH-funded registry yielded similar results. Technical success rate reported in this trial was 96.7%, with a peri-procedural complication rate of 6.2% *(25)*. These peri-procedural complications were more associated with posterior circulation lesions, low-volume centers, earlier time from qualifying event and stroke as the presenting symptom *(26)*. ISR reported by this group was 25% *(25)*.

Balloon-mounted stents, mainly developed for use in the coronary circulation, have also been utilized for ICAD. An example of a patient treated with a balloon-mounted stent is shown in Fig. 3. These may offer the advantage of the protection of the stent during angioplasty of the stenotic lesion, lessening the chances of dissection and perforation as compared to unprotected angioplasty. Technical results appear to be improved, with less residual stenosis as the conclusion of the procedure as compared to those reported for self-expanding stents *(27, 28)*. Restenosis also appears to be lower after placement of balloon-mounted stents as compared to self-expanding stents *(21)*. However, concerns remain with the complication rates with balloon-mounted stents *(29)*, particularly in the basilar artery and MCA, where significant numbers of perforating arteries are present.

Drug-eluting stents (DES) have also been explored for management of ICAD, particularly as high rates of ISR were noted with treatment with bare metal stents. However, DES are on a balloon-mounted stent platform and can be difficult to navigate in the intracranial circulation, and thus their role in the management of ICAD, at present, is limited. However, lower rates of ISR have been noted with these devices. In a report of the use of DES for extracranial and intracranial cerebral circulation, 29 patients were included with ICAD. In three patients the DES could not be placed, all three of whom

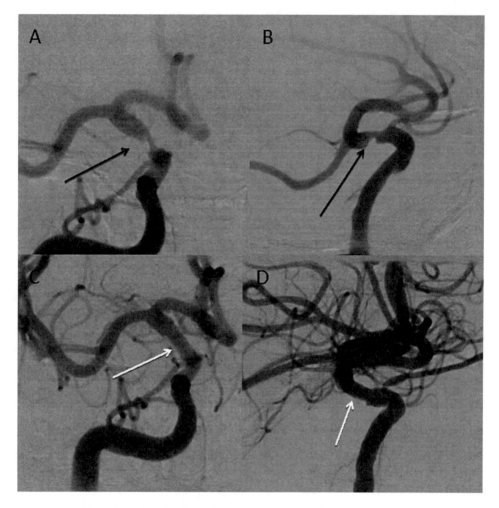

Fig. 3. (**A**, **B**) PA and lateral projections of a supraclinoid right ICA stenosis above the level of the ophthalmic artery (*black arrow*). (**C**, **D**) PA and lateral projections of the area of stenosis post-treatment with a balloon-mounted Minivision stent (*white arrow*).

had ICAD, yielding a technical failure rate of 10% *(30)*. As the device technology improves, these devices may have an increased role.

INDICATIONS FOR TREATMENT OF CEREBRAL ANEURYSMS

Introduction

The incidence of cerebral aneurysms in the United States is estimated to be 1–2% of the population *(31)*. The risk of rupture has been associated with the size, location, family history, and use of tobacco. A recent prospective study of 1,692 patients followed for 5 years has stratified the risk of aneurysm rupture based on size and location. Aneurysms smaller than 7 mm appear to have a very low rate of rupture, while posterior circulation aneurysms have higher rates of rupture compared to anterior circulation aneurysms *(31)*. The study has been criticized due to selection bias at individual centers, as well as other studies having showed higher rupture rates *(32)*. Selecting patients with non-ruptured aneurysms for treatment with coil embolization requires a team approach.

If an aneurysm is deemed appropriate for treatment, it is important to recognize the morbidity associated with the procedure with respect to the natural history. Given that the reported risks of rupture of a 7-mm anterior circulation aneurysm is 1% annually, the surgical complication rate must be less than 2% to justify treatment. MCA aneurysms tend to be more commonly treated with microsurgical clipping as these aneurysms typically are wide-necked and incorporate the divisions of the MCA along the base of the aneurysm. Basilar apex aneurysms tend to be treated with coil embolization due to rates of morbidity associated with microsurgical clipping. Treatment decisions should be based on discussions with an open vascular specialist as well as an endovascular specialist to achieve optimal results.

TECHNIQUE

Pre-procedure and post-procedure images of a patient treated with coil embolization are shown in Fig. 4. Most centers perform embolization of cerebral aneurysms under general anesthesia. For ruptured aneurysms, an external ventricular drainage catheter is

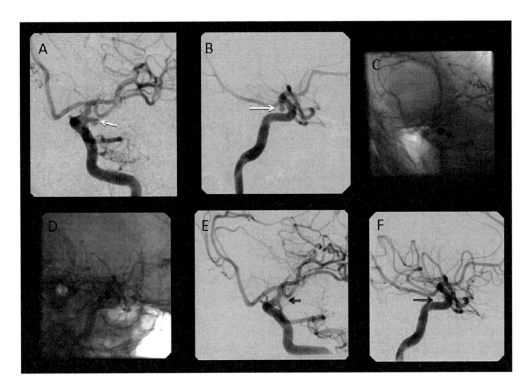

Fig. 4. (**A**) Oblique projection of a narrow-necked left PCOM aneurysm (*white arrow*) with a fetal type posterior cerebral artery near the neck of the aneurysm. (**B**) Lateral projection of left PCOM aneurysm (*white arrow*). (**C, D**) Following coil embolization, coil mass is visualized within the aneurysm (*black arrow*). (**E, F**) Subtracted images show complete obliteration with no residual filling (*black arrow*).

placed prior to the start of the procedure in many cases. This should be connected to a continuous monitor during the procedure to measure the intracranial pressure. A 6-Fr Sheath is placed in the common femoral artery and diagnostic images are acquired to visualize the neck of the aneurysm relative to the parent artery in two views. The guide catheter is then placed in the safest distal most point. Heparin is administered to obtain an activated clotting time of 250 s. The coils utilized for embolization are platinum and range in shapes from a three-dimensional geometry, spherical shape and helical shape. Selection of a particular coil requires an experienced operator to determine the best shape and size to place based on the geometry of the aneurysm.

Narrow-necked aneurysms can be embolized without adjunctive devices. Typically, a 2.3-Fr microcatheter is placed in the aneurysm over a 0.014″ microwire. Once positioned in the aneurysm, sequential coils are placed starting with a framing complex coil sized to the diameter of the aneurysm. The filling coils are softer and helical shaped to cover the spaces within the frame. Angiographic runs are performed intermittently after coil detachment. The aim of treatment is to obliterate the aneurysm without protrusion of coils into the parent artery.

For ruptured aneurysms, most operators will avoid the use of stents for wide-necked aneurysms as this will require anti-platelet medications to prevent platelet aggregation on the stent struts. For wide-necked aneurysms, the use of a Hyperglide or Hyperform balloon (EV3, Irvine, CA) is typically used in ruptured aneurysms. Through a 6-Fr guide, the balloon is navigated over a 0.010″ microwire and the balloon is positioned across the neck of the aneurysm. A 2.3-Fr microcatheter is navigated over a 0.014″ microwire under roadmapping assistance. Once the microcatheter is placed in the aneurysm, a framing coil is selected to match the diameter of the aneurysm. The coil is deployed in the aneurysm and the balloon is gently inflated to ensure the coil mass is retained in the aneurysm. A series of complex shaped or helical coils is then sequentially placed to create a stable coil mass prior to deflation of the balloon. Care must be taken to ensure inflation times are no longer than 5 min to minimize ischemic complications. The risk of this technique is that the coil mass is unstable and pulsates with each heartbeat thereby herniating into the parent artery. The technique requires experience given the potential pitfalls. In patients with non-ruptured, wide-necked aneurysms, the use of a nitinol self-expanding stent bridging the neck of the aneurysm can assist in prevention of coil herniation. Currently two stents are available: Enterprise (Cordis, Miami Lakes, FL) and Neuroform (Boston-Scientific, Natick, MA) for bridging of aneurysm necks. There may be additional theoretical benefit of the stent struts providing additional healing at the neck of the aneurysm with fibroblast growth along the interface of the coils and stent struts. After stent deployment, the 2.3-Fr microcatheter can be placed through the stent struts into the aneurysm to allow for coil embolization with parent artery protection.

Complications Associated with Coil Embolization

The most feared complications of treating cerebral aneurysms with endovascular techniques is aneurysm rupture and thromboembolic events. Although aneurysm rupture is not common, it is associated with a high mortality rate. If a rupture occurs, it is imperative to reverse all anti-coagulant medications (i.e., protamine is administered to reverse heparinization). A neurosurgeon should be contacted to place an emergent external ventricular drainage catheter, while the operator attempts to stop the extravasation through one of two techniques. Emergent rapid packing of the aneurysm with coils to prevent further bleeding can be performed. Alternatively, a balloon can be inflated across the neck of the aneurysm if this was already in place at the time of coiling. Monitoring the intracranial pressure and obtaining emergent radiographic imaging is also important once the aneurysm has been secured.

Thromboembolic events appear to be associated with the duration of catheter time, number of catheters being employed, and the use of a balloon to assist with coiling. Care must be taken to ensure the patient has adequate anti-coagulation during the procedure. Should an embolus develop during the procedure, several case series have described the use of abciximab or eptifibatide to help resolve the embolus as it has been felt to be related to platelet aggregation.

ACUTE STROKE INTERVENTIONS

Review of Natural History Data for Large Artery Occlusions

Large cerebral artery occlusion resulting in ischemic stroke is a devastating condition with high morbidity and mortality. Although therapy with recombinant tissue plasminogen activator (rt-PA) improves outcomes in ischemic stroke patients *(33, 34)*, recanalization rates for large vessel occlusion are low, particularly for the ICA terminus *(35)*. Clinical outcome for large vessel occlusion is also relatively poor, especially if recanalization is not achieved *(36, 37)*. Due to this, methods which promote recanalization safely and rapidly are under study and development.

Brief Overview of Imaging Techniques

Imaging is critical in assessment and management of the acute stroke patient. Non-contrast computed tomography (CT) of the brain should be performed as soon as possible after the patient presents to the emergency department. Guidelines from the American Stroke Association recommend that door to CT times should be less than 45 min *(37)*. The main purpose for this CT scan is to rule out intracerebral hemorrhage, an absolute contraindication for thrombolysis *(33)*. Early signs of cerebral ischemia can also be assessed, including hyperdense artery signs, sulcal effacement, and loss of gray-white differentiation. These early ischemic changes can be quantified using the Alberta Stroke Program Early CT score (ASPECTS) *(38)*. This 10-point scale gives 1 point for each intact predefined area on the CT scan. At the level of the basal ganglia, the head of caudate, internal capsule, lentiform nucleus, insula are assessed as well as the cortical areas within the MCA territory divided into the anterior (M1), middle (M2), and posterior (M3) sections. At the level above which the basal ganglia ends, the MCA territory is again divided into the anterior (M4), middle (M5), and posterior (M6) sections. The score has been validated retrospectively with the NINDS tPA dataset *(39)* and the PROACT dataset *(40)*, with ASPECTS > 7 shown to be related to better clinical outcome. Magnetic resonance imaging (MRI) has been shown to be more sensitive and specific for cerebral ischemia, particularly if diffusion-weighted sequences are utilized *(41)*. Diffusion-weighted sequences are particularly sensitive to ischemia, detecting areas of diffusion restriction within minutes of onset *(42)*. This can be particularly helpful if stroke mimics are suspected. However, practical issues of MRI screening and proximity to the emergency room limit the use of MRI in most stroke patients.

Assessment of the cerebral vasculature can also be useful in acute stroke patients, particularly if intra-arterial therapy is being considered. Transcranial Doppler ultrasound can be utilized at the bedside to assess for proximal vessel occlusion, and prolonged ultrasound may also be helpful to augment clot lysis *(43)*. While inexpensive and portable, its use is limited due to availability and that expertise with the technique is required, as inter-rater variability can be high *(44)*. CT angiography (CTA) can be performed at the same time as the non-contrast CT and provide useful information regarding the site of occlusion as well as tandem lesions. CTA has been shown to have high sensitivity and specificity for the detection of intra-arterial occlusions in acute stroke, close to that of digital subtraction angiography *(45)*. MR angiography (MRA) is another useful technique in selected stroke patients and can be performed in the same sitting as the standard MRI sequences. For certain conditions, such as dissections, MRA in conjunction with standard MRI may offer more useful information for triage and management *(37)*. DSA is the gold standard for assessment of the cerebral vasculature. This technique should be used with caution as it is invasive with the potential for serious complications, although evidence suggests that this risk is fairly low, with estimates ranging from 0.2 to 1% *(46)*. In addition to assessment for sites of stenosis, occlusion, and thrombus, the cerebral collateral circulation can be assessed. Done in the acute setting, DSA also offers the opportunity for intervention for intra-arterial stroke therapies by trained specialists *(47)*.

Cerebral perfusion assessed by MR perfusion (MRP) or CT perfusion (CTP) are gaining widespread interest as they offer the potential of assessing the amount of salvageable tissue present in acute stroke patients. Thorough reviews of these techniques are beyond the scope of this chapter but available *(41, 48, 49)*. By comparing areas of core infarct, as estimated by the areas of diffusion restriction on MRI and the areas of reduced cerebral blood volume on CTP, against areas of reduced perfusion, assessed by various time or flow maps from MRP or CTP, the "area at risk" of further infarction can be estimated. If recanalization does not occur in patients with this "mismatch" pattern, the core infarct typically increases in size until it approaches the area of perfusion deficit *(50, 51)*. To date, however, data on the selection of patients on the basis of "mismatch" has been conflicting, and not clearly shown to improve clinical outcome *(52, 53)*. This may be due to limitations inherent to the techniques. DWI and CBV lesions have been shown to be reversible, particularly if reperfusion occurs within 6 h of stroke onset *(54, 55)*. It has also not clearly been determined which time or flow maps from the MRP or CTP best estimate the true perfusion deficit, as these maps with include varying degrees of benign oligemia which will not go on to infarct *(56, 57)*. Thus, while selection of patients may be enhanced by utilizing MRP and CTP, more research into these techniques is required before recommending their widespread use.

BRIEF OVERVIEW OF CLINICAL TRIAL DATA

The treatment of MCA occlusions in the 3–6 h time window carries a level of evidence IB based on benefit being established with a single randomized controlled study. The PROACT II study was a randomized controlled study of 180 patients *(58)*. The treatment group received 9 mg of pro-urokinase directly placed into the thrombus and the medical group received heparin. The primary endpoint of a mRS of 0–2 was achieved in 40% of the treatment group and 25% in the medical group and achieved statistical significance. There was a 10% rate of symptomatic intracranial hemorrhage in the pro-urokinase group *(58)*. More recently, a randomized trial of intra-arterial urokinase for MCA occlusion was stopped early. The MELT trial enrolled 114 patients prior to being prematurely stopped and revealed a significantly higher proportion of urokinase patients achieved a mRS of 001 (42 vs. 23%, $p<0.045$) *(59)*. Based on a meta-analysis of these two trials, only 30% of patients in the non-treatment group achieved a favorable clinical outcome compared to 42% in the treatment group *(60)*.

Pharmacologic treatment with fibrinolytic treatment carries the theoretical higher risk of hemorrhage as well as longer durations of valuable time to achieve reperfusion. Mechanical interventions may reduce thrombus burden and aid with more rapid reperfusion. Currently there are two devices that have received 510K clearance from the FDA based on single-arm registry data *(61, 62)*. Both trials were similar in design testing the hypothesis of recanalization in the 3–8 h time window for large artery occlusion (MCA, basilar, ICA). These devices have undergone changes in iterations since their approval.

The Merci device (Fig. 5) is a corkscrew type device that is placed distal to thrombus and gently pulled back to engage the thrombus. The device is then retracted into the guide catheter while aspiration is applied on the guide catheter to remove the thrombus. The newer generation devices have been sized to the vessel diameter of the thrombus as well as different types of stiffness. The potential complications with this technique include device fractures, perforations of the vessel, and distal embolization in unaffected territories. The technique does require an experienced operator due to the number of steps involved as well as the recent introduction of a distal access catheter that is placed close to the thrombus to aid in aspiration. The Penumbra system is a thromboaspiration catheter. The catheter is navigated to the face of the thrombus and aspiration is performed via a vacuum suction pump. A separator device is placed through the catheter to help fragment the thrombus as aspiration is performed. The potential complication with this technique is the separator device causing a perforation and also of distal embolization as the thrombus is fragmented.

Technical Aspects Regarding Treatment of Large Artery Occlusion

After the decision is made to proceed with intra-arterial intervention, the patient should rapidly be taken to angiography suite. Controversy exists as to the best method of sedation. While general endotracheal anesthesia eliminates patient discomfort and movement which could potentially increase the risk of the procedure, recent data suggests that general anesthesia may be associated with worse clinical outcomes as compared to conscious sedation. Whichever method is employed, care should be taken to try to maintain a good cerebral perfusion pressure, with mean arterial pressures >80 mmHg and systolic blood pressure targets from 140 to 180 mmHg. After being placed under sedation or anesthesia, the groin sheath is placed. Heparinization may be considered if the patient did not receive intravenous tissue plasminogen activator (IV tPA) with an ACT target of 200–250. If the patient has received IV tPA, many operators do not use heparin, as the risk of hemorrhagic conversion is likely high. The artery should be accessed and the target vessel selected. We favor this approach as the thrombus can be more rapidly accessed, thereby salvaging more brain tissue, and collaterals have likely already been partially assessed from the previously performed non-invasive imaging. An exchange can then be performed for the guide catheter. Proper guide

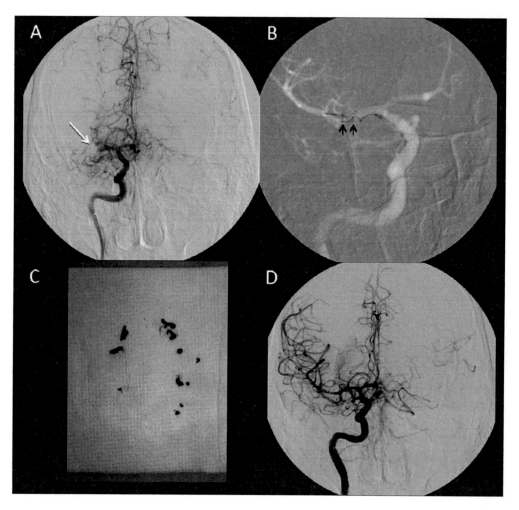

Fig. 5. Fifty-nine-year-old male with known severe cardiac disease presented with acute left-sided weakness. (**A**) Angiography at 2 h post-symptom onset revealed right M1 MCA occlusion (*white arrow*). (**B**) MERCI device deployed in thrombus (*short black arrows*). (**C**) Large amount of thrombus retrieved by MERCI device. (**D**) Final angiographic runs showing TIMI 3 flow in the right MCA.

catheter selection is critical in these patients, and it is important to remember that often these patients are older with multiple vascular risk factors, making their vascular anatomy more tortuous and difficult to navigate. The specific use of chemical ± mechanical intra-arterial therapies is very center dependent. In our center, we employ a multimodal approach, which has been assessed to have better rates of recanalization as compared to individual methods alone (63). After accessing the site of occlusion with a microwire and microcatheter, a small amount of intra-arterial (IA) tPA ± IA glycoprotein IIb/IIIa inhibitor is infused into the thrombus. The exact amounts depend on whether the patient has received intravenous IV tPA, with minimal amounts (1–2 mg) given if IV tPA has been administered, as risk of hemorrhagic conversion of the infarct increases substantially. If no IV tPA has been given, larger doses of intra-arterial tPA up to 20 mg have been reported. Many operators avoid use of thrombolytics during the procedure and utilize mechanical approaches as first-line therapy. The ultimate decision to utilize thrombolytics is often based on the degree of ischemia present prior to treatment as well as the time to treatment. Patients treated at later time points are deemed higher risk for thrombolytics. As a bailout if the above methods fail, many operators utilize angioplasty and stenting to achieve recanalization (Fig. 6). The use of stents appears to be associated with higher rates of recanalization, although devices have not been compared with each other in a randomized trial to date. Once recanalization is achieved, the blood pressure should be made normotensive as to reduce the risk of reperfusion injury *(15)*.

It is important to recognize that the intra-arterial management of acute stroke is highly dynamic and patient dependent. Rapid assessment in the emergency department is critical as outcome following intravenous or intra-arterial stroke therapy is highly time dependent *(64, 65)*. Patient selection is key as to intervene on patients who have

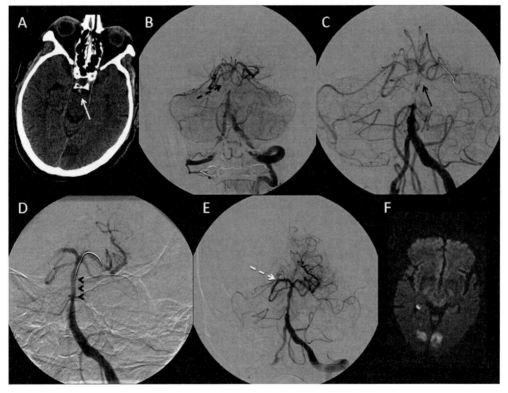

Fig. 6. Eighty-three-year-old male presenting with acute right-sided weakness and difficultly speaking, followed by decreasing level of consciousness. (**A**) CT revealing hyperdense basilar artery sign (*white arrow*) and subacute infarct in left occipital lobe. (**B**) Angiography revealed mid basilar sub-occlusive thrombus with likely underlying stenosis (*dashed black arrow*). (**C**) Magnified view showing thrombus (*black arrow*) in the distal portion of the basilar artery. (**D**) Following administration of intra-arterial eptifibatide and intra-arterial tissue plasminogen activator, the lesion was crossed and angioplasty with a Maverick 2×9 mm balloon followed by deployment of a balloon-mounted 3×12 mm Multi-link Vision stent (*black arrow heads*). (**E**) Final angiographic runs show TIMI 2 flow due to a persistent occlusion of the right posterior cerebral artery (*white dashed arrow*). (**F**) Post-intervention MRI shows bilateral acute occipital infarcts but no infarct in brainstem.

the best potential benefit and not perform intra-arterial stroke therapy on those in whom the infarct is completed. Rapid assessment and proper patient selection requires close collaboration between the emergency staff, neuroradiology, neurology, and the neurointerventional teams. The interventionalist must take care to keep in mind the objective of restoring flow to the penumbral areas, as it is easy to become overly aggressive in an attempt to obtain an excellent angiographic result. The pursuit of recanalization must be balanced against the risk of intracerebral hemorrhage. Post-interventional management is also of vital importance as these patients should be managed in a neurointensive care unit. Careful neurological assessment and tight control of glucose and blood pressure are important in the post-operative management.

REFERENCES

1. Osborn A. *Diagnostic Cerebral Angiography*. Philadelphia: Lippincott, Williams & Wilkins; 1999.
2. Schmahmann JD. Vascular syndromes of the thalamus. *Stroke*. 2003;34:2264–2278.
3. Osborn A. Circle of willis. *Diagnostic Cerebral Angiography*. Philadelphia: Lippincott Williams & Wilkins; 1999:105–116.
4. Liebeskind DS. Collateral circulation. *Stroke*. 2003;34:2279–2284.
5. Sacco RL, Kargman DE, Gu Q, Zamanillo MC. Race-ethnicity and determinants of intracranial atherosclerotic cerebral infarction. The northern Manhattan stroke study. *Stroke*. 1995;26:14–20.
6. Lee DK, Kim JS, Kwon SU, Yoo SH, Kang DW. Lesion patterns and stroke mechanism in atherosclerotic middle cerebral artery disease: early diffusion-weighted imaging study. *Stroke*. 2005;36:2583–2588.
7. Derdeyn CP, Powers WJ, Grubb RL Jr. Hemodynamic effects of middle cerebral artery stenosis and occlusion. *AJNR Am J Neuroradiol*. 1998;19:1463–1469.
8. Chimowitz MI, Lynn MJ, Howlett-Smith H, et al. Comparison of warfarin and aspirin for symptomatic intracranial arterial stenosis. *N Engl J Med*. 2005;352:1305–1316.
9. Kasner SE, Chimowitz MI, Lynn MJ, et al. Predictors of ischemic stroke in the territory of a symptomatic intracranial arterial stenosis. *Circulation*. 2006;113:555–563.
10. Derdeyn CP, Chimowitz MI. Angioplasty and stenting for atherosclerotic intracranial stenosis: Rationale for a randomized clinical trial. *Neuroimaging Clin N Am*. 2007;17:355–363, viii–ix
11. Famakin BM, Chimowitz MI, Lynn MJ, Stern BJ, George MG. Causes and severity of ischemic stroke in patients with symptomatic intracranial arterial stenosis. *Stroke*. 2009;40:1999–2003.
12. Gupta R. Symptomatic intracranial atherosclerotic disease: what is the best treatment option? *Stroke*. 2008;39:1661–1662.
13. Samuels OB, Joseph GJ, Lynn MJ, Smith HA, Chimowitz MI. A standardized method for measuring intracranial arterial stenosis. *AJNR Am J Neuroradiol*. 2000;21:643–646.
14. Mori T, Fukuoka M, Kazita K, Mori K. Follow-up study after intracranial percutaneous transluminal cerebral balloon angioplasty. *AJNR Am J Neuroradiol*. 1998;19:1525–1533.
15. Scozzafava J, Hussain MS, Yeo T, Jeerakathil T, Brindley PG. Case report: aggressive blood pressure management for carotid endarterectomy hyperperfusion syndrome. *Can J Anaesth*. 2006;53:764–768.
16. Abou–Chebl A, Reginelli J, Bajzer CT, Yadav JS. Intensive treatment of hypertension decreases the risk of hyperperfusion and intracerebral hemorrhage following carotid artery stenting. *Catheter Cardiovasc Interven*. 2007;69:690–696.
17. Leung TW, Kwon SU, Wong KS. Management of patients with symptomatic intracranial atherosclerosis. *Int J Stroke*. 2006;1:20–25.
18. Marks MP, Marcellus ML, Do HM, et al. Intracranial angioplasty without stenting for symptomatic atherosclerotic stenosis: Long-term follow-up. *AJNR Am J Neuroradiol*. 2005;26:525–530.
19. Marks MP, Wojak JC, Al-Ali F, et al. Angioplasty for symptomatic intracranial stenosis: clinical outcome. *Stroke*. 2006;37:1016–1020.

20. SSYLVIA Study Investigators. Stenting of symptomatic atherosclerotic lesions in the vertebral or intracranial arteries (ssylvia): study results. *Stroke.* 2004;35:1388–1392.
21. Groschel K, Schnaudigel S, Pilgram SM, Wasser K, Kastrup A. A systematic review on outcome after stenting for intracranial atherosclerosis. *Stroke.* 2009;40:e340–347.
22. Fiorella D, Levy EI, Turk AS, et al. Us multicenter experience with the wingspan stent system for the treatment of intracranial atheromatous disease: periprocedural results. *Stroke.* 2007;38:881–887.
23. Fiorella DJ, Levy EI, Turk AS, et al. Target lesion revascularization after wingspan: Assessment of safety and durability. *Stroke.* 2009;40:106–110.
24. Turk AS, Levy EI, Albuquerque FC, et al. Influence of patient age and stenosis location on wingspan in-stent restenosis. *AJNR Am J Neuroradiol.* 2008;29:23–27.
25. Zaidat OO, Klucznik R, Alexander MJ, et al. The NIH registry on use of the wingspan stent for symptomatic 70-99% intracranial arterial stenosis. *Neurology.* 2008;70:1518–1524.
26. Nahab F, Lynn MJ, Kasner SE, et al. Risk factors associated with major cerebrovascular complications after intracranial stenting. *Neurology.* 2009;72:2014–2019.
27. Kurre W, Berkefeld J, Sitzer M, Neumann-Haefelin T, du Mesnil de Rochemont R. Treatment of symptomatic high-grade intracranial stenoses with the balloon-expandable pharos stent: Initial experience. *Neuroradiology.* 2008;50:701–708.
28. Miao ZR, Feng L, Li S, et al. Treatment of symptomatic middle cerebral artery stenosis with balloon-mounted stents: Long-term follow-up at a single center. *Neurosurgery.* 2009;64:79–84; discussion 84–75.
29. Fiorella D, Chow MM, Anderson M, Woo H, Rasmussen PA, Masaryk TJ. A 7-year experience with balloon-mounted coronary stents for the treatment of symptomatic vertebrobasilar intracranial atheromatous disease. *Neurosurgery.* 2007;61:236–242; discussion 242–233.
30. Gupta R, Al-Ali F, Thomas AJ, et al. Safety, feasibility, and short-term follow-up of drug-eluting stent placement in the intracranial and extracranial circulation. *Stroke.* 2006;37:2562–2566.
31. Wiebers DO, Whisnant JP, Huston J III, et al. Unruptured intracranial aneurysms: natural history, clinical outcome, and risks of surgical and endovascular treatment. *Lancet.* 2003;362:103–110.
32. Juvela S, Porras M, Poussa K. Natural history of unruptured intracranial aneurysms: probability of and risk factors for aneurysm rupture. *J Neurosurg.* 2000;93:379–387.
33. Tissue plasminogen activator for acute ischemic stroke. The national institute of neurological disorders and stroke rt-pa stroke study group. *N Engl J Med.* 1995;333:1581–1587.
34. Hacke W, Kaste M, Bluhmki E, et al. Thrombolysis with alteplase 3 to 4.5 hours after acute ischemic stroke. *N Engl J Med.* 2008;359:1317–1329.
35. Saqqur M, Uchino K, Demchuk AM, et al. Site of arterial occlusion identified by transcranial doppler predicts the response to intravenous thrombolysis for stroke. *Stroke.* 2007;38:948–954.
36. Rha JH, Saver JL. The impact of recanalization on ischemic stroke outcome: a meta-analysis. *Stroke.* 2007;38:967–973.
37. Latchaw RE, Alberts MJ, Lev MH, et al. Recommendations for imaging of acute ischemic stroke: a scientific statement from the American Heart Association. *Stroke.* 2009;40:3646–3678.
38. Barber PA, Demchuk AM, Zhang J, Buchan AM. Validity and reliability of a quantitative computed tomography score in predicting outcome of hyperacute stroke before thrombolytic therapy. Aspects study group. Alberta stroke programme early ct score. *Lancet.* 2000;355:1670–1674.
39. Demchuk AM, Hill MD, Barber PA, Silver B, Patel SC, Levine SR. Importance of early ischemic computed tomography changes using aspects in ninds rtpa stroke study. *Stroke.* 2005;36:2110–2115.
40. Hill MD, Rowley HA, Adler F, et al. Selection of acute ischemic stroke patients for intra-arterial thrombolysis with pro-urokinase by using aspects. *Stroke.* 2003;34:1925–1931.
41. Muir KW, Buchan A, von Kummer R, Rother J, Baron JC. Imaging of acute stroke. *Lancet Neurol.* 2006;5:755–768.
42. Hjort N, Christensen S, Solling C, et al. Ischemic injury detected by diffusion imaging 11 minutes after stroke. *Ann Neurol.* 2005;58:462–465.
43. Alexandrov AV, Molina CA, Grotta JC, et al. Ultrasound-enhanced systemic thrombolysis for acute ischemic stroke. *N Engl J Med.* 2004;351:2170–2178.
44. Demchuk AM, Saqqur M, Alexandrov AV. Transcranial doppler in acute stroke. *Neuroimaging Clin N Am.* 2005;15:473–480, ix.

45. Lev MH, Farkas J, Rodriguez VR, et al. Ct angiography in the rapid triage of patients with hyperacute stroke to intraarterial thrombolysis: accuracy in the detection of large vessel thrombus. *J Comput Assist Tomogr.* 2001;25:520–528.
46. Kaufmann TJ, Huston J III, Mandrekar JN, Schleck CD, Thielen KR, Kallmes DF. Complications of diagnostic cerebral angiography: Evaluation of 19,826 consecutive patients. *Radiology.* 2007;243:812–819.
47. Nogueira RG, Yoo AJ, Buonanno FS, Hirsch JA. Endovascular approaches to acute stroke, part 2: A comprehensive review of studies and trials. *AJNR Am J Neuroradiol.* 2009;30:859–875.
48. Shetty SK, Lev MH. Ct perfusion in acute stroke. *Neuroimaging Clin N Am.* 2005;15:481–501, ix.
49. Harris AD, Coutts SB, Frayne R. Diffusion and perfusion MRI imaging of acute ischemic stroke. *Magn Reson Imaging Clin N Am.* 2009;17:291–313.
50. Davis SM, Donnan GA, Parsons MW, et al. Effects of alteplase beyond 3h after stroke in the echoplanar imaging thrombolytic evaluation trial (epithet): a placebo-controlled randomised trial. *Lancet Neurol.* 2008;7:299–309.
51. De Silva DA, Fink JN, Christensen S, et al. Assessing reperfusion and recanalization as markers of clinical outcomes after intravenous thrombolysis in the echoplanar imaging thrombolytic evaluation trial (epithet). *Stroke.* 2009;40:2872–2874.
52. Hacke W, Furlan AJ, Al-Rawi Y, et al. Intravenous desmoteplase in patients with acute ischaemic stroke selected by MRI perfusion-diffusion weighted imaging or perfusion ct (dias-2): A prospective, randomised, double-blind, placebo-controlled study. *Lancet Neurol.* 2009;8:141–150.
53. Donnan GA, Baron JC, Ma H, Davis SM. Penumbral selection of patients for trials of acute stroke therapy. *Lancet Neurol.* 2009;8:261–269.
54. Olivot JM, Mlynash M, Thijs VN, et al. Relationships between cerebral perfusion and reversibility of acute diffusion lesions in defuse: Insights from radar. *Stroke.* 2009;40:1692–1697.
55. McKinney A, Truwit CL, Kieffer S. Reversibility of an "apparent" infarct on dynamic perfusion ct after lytic therapy: comment regarding cerebral blood flow and blood volume thresholds. *AJNR Am J Neuroradiol.* 2006;27:1391–1392; author reply 1392–1393.
56. Sobesky J, Zaro Weber O, Lehnhardt FG, et al. Does the mismatch match the penumbra? Magnetic resonance imaging and positron emission tomography in early ischemic stroke. *Stroke.* 2005;36:980–985.
57. Heiss WD, Sobesky J. Comparison of pet and dw/pw-MRI in acute ischemic stroke. *Keio J Med.* 2008;57:125–131.
58. Furlan A, Higashida R, Wechsler L, et al. Intra-arterial prourokinase for acute ischemic stroke. The PROACT II study: a randomized controlled trial. Prolyse in acute cerebral thromboembolism. *J Am Med Assoc.* 1999; 282: 2003–2011.
59. Ogawa A, Mori E, Minematsu K, et al. The MELT Japan Study Group. *Stroke.* 2007;38:2633–3639.
60. Saver J. Intra-arterial fibrinolysis for acute ischemic stroke. The message of MELT. *Stroke.* 2007;38:2627.
61. Smith WS, Sung G, Starkman S, et al. Safety and efficacy of mechanical embolectomy in acute ischemic stroke: results of the MERCI trial. *Stroke.* 2005;36:1432–38.
62. Bose A, Henkes H, Alfke K, et al. The Penumbra System: a mechanical device for the treatment of acute stroke due to thromboembolism. *AJNR Am J Neuroradiol.* 2008;29:1409–13, Epub 2008 May 22
63. Gupta R, Vora NA, Horowitz MB, et al. Multimodal reperfusion therapy for acute ischemic stroke: Factors predicting vessel recanalization. *Stroke.* 2006;37:986–990.
64. Hacke W, Donnan G, Fieschi C, et al. Association of outcome with early stroke treatment: Pooled analysis of atlantis, ecass, and ninds rt-pa stroke trials. *Lancet.* 2004;363:768–774.
65. Khatri P, Abruzzo T, Yeatts SD, Nichols C, Broderick JP, Tomsick TA. Good clinical outcome after ischemic stroke with successful revascularization is time-dependent. *Neurology.* 2009;73:1066–1072.

8 Abdominal and Thoracic Aortic Aneurysms*

Aravinda Nanjundappa, MD, *Bryant Nguyen,* MD, *Robert S. Dieter,* MD, RVT, *John J. Lopez,* MD, *and Akhilesh Jain,* MD

CONTENTS

ENDOVASCULAR REPAIR OF THE THORACO-ABDOMINAL AORTA
ABDOMINAL AORTIC ANEURYSM
DETECTION OF ABDOMINAL AORTIC ANEURYSM
SCREENING FOR ABDOMINAL AORTIC ANEURYSM
INDICATIONS FOR INTERVENTION
CONTRAINDICATIONS
EVAR
TYPES OF DEVICES AVAILABLE
PRE-OPERATIVE IMAGING AND EVALUATION
ANATOMICAL CONSIDERATIONS FOR EVAR
SURVEILLANCE AFTER EVAR
OPEN SURGICAL VERSUS ENDOVASCULAR REPAIR
CONCLUSION
THORACIC ENDOVASCULAR AORTIC REPAIR (TEVAR)
TEVAR TECHNIQUE
CASE 1 (SEE FIGS. 20–23)
REFERENCES

ENDOVASCULAR REPAIR OF THE THORACO-ABDOMINAL AORTA

Developed in the early 1990s, endovascular techniques of aortic repair offer a novel alternative to open surgical repair. Despite the initial concerns about safety and efficacy of Endovascular Aneurysm Repair (EVAR), progressive improvement in technology

---

*This chapter is dedicated to my late beloved mother Muniswamy Lakshmidevamma who was my lifetime inspiration and motivation.

From: *Peripheral and Cerebrovascular Intervention*, Contemporary Cardiology
Edited by: D. L. Bhatt, DOI 10.1007/978-1-60327-965-9_8
© Springer Science+Business Media, LLC 2012

and increased experience has led to its emergence as a dominant method of infrarenal abdominal aortic aneurysm (AAA) repair. The subsequent sections discuss the various aspects of evaluation, decision making, technique, and outcomes following EVAR.

ABDOMINAL AORTIC ANEURYSM

An aneurysm is defined as a permanent localized dilatation of an artery, having at least a 50% increase in diameter compared with the expected normal diameter (1). A practical working definition of an AAA is a transverse diameter 3 cm or greater. AAAs are largely a disease of elderly white men with a prevalence of 5–7% in patients greater than 65 years of age. AAAs represent a degenerative process that has often been attributed to atherosclerosis, although further research is being conducted to better elucidate its etiology (2). Degenerative connective tissue disorders, such as Marfan's syndrome and Ehler-Danlos syndrome, also account for a minority of cases. Female gender, African-American ethnicity, and diabetes mellitus are factors associated with a lower risk of developing AAAs (3, 4).

DETECTION OF ABDOMINAL AORTIC ANEURYSM

Majority of aortic aneurysms are in fact diagnosed incidentally, in their asymptomatic stage, on abdominal imaging performed for unrelated reasons. Although, most clinically significant AAAs should be palpable by physical examination, it is not considered to be an accurate way to rule in or out an aortic aneurysm. In a pooled analysis of 15 studies, Lederle et al. (5) determined the diagnostic sensitivity of physical examination to be 29% for AAAs 3–3.9 cm, 50% for AAAs 4–4.9 cm, and 75% for AAAs 5 cm or larger. The positive predictive value of palpation for AAAs of 3 cm or greater in size was 43% in these studies.

Abdominal B-mode ultrasound is frequently used as an imaging modality of choice for the initial diagnosis and subsequent follow-up on the size of AAAs (Fig. 1). Besides being relatively inexpensive, it is non-invasive and free of the hazard of ionizing radiation and nephrotoxic contrast as seen in a computed tomographic scan. When compared to a CT scan, ultrasound typically underestimates the diameter of AAAs by approximately 2–4 mm in the anteroposterior direction (6). When doing a serial follow-up in the size of an AAA, it is hence advised to use identical modality for size measurements to avoid inaccuracies in estimating the growth rate.

Computed tomography scans, despite the associated risk of contrast nephropathy and ionizing radiation, is the imaging modality of choice for preoperative planning for AAAs (Fig. 2). It offers low inter observer variability, easy reproducibility, and detailed vascular anatomy essential for preoperative planning. CT is also the gold standard modality for determining anatomic eligibility for an endovascular repair.

SCREENING FOR ABDOMINAL AORTIC ANEURYSM

Even though AAAs may be asymptomatic for years, left untreated, a significant proportion of these eventually rupture. Due to unacceptably high mortality of a ruptured aortic aneurysm, it is desirable to make a diagnosis in every patient prior to rupture/leak to allow an elective repair.

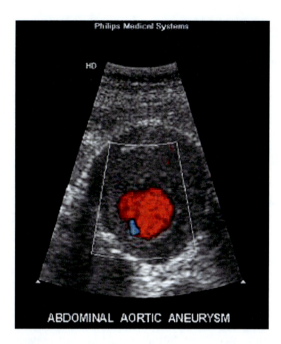

Fig. 1. Duplex ultrasound of abdomen demonstrating a AAA. Notice a small lumen compared to the size of the aneurysm indicating presence of large amount of thrombus.

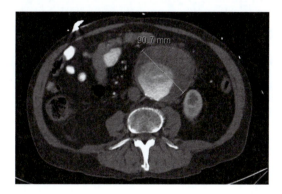

Fig. 2. AAA of 9 cm identified in a patient presenting with new onset back and abdominal pain with a prominent aortic pulsation on examination.

In 2005, United States Preventive Services Task Force (USPSTF) revised its earlier guidelines and made a recommendation for one-time screening for AAA by ultrasonography in men aged 65–75 who have ever smoked (7). Based on their meta-analysis, USPSTF determined that an invitation to attend screening was associated with a significant reduction in the AAA-related mortality (odds ratio, 0.57 (95% CI, 0.45–0.74)) without any significant reduction in the all-cause mortality. Ultrasound has been shown to have 95% sensitivity and nearly 100% specificity in the detection of AAA (8). In a cohort-based screening study, Crow et al. concluded that a single normal ultrasonographic scan at age of 65 years in men rules out significant aortic aneurysm disease for life (9).

As part of the same guideline, USPSTF recommended against routine screening for AAA in women. This was based on the results of a single available trial at that time *(7, 10)*. The rationale being a low prevalence of AAA in women, in which case, the screening and early treatment of AAA in women would lead to increasing number of unnecessary surgeries with associated morbidity and mortality. In a consensus statement, Society of Vascular Surgery (SVS) published screening guidelines on AAA in 2004 *(11)*. The consensus statement, while essentially similar to USPSTF guidelines for men, also recommended AAA screening in women 60–85 years of age with cardiovascular risk factors and AAA screening in both men and women older than 50 years with a family history of AAA. Derubertis et al., in their efforts to further clarify this issue, also concluded that women >65 years of age with multiple atherosclerotic risk factors were at substantially high risk of developing a AAA with prevalence rate as high as 6.4% *(12)*.

Ferket et al. *(13)* conducted a systemic review of seven guidelines, published between 2003 and 2010, on AAA screening. They concluded that consensus existed across guidelines on one-time screening of elderly men to detect and treat AAAs > 5.5 cm. Four guidelines, of which three were less rigorously developed, based on Appraisal of Guidelines Research and Evaluation instrument (AGREE scores) scores of less than 40%, contained disparate recommendations on screening of women and middle-aged men at elevated risk. Better prediction model and cost-effectiveness analyses are needed to provide guidance for screening recommendations in these groups.

INDICATIONS FOR INTERVENTION

Recommendation for repair of an aortic aneurysm is based on the premise that surgical repair (open or endovascular) prevents aneurysm rupture, a condition associated with 80–90% mortality rate, which has shown only marginally improvement over past 6 decades of experience *(14–16)*.

Symptomatic Aneurysm

Most aortic aneurysms are asymptomatic, however, when symptoms occur, they can be classified into: (1) rupture or impending rupture, (2) embolic or thrombotic complications, and (3) mass effect.

Sudden onset of severe abdominal/back pain, hypotension, and palpable pulsatile abdominal mass comprise the classical triad associated with ruptured AAA *(17)*. The triad is, however, present in only a minority of patients *(18)* and an accurate diagnosis requires a high index of suspicion in appropriate clinical setting in conjunction with expeditious imaging for confirmation. Common misdiagnoses associated with ruptured AAA include renal colic, perforated viscus, diverticulitis, and ischemic bowel *(18)*.

Ischemic/thrombotic symptoms are relatively rare but catastrophic manifestations of a symptomatic AAA. In a review of 302 patients undergoing open repair of AAA, Baxter et al. *(19)* identified 15 patients (5%) presenting with distal embolization as the first manifestation of their AAA. Out of these, only two aneurysms were larger than 5 cm indicating a potentially dangerous nature of small AAAs, which are more likely to present with ischemic/thrombotic symptoms.

Rarely, large AAAs may cause symptoms like vague abdominal or back pain, early satiety, urinary symptoms from ureteral compression or venous thrombosis from iliocaval compression.

Asymptomatic Aneurysm

It is estimated that 80% of mortality from AAA is secondary to rupture. Since, the intervention in patients with asymptomatic AAAs is intended to prevent rupture, the decision to intervene should be based on a favorable risk-to-benefit ratio. The factors under consideration include: (1) estimated risk of rupture under observation, (2) the operative risk involved, (3) life expectancy of the patient, and (4) patient's personal preferences.

Maximum aneurysm diameter is currently the most accepted primary determinant of the risk of rupture. In 1966, Szilagyi et al. *(20)* were the first to highlight the importance of aneurysm diameter in predicting the risk of rupture. Multiple authors have subsequently validated above findings *(21–34)*. These and other studies, however, have projected substantially varied risks of rupture associated with various aneurysm sizes. The factors contributing to this variability are related to different referral patterns, inconsistent measurement techniques (major axis vs. minor axis), and imaging modalities (ultrasound vs. CT scan). However, despite of differences in precise estimates, there is general consensus across board that the rupture risk increases substantially with AAA diameters 5–6 cm *(23, 25)*.

In addition, rapidly expanding AAAs, defined as growth by more than 1 cm in diameter over 12 months or 0.5 cm over 6 months, is an indication for repair *(26)*.

Laplace's law indicates that wall tension of a symmetric shape is directly proportional to its radius and intraluminal pressure and inversely proportional to the wall thickness. Actual AAAs, however, are not ideal symmetric shapes and have walls of variable thickness and strength. Based on more recent studies, a biomechanical tool like Finite Element Analysis of the aneurysm, may be more accurate than size alone in predicting the risk of rupture *(27)*. These tools are still investigational and until then the maximal aneurysmal diameter remains the "gold standard" in predicting the rupture risk for AAAs.

The operative mortality of elective AAA repair has been reported to range from 5 to 8% in various studies *(28, 29)*. Co-morbid conditions like cardiac disease (ischemia, cardiomyopathy), pulmonary disease, and renal insufficiency have been shown to dramatically increase the mortality from an elective AAA repair *(30)* and should be kept in consideration when offering an elective repair.

CONTRAINDICATIONS

Since elective EVAR is performed with intent to prevent a rupture and thus prolong life, any condition that limits patient's life expectancy to less than 6 months is a contraindication for elective EVAR.

In cases of elderly debilitated patients with mental deterioration, it is important to consider patient's quality of life before a decision is made to prolong such life. In-depth unbiased decision, with patient's family and primary care physician, focused towards patient's best interest is helpful in such situations.

Presence of active systemic infection is a high risk of seeding the endoprosthesis and thus a relative contraindication for EVAR.

Patients with high-grade stenosis/occlusion of superior mesenteric and celiac arteries have their bowel supply dependent on inferior mesenteric artery (IMA) via collaterals. In such cases, covering the IMA would lead to a fatal acute mesenteric ischemia and thus is a contraindication to EVAR.

Other relative contraindications for EVAR include anatomical considerations that increase the complications associated with EVAR. These considerations are discussed in later in the chapter (see Anatomical Considerations).

EVAR

Since its inception by Juan Parodi in 1991, EVAR has seen progressive improvements in technique and stent technology. Conceptually, during an EVAR, an endoluminal impervious stent graft connects the non-dilated arteries proximal to the aneurysm sac to the non-dilated arteries distal to the aneurysm, thereby excluding the aneurysm from the circulation. This decreases the pressure on the aneurysm wall thereby reducing/eliminating the risk of rupture.

A rapid and progressive improvement in the stent technology like a narrower profile device delivery systems, improved fixation in association with improved experience with EVAR has led to progressively increase in the percentage of AAAs being repaired with endovascular techniques. According to nationwide hospital databases, there has been a 600% increase in the annual number of EVAR procedures performed in the United States since 2000 *(31)*. EVAR now accounts for more than half of all AAA repairs.

TYPES OF DEVICES AVAILABLE

Presently, four EVAR device systems have received FDA approval in the United States for the treatment of AAA *(32)*:

- Zenith FLEX AAA endograft (Cook Medical Inc., Bloomington, IN) (Fig. 3)
- Gore Excluder (W.L. Gore and Associates, Inc., Flagstaff, AZ) (Fig. 4)
- Endologix Powerlink (Endologix, Inc, Irvine, CA)
- Medtronic Talent and AneuRx (Medtronic Corp., Minneapolis, MN) (Fig. 5)
- Ancure device (Guidant<Menlo Park, CA) *(withdrawn from the US market in 2003).

The basic EVAR system comprises three components: delivery system, stent graft, and fabric sleeve for exclusion of the aneurysm. Early endografts created by Parodi et al. utilized either an aorto–aortic design or an aorto–unifemoral design that necessitated femoral–femoral bypass and coil embolization of the contralateral iliac artery. Due to the lack of normal aorta at the aortic bifurcation in most AAA patients, the aortoaortic endograft design was abandoned in 1994. Modern grafts rely on distal fixation in the iliac arteries and proximal fixation in the infrarenal or suprarenal aorta. The modular design has also been incorporated, with three of the four current grafts composed of a main body with "ipsilateral" iliac endograft as the first component, and a smaller "contralateral" graft attached to the main body as the second component. The Powerlink

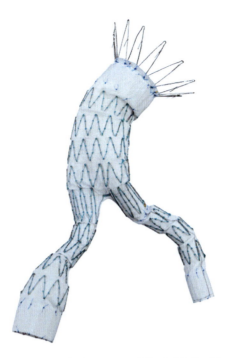

Fig. 3. Zenith FLEX AAA endograft (Courtesy of Cook Medical Inc., Bloomington, IN).

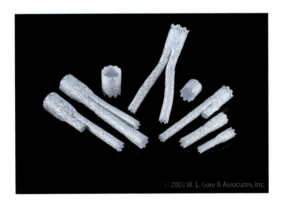

Fig. 4. Gore Excluder (Courtesy of W.L. Gore and Associates, Inc., Flagstaff, AZ).

(Endologix, Inc., Irvine, California, USA) endograft is a unique unibody endograft, which contains the main body and bilateral iliac grafts for fixation. The Powerlink device does not require bilateral femoral cutdown, as percutaneous 9 Fr access can be used on the contralateral side for stent positioning.

PRE-OPERATIVE IMAGING AND EVALUATION

Contrasted computed tomography scan using fine cuts (<3 mm) is the imaging of choice for pre-operative evaluation of the AAA prior to EVAR. CT scan without intravenous contrast may be used in patients with severe renal insufficiency although this

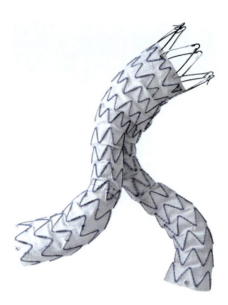

Fig. 5. Medtronic Endurant stent graft (Courtesy of Medtronic Corporation, Minneapolis, MN, USA).

Table 1
Characteristics that Should be Studied on a CT Angiogram Prior to EVAR

Aortic neck	Diameter	Measure at the level of lowest renal artery and 15 mm caudal (10 mm for newer Medtronic devices)	Should be 19–32 mm
	Length	Level of renal arteries to the beginning of the aneurysm	>15 mm for most devices (>10 mm for Talent and Endurant devices)
	Angulation	Between the central line of aorta and aneurysm	Less than 60°
	Thrombus	Should be <25% of vessel circumference	
	Calcification	Extensive/circumferential predicts problems with good seal	
	Taper	Look for reverse taper (>4 mm diameter increase over 10 mm aortic length)	Increase chances of proximal type I endoleak
Aortic bifurcation		Look for narrowing that may preclude passage of device	
External iliacs		Should be able to accommodate 14–20-Fr sheath depending on the type of device	
Hypogastrics		For patency and aneurysms	
Femoral arteries		For anterior calcium/atherosclerosis	

may miss important anatomical information like laminated thrombus, patent IMA, and severe iliofemoral occlusive disease. Besides the axial cuts, a review of saggital, coronal, and three-dimensional reconstructions is necessary to fully understand the aneurysm anatomy including its angulation. *See* Table 1 for various characteristics that should be evaluated on the pre-operative CT angiogram of an AAA.

In patients with severe renal insufficiency, contraindicating intravenous contrast, intravascular ultrasound can be used to size the aortic and iliac seal zones, evaluate potential eccentric thrombus in the aortic neck, and evaluate the external iliacs for occlusive disease.

ANATOMICAL CONSIDERATIONS FOR EVAR

Anatomical considerations for selecting a patient for EVAR relate to: (1) suitability of proximal and distal attachment sites, (2) adequacy of access arteries, and (3) the presence of side-branches of aortoiliac circulation to be excluded from the systemic circulation.

Proximal Attachment Site (Aortic Neck)

The major anatomic factor in predicting suitability for EVAR is the character of the aortic neck. The most acceptable method of proximal endograft fixation is deployment at the level of renal arteries also known as infrarenal fixation. This is performed in the nondilated portion of the infrarenal aorta proximal to the aneurysm sac commonly known as the aortic neck. According to the instructions for use of endografts with infrarenal fixation, an infrarenal neck at least 15 mm in length and less than 32 mm in diameter with an angulation <60° is required for optimal sealing (Figs. 6 and 7) *(33)*. The recommendations for Talent or Endurant stent graft system (Medtronic, Inc., Santa Rosa, CA) require a minimum 10 mm of infrarenal aorta neck for adequate proximal fixation *(34)*.

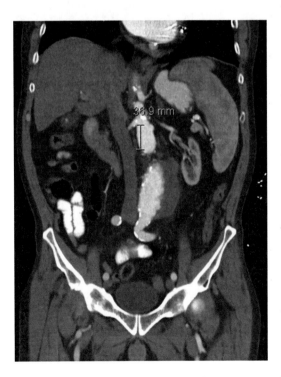

Fig. 6. Coronal reformatted image of a CT scan demonstrating a >15-mm-long aortic neck with minimal angulation. Also note absence of significant thrombus (abundance of which can cause poor sealing and embolic complications at the time of graft deployment).

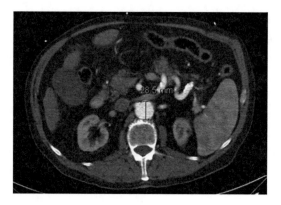

Fig. 7. Axial cut of a CT scan at the level of lowest renal artery (right in this patient) demonstrating short axis diameter of 28.5 mm suitable for EVAR. Again, there is minimal calcification and minimal thrombus lining the walls both of which are favorable factors.

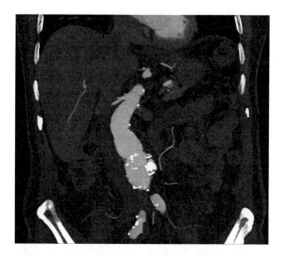

Fig. 8. Coronal reformatted image demonstrating significant angulation of aortic neck (measured between the center axis of aorta and the aneurysm). Also note a progressive increase in aortic diameter in the distal aortic neck (reverse taper), which is predictive of increased proximal type I endoleak and early intervention.

Since aortic neck is the first place where the endograft excludes the aneurysm from systemic circulation, it is imperative to have a suitable aortic neck for effective device deployment. The most common reason (>50%) for patients with AAA to be considered ineligible for endovascular repair is unsuitable anatomy of proximal aortic neck *(35)*. The considerations that may make a patient unsuitable for EVAR include, an aortic neck that is too short, too tortuous or too wide, or conditions like presence of excessive calcification or a thick layer of thrombus at the level of aortic neck (Figs. 8 and 9) *(36, 37)*. In a review of 258 patients, EVAR performed in patients with a hostile neck defined by, any or all of, length of <10 mm, angle of >60°, diameter of >28 mm, ≥50% circumferential thrombus, ≥50% calcified neck, and reverse taper, is accompanied by higher rates of early (intraoperative) type I endoleak and intervention *(38)*. The midterm outcomes

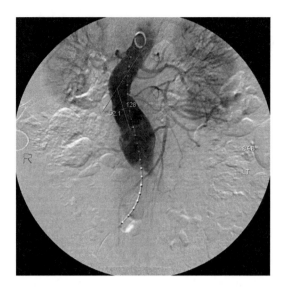

Fig. 9. Angiogram of the patient in Fig. 8 confirming significant angulation (although <60°) and reverse taper. Patient underwent EVAR and ended up with a proximal type I endoleak requiring additional proximal cuff.

were similar to those with favorable neck anatomy. The findings, however, need to be validated by larger multicenter randomized studies.

Suprarenal fixation has been proposed as more effective means of proximal fixation especially when morphological features of aortic neck are unfavorable. Despite the potential advantages of suprarenal fixation, there have been concerns regarding short- and long-term risks of renal or mesenteric artery embolization and occlusion.

Distal Attachment Site

Bifurcated endografts are currently used in more than 95% of abdominal EVAR cases. In these the distal attachment, also known as the distal landing zone, is preferably in common iliac arteries, allowing antegrade perfusion of hypogastric vessels. However, in cases of too short or aneurysmal common iliac arteries, distal attachment can be at the level of external iliac vessels, in which case hypogastric coil embolization is recommended to decrease the chance of type II endoleak (discussed later) *(39, 40)*.

Access Arteries

The common femoral artery is the vessel used most commonly for introduction of the delivery sheath. Access to the aorta may be hampered by severe atherosclerotic narrowing of the iliacs, excessive tortuosity especially with heavy calcification, or small-diameter native iliacs. A focal iliac stenosis amenable to angioplasty should undergo angioplasty without stenting prior to any attempts to advance the device. One of the major intraoperative catastrophes in EVAR is disruption of external iliac artery, which can occur, following forceful introduction of a large sheath through a narrow/diseased iliac artery.

A narrow aortic bifurcation, despite adequate iliac vessels, may also preclude a safe delivery of the endograft. For this reason, the iliac vessels and the aortic bifurcation should be carefully studied preoperatively with a contrasted CT scan for adequate risk assessment and planning. Delivery catheters of aortic endografts from most manufacturers have an outer diameter ranging from 18 to 26 Fr, and easily traverse iliac segments as narrow as 5.5–7.5 mm in diameter.

The access to the femoral arteries can be obtained in an open or percutaneous fashion. Open access to bilateral femoral arteries using bilateral groin incision is a well-established and time-tested method. It also allows for the possibility of performing an endarterectomy or patch angioplasty to gain access in cases of femoral arterial occlusive disease.

With the advent of vascular access closure devices, percutaneous access to femoral arteries is increasingly being used with a low incidence of early and late access site complications *(41, 42)*. The "preclose" technique of percutaneous access, described by Lee et al., uses two Perclose Proglide (Abbott Laboratories, Illinois, USA) devices *(43)*. The first device is deployed with a 30° medial rotation and the second with 30° lateral rotation, while maintaining wire access. This technique places a single monofilament suture proximal and distal to the puncture site. The sutures are exteriorized and tagged for closure of the arteriotomy at the completion of EVAR. Anterior wall calcification and severe fibrosis of the access vessel are predictors of primary failure of this technique, whereas obesity and sheath size are not *(44)*.

Aortic Side Branches

Pelvic ischemia from obliteration of hypogastric vessels and Type II endoleak (explained later), mainly from patent lumbar arteries, are two main issues related to obliteration of aortic side branches.

As mentioned earlier, exclusion of hypogastric artery (HA) is usually required during endovascular repair of aortoiliac aneurysms that involve either the distal common iliac artery or the HA itself. Buttock claudication and erectile dysfunction are two complications most commonly associated with interruption of unilateral or bilateral hypogastric arteries during EVAR. One of the largest series of patients undergoing HA interruption during AAA repair revealed that persistent buttock claudication developed in 12% of unilateral and 11% of bilateral HA interruptions, whereas impotence occurred in 9% of unilateral and 13% of bilateral HA occlusions *(44)*.

The most feared complication, ischemic colitis, occurs in less than 2% of elective EVAR cases *(45)*. The risk for colon necrosis is higher if EVAR occludes a previously patent IMA, previous colon surgery has interrupted the collateral pathways from the superior mesenteric artery, or the superior mesenteric and celiac arteries are stenotic or occluded. In practice, colon ischemia is more likely to result from atheroembolism to the pelvic circulation than from proximal internal iliac artery occlusion *(46, 47)* (Fig. 10).

Endoleaks

One of the factors that threaten the durability of an endovascular repair is persistent blood flow and resultant pressure in the aneurysm sac, termed as endoleak. Contrast-enhanced CT scan is currently the "gold standard" modality for detection and categorization of endoleaks although MR angiography and contrast-enhanced ultrasound are being studied as well *(48)*. Different types of endoleaks are classified according to the site and origin of blood flow into the aneurysm sac (Table 2) *(49)*.

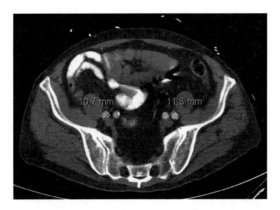

Fig. 10. Axial cut on CT scan showing the size of external iliacs just distal to the hypogastric take off. Minimal calcification and large size with absence of tortuosity of iliacs ensures a trouble-free passage of sheaths across iliacs.

Table 2
Types of Endoleaks and their Treatment

Classification	Features	Treatment
Type I	Proximal or distal graft attachment zone	Proximal or distal extension or cuff Embolization in case of patent hypogastric artery
Type II	Patent lumbar vessels or inferior mesenteric artery	Conservative Coil embolization in case of sac expansion
Type III	Graft component separation or graft erosion	Secondary endograft
Type IV	Graft porosity	Conservative

Type 1 Endoleaks

Type 1 endoleaks occur due to imperfect sealing of the endograft at its proximal or distal landing zone. This leads to antegrade flow of blood at systemic pressure into the aneurysm sac resulting in a high risk of rupture. Consequently, there is no role of conservative management in these types of endoleaks and most of these should be identified and treated at the time of stent graft implantation (Figs. 11 and 12). Distal type I endoleaks can easily be repaired by placement of distal extension leading to a seal at the level of external iliac artery. Proximal type I endoleaks are mostly secondary to less than ideal aortic neck anatomy or poor patient selection. Studies have shown that a hostile neck anatomy (defined earlier) results in a higher incidence of early (intraoperative) proximal type I endoleak and intervention *(38)*. Deployment of proximal cuff or bare metal "palmaz" type stent at the site of proximal landing zone can be used to correct these types of endoleaks, although failure of endovascular techniques would frequently result in an open repair *(50, 51)*.

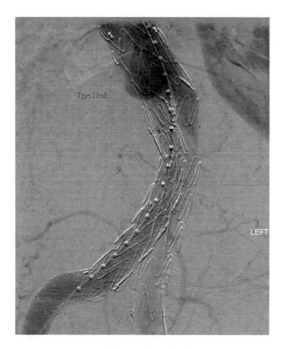

Fig. 11. Proximal type I endoleak seen on completion angiogram as demonstrated by presence of contrast outside the graft on the right side.

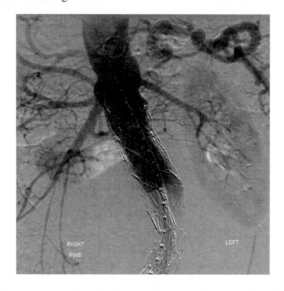

Fig. 12. Angiogram of the patient in Fig. 11 after deployment of proximal cuff, showing the resolution of type I endoleak (contrast confined within the graft).

Type II Endoleaks

Type II endoleaks result from retrograde perfusion of the aneurysm sac, frequently from the patent lumbar arteries or the patent IMA. Early post-operative follow-up CT scans demonstrate the presence of a type II endoleak in 10–20% of cases, of which, up

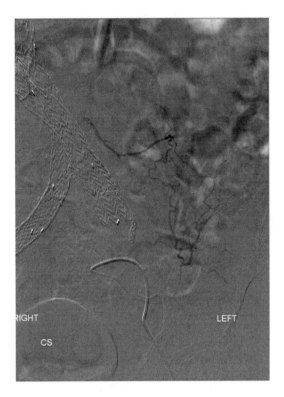

Fig. 13. Angiogram performed for a type II endoleak persistent at 6 months post-EVAR. Note the tip of catheter in left internal iliac artery and a meandering collateral coming off this vessel and going towards the AAA sac. The leak was confirmed on delayed images and the subsequently embolized (Fig. 14).

to 80% resolve spontaneously within 6 months of the endograft implantation (52, 53). As compared to the direct type I and type III endoleaks, type II endoleaks are indirect and consequently low-pressure leaks that are considered relatively benign with low likelihood of sac expansion and rupture. As mentioned earlier, majority of these resolve spontaneously and it is prudent to follow these with serial surveillance CT scans. Aneurysm sac expansion and/or persistence of the endoleak are indications for intervention for a type II endoleak (Figs. 13 and 14). Transarterial coil embolization, open or laparoscopic suture ligation, and polymer embolization of the aneurysm cavity are the various treatment options described in literature (54).

Type 3 Endoleaks

Type 3 endoleaks are secondary to either tear in the fabric of the endograft or due to separation of its components leading to a high-pressure leak into the aneurysm cavity with high risk of rupture in short term. As for type I leaks, these mandate an intraoperative correction although a progressive refinement of stent graft technology has made these leaks relatively rare. Imprecise sizing of the limbs leading to kinks is another cause of type III endoleaks (Figs. 15 and 16). Treatment of type III endoleak requires deployment of an additional endograft at the site of component separation or fabric tear.

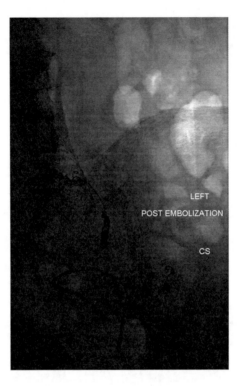

Fig. 14. Coils deployed in left internal iliac artery at the site of origin of collateral causing the endoleak. Subsequent follow-up confirmed resolution of endoleak.

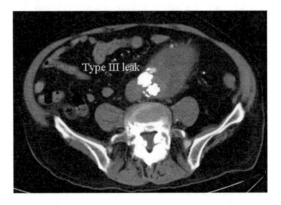

Fig. 15. One-month follow-up CT angiogram following EVAR, demonstrating a type III endoleak. Subsequent angiogram revealed a kink in right limb of the prosthesis (Fig. 16).

Type 4 Endoleaks

Type 4 endoleak is the term used for temporary oozing of blood into the aneurysm sac that occurs secondary to the porosity of the endograft fabric. This was something which was seen with earlier generation of stent grafts and is now rare due to improvements in the design and fabric of the endograft.

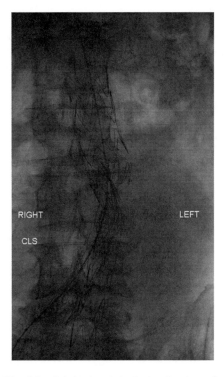

Fig. 16. Kink in the right limb of endograft.

Endotension

Endotension is the term used to describe aneurysm sac pressurization in the absence of endoleak. The precise etiology of endotension is unknown. Transmission of pressure from aorta to the aneurysm sac via thrombus layered between the aortic wall and the stent graft is one of the postulated mechanism of endotension *(55)*. Until recently, direct aneurysm sac pressure measurement, performed by translumbar puncture or by the selective catheterization through the IMA, superior mesenteric artery, or internal iliac artery, was the only way of demonstrating endotension *(56)*. More recently, a concise radiofrequency sensor (EndoSensor; Cardio-MEMS Inc., Atlanta, GA, USA) has been newly developed and is being used in clinical setting. In a multicenter APEX trial using this device, an accurate pressure measurement was obtained in 93% of patients *(57)*.

SURVEILLANCE AFTER EVAR

EVAR offers the advantage of lower perioperative morbidity and mortality but carries the cost of device-related complications such as endoleak, graft migration, graft thrombosis, and structural graft failure. These complications mandate lifelong surveillance following EVAR. The primary goal of follow-up is to identify impending failure while it is still amenable to treatment, preferably catheter-based. Current standard of care EVAR surveillance regimen includes serial contrasted CT scans at 1, 6, and 12 months and yearly thereafter. These recommendations were developed based on initial multicenter studies and as part of standard approval process. Besides being impractical, other concerns expressed with such a regimen include: cumulative contrast load from CT scans *(58)*, potential carcinogenic effects of radiation *(59)*, contrast nephrotoxicity and high costs. In a long-term follow-up cost study following EVAR, Noll et al. identified that current EVAR surveillance regimen comprises 30–35% of the total costs of EVAR follow-up during a 5-year period *(60)*. Based on 5-year follow-up in the US Zenith multicenter trial, Sternbergh et al. *(61)* identified a greatly improved long-term freedom from aneurysm-related morbidity (ARM) in absence of endoleak at 30 and 365 days. In a new EVAR surveillance regimen, authors recommended that in the absence of early endoleak, the 6-month surveillance be eliminated, and suggested aortic ultrasound for long-term surveillance >1 year. Such recommendations, although attractive, are yet to be validated in a randomized, prospective trial. Until such time, periodic contrasted CT scans remains the standard surveillance method.

OPEN SURGICAL VERSUS ENDOVASCULAR REPAIR

Non-randomized comparison of the outcomes from EVAR and open repair demonstrates that the incidence of most systemic complications is lower with EVAR. In their meta-analysis of observational studies conducted prior to 2002, Adriaensen et al. *(62)* found a mean incidence of systemic complications of 9% for EVAR, compared with 25% in the combined studies on open surgery. This, reduced rate of systemic events has been attributed primarily to lower incidences of cardiac and pulmonary complications secondary to lower physiological stress associated with EVAR.

Multiple studies have consistently demonstrated that, compared to open repair, EVAR results in fewer complication, shorter stay in the intensive care unit, shorter hospital stay, and overall more rapid recovery with decreased blood loss *(63–67)*. The operative mortality is reduced from 4.7% (open repair) to 1.7% (EVAR) in two European prospective randomized trials: Endo-Vascular Aneurysm Repair trial (EVAR-I) *(68)* and the Dutch Randomized Endovascular Aneurysm Management trial (DREAM) *(69)*. Recently published U.S. Open versus Endovascular Repair trial (OVER) *(70)* also showed similar outcomes with lower perioperative mortality for EVAR (0.5 vs. 3.0%; $p=0.004$), without significant difference in mortality at 2 years (7.0 vs. 9.8%; $p=0.13$). Unlike DREAM and EVAR-I trials, the early advantage of endovascular repair, in OVER trial, was not offset by increased morbidity or mortality in the first 2 years after repair.

While the short and midterm data validates the safety of EVAR, the long-term data confirming the prolonged efficacy of newer devices is still limited. Although DREAM trial reported that quality of life scores were greater for those patients treated by EVAR, within 6 months, differences were no longer apparent and sexual function scores were similar or better for those who underwent open surgical repair *(71)*. Six-year follow-up results from the DREAM trial *(72)* showed similar long-term survival, for both open and EVAR group, 6 years after randomization with higher rate of secondary interventions in the endovascular group. Cumulative rates of freedom from secondary interventions were 81.9% for open repair and 70.4% for endovascular repair, for a difference of 11.5% points (95% CI, 2.0–21.0; $p=0.03$). After open repair, the most frequent re-intervention was correction of abdominal incisional hernia, whereas EVAR re-interventions were most often performed because of endograft-related complications, such as endoleak and endograft migration.

CONCLUSION

Endovascular repair of aortic aneurysm is a safe modality of treatment with lower perioperative morbidity and mortality compared to open surgical repair. However, this comes at the cost of increased secondary, device-related, complications and interventions. Lifelong surveillance with periodic contrast-enhanced CT scans is mandatory following EVAR since delayed endograft-related complications are known to occur. The early survival advantage of EVAR over open surgical repair is lost by 3 years of follow-up and survival at the end of 6 years remains similar for both procedures. The decisions between open versus EVAR for a AAA must be made by a nonbiased surgeon who is well experienced with both approaches. The patient and family members should also be well educated about the risk of rupture and the morbidity and mortality of each approach and encouraged to participate actively in the decision-making process. Proper patient selection for EVAR, preoperative planning, and surgeon training minimize the perioperative and long-term morbidity and mortality. It is recommended that elective EVAR is best performed at centers that have a documented in-hospital mortality of less than 3% and a primary conversion rate to open surgical repair of less that 2% for elective repair. Further research is needed to study the long-term impact and durability of EVAR as compared to open repair.

THORACIC ENDOVASCULAR AORTIC REPAIR (TEVAR)

Background

Thoracic endovascular aortic repair (TEVAR) is an alternative to open surgical repair that has garnered significant interest since Dake et al. first performed the procedure in 1992 at Stanford University Medical School *(73)*. First generation devices comprised of, stainless-steel Z stents and fabric Dacron sleeves delivered through 24 Fr sheath delivery systems. Early results of the first 103 cases demonstrated the feasibility of TEVAR, with a 5-year mortality of $9 \pm 3\%$ even though 60% of patients were deemed too high risk for open surgical repair. Mulitvariate analysis showed that prior MI and stroke increased the risk of death by 8 and 9-fold respectively *(74)*. Presently, three companies offer FDA-approved available TEVAR devices in the United States:

- Gore TAG (W.L. Gore and Associates, Flagstaff, AZ) (Fig. 17)
- Medtronic Talent, Medtronic Valiant and Captiva (Medtronic Corp., Sunnyvale, CA) (Fig. 18)
- Cook Zenith TX1 and TX2 endografts (Cook Medical, Bloomington, IN, USA) (Fig. 19)

Indications for the Use of TEVAR (See Table 3)

Indications for TEVAR include all symptomatic descending aortic aneurysms and asymptomatic descending aortic aneurysm measuring >6 cm in diameter in patients who are at high risk for open surgical repair. Traumatic transection of the aorta, thoracic dissection with aneurysmal degeneration, and pseudoaneurysms of aorta are newly emerging indications for TEVAR *(75)*. Despite of paucity of clinical data, one important area of use of TEVAR is descending aortic dissection of Stanford Type B (DeBakey III) classification for both acute and chronic presentations.

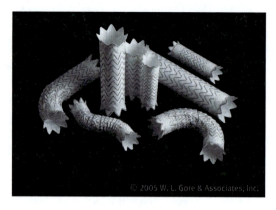

Fig. 17. Gore TAG thoracic stent graft (Courtesy of W.L. Gore and Associates, Flagstaff, AZ).

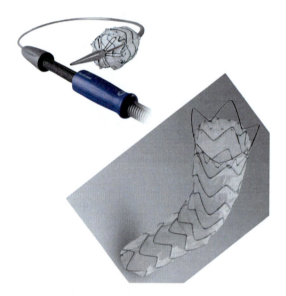

Fig. 18. Medtronic Captiva thoracic stent graft (Courtesy of Medtronic Corporation, Minneapolis, MN, USA).

Descending Thoracic Aorta Aneurysms

The timing of intervention in management of a descending thoracic aortic aneurysm (DTAA), whether endovascular or surgical, is generally based on aneurysm size and/or presence of symptoms. Thoracic aneurysm revascularization guidelines are based upon the natural history of untreated DTAA and corresponding rates of rupture or dissection *(76)*. In descending aorta, the lifetime risk of rupture or dissection for a 7 cm aneurysm is 43%, in contrast to a less than 5% risk when aneurysm is less than 5 cm *(77)*. A currently accepted cut-off for intervention for DTAA is 6 cm or two times the diameter of the normal aortic arch (if present). Adjustments for smaller or larger body sizes have been described, such as, adding 0.6 cm for individuals greater than 6 ft tall, or subtracting the same amount for those less than 5 ft tall. Symptomatic patients include those with backache, pain, and/or discomfort. Aortic dissection can present with sudden

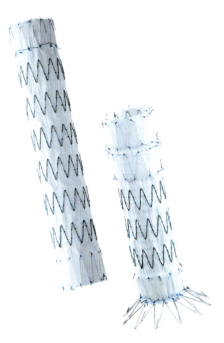

Fig. 19. Cook Zenith thoracic stent graft (Courtesy of Cook Medical Inc., Bloomington, IN, USA).

Table 3
Indications for Thoracic Endovascular Aneurysm Repair

Symptomatic	Descending thoracic aneurysm of any size
	Aortic transaction
	Acute type B dissection
Asymptomatic	Descending thoracic aneurysm >6 cm diameter
	Pseudoaneurysm (traumatic/co-arctation)
	Chronic type B dissection
	Aortic dissection with aneurysmal degeneration

tearing back pain or pain between the shoulder blades. Difficulty in walking and speaking can also accompany the acute event. Thus symptomatic patients should be evaluated for intervention, regardless of aneurysm size *(78)*. Post-infectious pseudoaneurysms such as squeal of tuberculosis are also being treated with endovascular stent graft placement *(79)*. Pseudoaneurysms and saccular aneurysms following dissection or balloon angioplasty for co-arctation probably pose a higher risk for rupture and should be considered for repair *(80)*.

There is no randomized controlled data comparing TEVAR and open surgical repair in the treatment of DTAA. Comparative data in the form of non-randomized trials and use of historical controls has shown that TEVAR may offer lower operative mortality and morbidity when compared to surgical aortic repair for DTA *(81, 82)*. Intermediate and long-term follow-up do not show a clear advantage of one approach over the other in terms of survival *(83)*. Similar to EVAR, the complications of TEVAR including endoleak, endograft migration, and stent fracture and may negate the "up-front" benefit of lower surgical mortality and morbidity. Post-procedure surveillance after TEVAR is also more frequent than with open repair secondary to the possibility of late complications *(84)*.

Acute Type B Aortic Dissection

Prior to the advent of TEVAR, patients with life-threatening complications due to acute Type B or "retro" Type A aortic dissection fared no better with open surgical repair vs. medical therapy *(85)*. TEVAR offers a less invasive intervention to prevent rupture or complications of an expanding dissection. In the earliest series of patients undergoing emergency TEVAR for acute Type B or "retro" Type A dissections, operative mortality was 16% with survival of 73% at 5 years *(86)*. Key to successful outcome in treatment of acute type B aortic dissection includes deployment of the endovascular graft at the site of an intimal tear while keeping the endograft length to a minimum. Low-volume case series have shown benefit of stent graft placement for acute type B dissection *(87)*. However, a recent randomized clinical trial comparing conservative management vs. stent grafting for type B acute dissection showed no additional benefit. INSTEAD (The Investigation of Stent grafts in patients with type B Aortic Dissection) – in this trial medical treatment and endovascular grafts for uncomplicated type B dissection showed equivalent mortality at 1 year *(88)*.

Chronic Type B Aortic Dissection

Treatment of Type B or DeBakey III aortic dissection has been primarily medical, through the attempts to decrease arterial wall tension (dP/dT) using beta-blockade and or other anti-hypertensives *(89)*. Emergent stent grafting in Type B aortic dissections have been performed for rupture, visceral or limb malperfusion, persistent and refractory back pain *(89)*.

Open surgical repair in these cases is usually reserved for patients experiencing late complications including recalcitrant pain, visceral, renal and limb mal-perfusion, uncontrolled hypertension, continuing aortic dilatation, or those patients who are at high risk of rupture *(90)*. Mortality and presence of late complications are related to patency of the false aortic lumen *(91)*. Additionally, patients with spontaneous thrombosis of the false lumen (4% of all Type B dissections) have been shown to have improved long-term outcomes. The use of TEVAR was proposed as a way to exclude the false lumen and improve aortic remodeling, thereby improving patient survival and decrease the occurrence of late complications *(92)*. The INSTEAD trial was a prospective randomized trail comparing optimal medical therapy to stent graft placement. This trial demonstrated that thoracic stent graft (TEVAR) placement failed to improve the rates of 2-year survival and adverse events when compared with optimal medical treatment. The frequency of aortic remodeling was significantly higher in the TEVAR group than the medical therapy group (91 vs. 14%) *(93)*. Preliminary results, from non-randomized trials and registries, suggested that TEVAR might be safer than open surgical repair, primarily due to lower rates of death and stroke *(83, 94)*.

Other Indications

Given the lower morbidity and mortality associated with the procedure and presence of landing zones of relatively normal aorta, the use of TEVAR in localized disease of the aorta is attractive. Penetrating aortic ulcers, first described in the medical literature as "dissection without intimal tear," occur in a patient population with high surgical risk and may most benefit from a less-invasive procedure. The treatment of acute, traumatic aortic transaction using TEVAR also offers the benefit of lower procedural mortality and morbidity in patients who may also be at high surgical risk due to concurrent trauma injury.

The RESCUE trial is an ongoing clinical trial to evaluate the clinical safety and effectiveness of the Valiant Thoracic Stent Graft with the Captivia Delivery System (Medtronic) in the endovascular treatment of blunt thoracic aortic injury in adult patients. This study will enroll 50 patients in up to 25 sites and patients will be followed for next 5 years.

TEVAR TECHNIQUE

Case Planning

TEVAR cases are done in hybrid labs under adequate fluoroscopy that allows digital subtraction imaging and large field image intensifier. The air exchange in the room should suffice for common femoral artery cut down in case a conduit placement is desired. Multidisciplinary approach to patient care involving the endovascular operators from vascular surgery or cardiology or interventional radiology and anesthesia should coordinate together for optimal outcomes. CT angiogram with 3D reconstruction is desirable modality for case planning. Magnetic resonance angiogram is also acceptable and conventional angiogram with intravascular ultrasound can be complimentary.

Aortic Arch Anatomy

Knowledge of five zones in the aortic arch is helpful in planning TEVAR cases:

Zone 0: Proximal to innominate artery
Zone 1: Between the innominate and left carotid
Zone 2: Between left carotid and left subclavian
Zone 3: From left subclavian orifice to 2 cm distal to it
Zone 4: Thoracic aorta >2 cm distal to the left subclavian artery

Left Subclavian Artery Coverage and Revascularization

Left subclavian artery coverage is needed when there is <2 cm of proximal landing zone for the thoracic endograft to achieve adequate seal. Carotid to subclavian bypass is recommended in patients with dominant left vertebral artery, patent LIMA to LAD bypass, anomalous origin of left vertebral artery from the aortic arch and left arm AV fistula.

Spinal Drainage

Indications for preoperative spinal drainage include planned extensive coverage of the thoracic aorta, use of two devices, previous infrarenal AAA repair, coverage of left subclavian artery, and cases of aortic dissection with visceral malperfusion.

Vascular Access

The common femoral access arteries should be free of significant calcification and external iliac artery diameters should be able to accommodate at least 20–24 Fr devices. Severe tortuosity, calcification, atherosclerosis, and stenosis of the iliac arteries can be potential barriers to passage of large bore TEVAR devices. In difficult access cases conduit of at least 10–12 mm can be sutured into the common femoral artery.

CONTRAINDICATIONS

General

Patients with life expectancy less than 6 months, patients with active sepsis and infectious aneurysms.

Aortic Arch

Tortuous aortic arch that will impede the delivery of thoracic stent graft, severe atherosclerosis of the aortic arch, significant thrombus and localized dissection preventing proper seal of the proximal and distal thoracic stent graft.

Vascular Access

Small caliber iliac artery, severe atherosclerotic disease of the iliac artery with calcification.

Branches

Inability to provide adequate perfusion of vital organs and cerebral vessels post-stent grafting.

COMPLICATIONS

Vascular access complications include bleeding, hematoma retroperitoneal bleed and infection. Forceful insertion of large caliber devices, through narrow/diseased external iliac arteries, can cause a catastrophic rupture or dissection. Inadvertent coverage of large cervical branches by the device can lead to stroke, myocardial infarction, endoleaks, and death.

PROCEDURAL STEPS

1. Patient is placed supine in a hybrid endovascular laboratory under general anesthesia.
2. Ipsilateral femoral artery cut down or pre-closure using the Perclose (Abbott Laboratories, California) is achieved to accommodate large-bore thoracic stent graft. Ipsilateral side is chosen based on less tortuosity of and larger caliber of the iliac artery.
3. Systemic heparanization, to achieve an activated clotting time of >250 s.
4. A super stiff wire of 0.035 in. is placed over a pigtail catheter across the aortic arch with the tip of the wire in the ascending aorta.
5. Contra lateral femoral access is obtained using a percutaneous technique and a 5 Fr sheath is placed.
6. A pigtail catheter is placed from the contra lateral limb for imaging and intravascular ultrasound if needed.
7. The device is advanced over the super stiff wire and the fabric of the graft is placed at the proximal landing zone. Imaging of the aneurysm, proximal, and distal portions of the aorta is obtained on a digital subtraction mode.

8. Breathing is suspended in intubated patients to minimize movement. Adenosine is simultaneously given at a dose of 32 mg to obtain cardiac arrest for 4–5 s. An alternative technique is to use pacing at 250–300 beats/min. The systolic BP should be around 100 mmHg for precise device deployment.
9. Post-dilatation is performed, following the device deployment, using large volume, device-specific, balloon that will mold the stent graft to the aorta.
10. The pig tail catheter is withdrawn prior to post-dilatation and the graft is re-cannulated using a soft tip 0.035 in. wire.
11. Final angiogram is obtained and special attention is paid for endoleak and exclusion of the aneurysmal sac.
12. Vascular closure is performed using the pre-placed Perclose system (Abbott Laboratories, California).

POST-IMPLANT CARE

Aggressive risk factor reduction is instituted in the post-operative phase and continued following discharge from the hospital. Risk factor reduction for atherosclerosis includes Aspirin, ACE inhibitors or angiotensin-II receptor blockers, statins and tobacco cessation.

DISCHARGE

Patients with spinal drain are observed for 48–72 h and sent home when stable after removing the spinal drain. If no spinal drain was placed prior to procedure, patients are ambulated within 24 h, if stable, followed by a discharge within 24–48 h of TEVAR implantation.

FOLLOW-UP

One week for groin check to evaluate for access site complications.

One month with CT scan to evaluate size of aneurysm and endoleaks.

If there is no increase in size of the aneurysm at 6-month follow-up CT scan, then annual evaluation using a contrasted CT scan is instituted.

CONCLUSION

Thoracic aortic aneurysms are co-existent in some patients with AAAs. Symptomatic and large aneurysms greater than 6 cm need intervention. TEVAR has demonstrated promising results and efficacy in management of DTAA. Emergent indications include traumatic transaction, pseudo aneurysms, and type B dissections. Early vascular access complications, endoleaks, and device fracture continue to be the Achilles heel of TEVAR.

CASE 1 (SEE FIGS. 20–23)

A 48-year-old patient presented to us with a past history open surgical repair for co-arctation of aorta at ages of 9 months and at 9 years. He had subsequently undergone a balloon angioplasty for recurrent co-arctation of aorta at the age of 18 years. Patient now presented to us with back pain at age of 48 years. CT scan of abdomen and pelvis showed descending aortic pseudoaneurysm measuring 6×4 cm distal to the left subclavian artery. Patient underwent left subclavian to left carotid bypass followed by an elective thoracic aortic stent graft placement using a Medtronic thoracic CAPTIVA endograft for exclusion of the pseudoaneurysm. Spinal drainage for 48 h was also performed. Patient was discharged home following an uneventful hospital course.

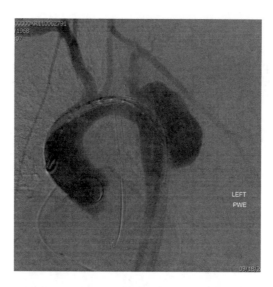

Fig. 20. Baseline angiogram following a pre-TEVAR carotid-subclavian bypass, demonstrating a large pseudoaneurysm distal to the left subclavian artery.

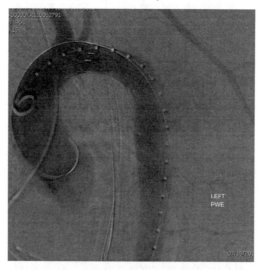

Fig. 21. Successful deployment of thoracic stent graft.

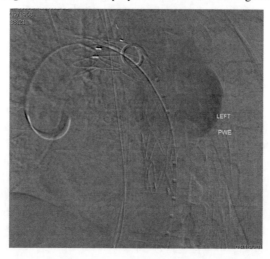

Fig. 22. Endoleak noted on the completion angiogram.

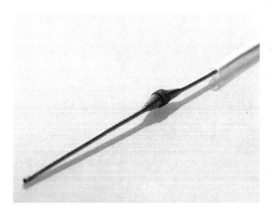

Fig. 23. Pigtail stationed inside the endoprosthesis demonstrating type IV endoleak in absence of proximal or distal endoleak (Courtesy of Medtronic Corporation, Minneapolis, MN).

REFERENCES

1. Johnston KW, Rutherford RB, Tilson MD, et al. Suggested standards for reporting on arterial aneurysms. Subcommittee on Reporting Standards for Arterial Aneurysms, Ad Hoc Committee on Reporting Standards, Society of Vascular Surgery and North American Chapter, International Society for Cardiovascular Surgery. *J Vasc Surg.* 1991;13:452.
2. Ailawadi G, Eliason JL, Upchurch GR Jr. Current concepts in the pathogenesis of abdominal aortic aneurysm. *J Vasc Surg.* 2003;38:584.
3. Lederle FA, Johnson GR, Wilson SE, et al. The aneurysm detection and management study screening program: validation cohort and final results. Aneurysm Detection and Management Veterans Affairs Cooperative Study Investigators. *Arch Intern Med.* 2000;160:1425.
4. Shantikumar S, Ajjan R, Porter KE, Scott DJ, et al. Diabetes and the abdominal aortic aneurysm. *Eur J Vasc Endovasc Surg.* 2010;39(2):200–207.
5. Lederle FA, Simel DL. The rational clinical examination. Does this patient have abdominal aortic aneurysm? *JAMA.* 1999;281:77–82.
6. Jaakkola P, Hippelainen M, Farin P, et al. Interobserver variability in measuring the dimensions of the abdominal aorta: comparison of ultrasound and computed tomography. *Eur J Vasc Endovasc Surg.* 1996;12:230–237.
7. Fleming C, Whitlock EP, Beil TL, Lederle FA. Screening for abdominal aortic aneurysm: a best-evidence systematic review for the U.S. Preventive Services Task Force. *Ann Intern Med.* 2005;142:203–211.
8. Wilmink AB, Forshaw M, Quick CR, Hubbard CS, Day NE. Accuracy of serial screening for abdominal aortic aneurysms by ultrasound. *J Med Screen.* 2002;9:125–127.
9. Crow P, Shaw E, Earnshaw JJ, Poskitt KR, Whyman MR, Heather BP. A single normal ultrasonographic scan at age 65 years rules out significant aneurysm disease for life in men. *Br J Surg.* 2001;88:941–944
10. Scott RA, Bridgewater SG, Ashton HA. Randomized clinical trial of screening for abdominal aortic aneurysm in women. *Br J Surg.* 2002;89:283–285.
11. Kent KC, Zwolak RM, Jaff MR, et al. Screening for abdominal aortic aneurysm: a consensus statement. *J Vasc Surg.* 2004;39:267–269.
12. Derubertis BG, Trocciola SM, Rayer EJ, et al. Abdominal aortic aneurysm in women: prevalence, risk factors, and implications of screening. *J Vasc Surg.* 2007;46:630–635.
13. Ferket BS, Grootenboer N, Colkesen EB, et al. Systematic review of guidelines on abdominal aortic aneurysm screening. *J Vasc Surg.* 2011.
14. Bengtsson H, Bergqvist D. Ruptured abdominal aortic aneurysm: a population-based study. *J Vasc Surg.* 1993;18:74–80.

15. Bown MJ, Sutton AJ, Bell PR, Sayers RD. A meta-analysis of 50 years of ruptured abdominal aortic aneurysm repair. *Br J Surg.* 2002;89:714–730.
16. Hoornweg LL, Storm-Versloot MN, Ubbink DT, et al. Meta analysis on mortality of ruptured abdominal aortic aneurysms. *Eur J Vasc Endovasc Surg.* 2008;35:558–570.
17. Marston WA, Ahlquist R, Johnson G Jr, Meyer AA. Misdiagnosis of ruptured abdominal aortic aneurysms. *J Vasc Surg.* 1992;16:17–22.
18. Akkersdijk GJ, van Bockel JH. Ruptured abdominal aortic aneurysm: initial misdiagnosis and the effect on treatment. *Eur J Surg.* 1998;164:29–34.
19. Baxter BT, McGee GS, Flinn WR, et al. Distal embolization as a presenting symptom of aortic aneurysms. *Am J Surg.* 1990;160:197–201.
20. Szilagyi DE, Smith RF, DeRusso FJ, et al. Contribution of abdominal aortic aneurysmectomy to prolongation of life. *Ann Surg.* 1966;164:678–699.
21. Foster JH, Bolasny BL, Gobbel WG Jr, Scott HW Jr. Comparative study of elective resection and expectant treatment of abdominal aortic aneurysm. *Surg Gynecol Obstet.* 1969;129:1–9.
22. Darling RC, Messina CR, Brewster DC, Ottinger LW. Autopsy study of unoperated abdominal aortic aneurysms, The case for early resection. *Circulation.* 1977;56(3suppl):II161–II164.
23. Brewster DC, Cronenwett JL, Hallett JW Jr, Johnston KW, Krupski WC, Matsumura JS. Guidelines for the treatment of abdominal aortic aneurysms. Report of a subcommittee of the Joint Council of the American Association for Vascular Surgery and Society for Vascular Surgery. *J Vasc Surg.* 2003;37:1106–1117.
24. Brown LC, Powell JT. Risk factors for aneurysm rupture in patients kept under ultrasound surveillance. UK Small Aneurysm Trial Participants. *Ann Surg.* 1999;230:289–296.
25. Hirsch AT, Haskal ZJ, Hertzer NR, et al. ACC/AHA 2005 Practice Guidelines for the management of patients with peripheral arterial disease (lower extremity, renal, mesenteric, and abdominal aortic): a collaborative report from the American Association for Vascular Surgery/ Society for Vascular Surgery, Society for Cardiovascular Angiography and Interventions, Society for Vascular Medicine and Biology, Society of Interventional Radiology, and the ACC/AHA Task Force on Practice Guidelines (Writing Committee to Develop Guidelines for the Management of Patients With Peripheral Arterial Disease): endorsed by the American Association of Cardiovascular and Pulmonary Rehabilitation; National Heart, Lung, and Blood Institute; Society for Vascular Nursing; TransAtlantic Inter-Society Consensus; and Vascular Disease Foundation. *Circulation.* 2006;113: e463–e654.
26. Cronenwett JL, Sargent SK, Wall MH, et al. Variables that affect the expansion rate and outcome of small abdominal aortic aneurysms. *J Vasc Surg.* 1990;11:260–268.
27. Stringfellow MM, Lawrence PF, Stringfellow RG. The influence of aorta-aneurysm geometry upon stress in the aneurysm wall. *J Surg Res.* 1987;42:425–433.
28. Brady AR, Fowkes FG, Greenhalgh RM, et al. Risk factors for postoperative death following elective surgical repair of abdominal aortic aneurysm: results from the UK Small Aneurysm Trial. On behalf of the UK Small Aneurysm Trial participants. *Br J Surg.* 2000;87:742–749.
29. Blankensteijn JD, Lindenburg FP, Van der Graaf Y, Eikelboom BC. Influence of study design on reported mortality and morbidity rates after abdominal aortic aneurysm repair. *Br J Surg.* 1998;85:1624–1630.
30. Steyerberg EW, Kievit J, de Mol Van Otterloo JC, et al. Perioperative mortality of elective abdominal aortic aneurysm surgery. A clinical prediction rule based on literature and individual patient data. *Arch Intern Med.* 1995;155:1998–2004.
31. Nowygrod R, Egorova N, Greco G, Anderson P, Gelijns A, Moskowitz A, et al. Trends, complications, and mortality in peripheral vascular surgery. *J Vasc Surg.* 2006;43:205–216.
32. Tan JWC, Yeo KK, Laird JR. Food and Drug Administration–approved endovascular repair devices for abdominal aortic aneurysms: a review. *J Vasc Interv Radiol.* 2008;19:S9–S17.
33. Chaikof EL, Brewster DC, Dalman RL, et al. The care of patients with an abdominal aortic aneurysm: The Society for Vascular Surgery practice guidelines. *J Vasc Surg.* 2009;50 (8S):1S–49S.
34. http://www.medtronic.com/your-health/abdominal-aortic-aneurysm/important-safety-information/index.htm#talent.
35. Dillavou ED, Muluk SC, Rhee RY, Tzeng E, Woody JD, Gupta N, et al. Does hostile neck anatomy preclude successful endovascular aortic aneurysm repair? *J Vasc Surg.* 2003;38:657–663.

36. Stanley BM, Semmens JB, Mai Q, et al. Evaluation of patient selection guidelines for endoluminal AAA repair with the Zenith stent-graft: the Australasian experience. *J Endovasc Ther.* 2001;8:457–464.
37. Wolf YG, Fogarty TJ, Olcott C IV, et al. Endovascular repair of abdominal aortic aneurysms: eligibility rate and impact on the rate of open repair. *J Vasc Surg.* 2000;32:519–523.
38. AbuRahma AF, Campbell JE, Mousa AY, et al. Clinical outcomes for hostile versus favorable aortic neck anatomy in endovascular aortic aneurysm repair using modular devices. *J Vasc Surg.* 2011;54(1):13–21.
39. Lee WA, O'Dorisio J, Wolf YG, Hill BB, Fogarty TJ, Zarins CK. Outcome after unilateral hypogastric occlusion during endovascular aneurysm repair. *J Vasc Surg.* 2001;33:921–926.
40. Rhee RY, Muluk SC, Tzeng E, Missig-Carroll N, Makaroun MS. Can the internal iliac artery be safely covered during endovascular repair of abdominal aortic and iliac artery aneurysms? *Ann Vasc Surg.* 2002;16:29–36.
41. Torsello G, Tessarek J, Kasprzak B, Klenk E. Treatment of aortic aneurysm with a complete percutaneous technique. *Dtsch Med Wochenschr.* 2002;127:1453–1457.
42. Lee WA, Brown MP, Nelson PR, Huber TS, Seeger JM. Midterm outcomes of femoral arteries after percutaneous endovascular aortic repair using the Preclose technique. *J Vasc Surg.* 2008;47:919–923.
43. Lee WA, Brown MP, Nelson PR, Huber TS. Total percutaneous access for endovascular aortic aneurysm repair ("Preclose" technique). *J Vasc Surg.* 2007;45:1095–1101.
44. Elsenack M, Umscheid T, Tesserek J, Torsello GF, Torsello GB. Percutaneous endovascular aortic aneurysm repair: a prospective evaluation of safety, efficiency, and risk factors. *J Endovasc Ther.* 2009;16:708–713.
45. Mehta M, Veith FJ, Ohki T, Cynamon J, Goldstein K, Suggs WD, et al. Unilateral and bilateral hypogastric artery interruption during aortoiliac aneurysm repair in 154 patients: a relatively innocuous procedure. *J Vasc Surg.* 2001;33:S27–S32.
46. Geraghty PJ, Sanchez LA, Rubin BG, et al. Overt ischemic colitis after endovascular repair of aortoiliac aneurysms. *J Vasc Surg.* 2004;40:413–418.
47. Dadian N, Ohki T, Veith FJ, et al. Overt colon ischemia after endovascular aneurysm repair: the importance of microembolization as an etiology. *J Vasc Surg.* 2001;34:986–996.
48. Stavropoulos SW, Chandragundla SR. Imaging techniques for detection and management of endoleaks after endovascular aortic aneurysm repair. *Radiology.* 2007;243:641–655.
49. White GH, Yu W, May J, et al. Endoleak as a complication of endoluminal grafting of abdominal aortic aneurysms: classification, incidence, diagnosis and management. *J Endovasc Surg.* 1997;4:152–168.
50. Kim JK, Noll RE Jr, Tonnessen BH, Sternbergh 3rd WC: A technique for increased accuracy in the placement of the "giant" Palmaz stent for treatment of type IA endoleak after endovascular abdominal aneurysm repair. *J Vasc Surg.* 2008;48:755–757.
51. Varcoe RL, Laird MP, Frawley JE. A novel alternative to open conversion for type 1 endoleak resulting in ruptured aneurysm. *Vasc Endovascular Surg.* 2008;42:391–393.
52. Chuter TA, Faruqi RM, Sawhney R, et al. Endoleak after endovascular repair of abdominal aortic aneurysm. *J Vasc Surg.* 2001;34:98–105.
53. Brewster DC, Jones JE, Chung TK, et al. Long-term outcomes after endovascular abdominal aortic aneurysm repair: the first decade. *Ann Surg.* 2006;244:426–438.
54. Jonker FH, Aruny J, Muhs BE. Management of type II endoleaks: preoperative versus postoperative versus expectant management. *Semin Vasc Surg.* 2009;22:165–171.
55. Naoki T, Tetsuji F, Yuji K and Takao O. Endotension following endovascular aneurysm repair. *Vasc Med.* 2008;13:305–311.
56. Lin, PH, Bush, RL, Katzman, JB, et al. Delayed aortic aneurysm enlargement due to endotension after endovascular abdominal aortic aneurysm repair. *J Vasc Surg.* 2003;38:840–842.
57. Ohki T, Ouriel K, Silveria PG, Katzen B, White R, Diethrich E. Initial results of wireless pressure sensing for EVAR: the APEX trial—Acute Pressure Measurement to Confirm Aneurysm Sac Exclusion. *J Vasc Surg.* 2007;45:236–242.
58. Alsac JM, Zarins CK, Heikkinen MA, et al. The impact of aortic endografts on renal function. *J Vasc Surg.* 2005;41:921–930.

59. Brenner DJ and Hall EJ. Computed tomography—an increasing source of radiation exposure. *N Engl J Med.* 2007;357:2277–2284.
60. Noll RE Jr, Tonnessen BH, Mannava K, Money SR, Sternbergh WC III. Long-term follow-up cost after endovascular aneurysm repair. *J Vasc Surg.* 2007;46:9–15.
61. Sternbergh WC 3rd, Greenberg RK, Chuter TA, Tonnessen BH. Redefining postoperative surveillance after endovascular aneurysm repair: recommendations based on 5-year follow-up in the US Zenith multicenter trial. *J Vasc Surg.* 2008;48:278–284.
62. Adriaensen MEAP, Bosch JL, Halpern EF, Myriam Hunink MG, Gazelle GS. Elective endovascular versus open surgical repair of abdominal aortic aneurysms: systematic review of short-term results. *Radiology.* 2002;224:739–747
63. Moore WS, Rutherford RB. Transfemoral endovascular repair of abdominal aortic aneurysms: results of the North American EVT phase 1 trial. *J Vasc Surg.* 1996;23:543–553.
64. Matsumura JS, Brewster DC, Makaroun MS, Naftel DC. A multicenter controlled clinical trial of open versus endovascular treatment of abdominal aortic aneurysm. *J Vasc Surg.* 2003;37:262–271.
65. Becquemin JP, Bourriez A, D'Audiffret A, et al. Mid-term results of endovascular versus open repair for abdominal aortic aneurysm in patients anatomically suitable for endovascular repair. *Eur J Vasc Endovasc Surg.* 2000;19:656–661.
66. May J, White GH, Waugh R, et al. Improved survival after endoluminal repair with second-generation prosthesis compared with open repair in the treatment of abdominal aortic aneurysms: a five-year concurrent comparison using life-table method. *J Vasc Surg.* 2001;33:S21–S26.
67. Hua HT, Cambria RP, Chuang SK et al. Early outcomes of endovascular versus open abdominal aortic aneurysm repair in the National Surgical Quality Improvement Program-Private Sector (NSQIP-PS). *J Vasc Surg.* 2005;41:382–389.
68. EVAR trial participants. Endovascular aneurysm repair versus open repair in patients with abdominal aortic aneurysm (EVAR trial 1): randomized controlled trial. *Lancet.* 2005;365:2179–2186.
69. Prinssen M, Verhoeven EL, Buth J, et al. Dutch Randomized Endovascular Aneurysm Management (DREAM) Trial Group. A randomized trial comparing conventional and endovascular repair of abdominal aortic aneurysms. *N Engl M Med.* 2004;351:1607–1618.
70. Lederle FA, Freishlag JA, Kyriakides TC, et al. Open Versus Endovascular Repair (OVER) Veterans Affairs Cooperative Study Group. Outcomes following endovascular vs open repair of abdominal aortic aneurysm: a randomized trial. *JAMA.* 2009;302: 1435–1442.
71. Blankensteijn JD, de Jong SE, Prinssen M, et al. Two-year outcomes after conventional or endovascular repair of abdominal aortic aneurysms. *N Engl J Med.* 2005;352:2398–2405.
72. De Bruin JL, Bass AF, Buth J, et al. For the DREAM Study group. Long-term outcome of Open or Endovascular Repair of Abdominal Aortic Aneurysm. *N Engl J Med.* 2010;362:1881–1889.
73. Dake MD, Kato N, Mitchell RS, et al. Endovascular stentgraft placement for the treatment of acute aortic dissection. *N Engl J Med.* 1999;340:1546 –1552.
74. Nienaber CA, Fattori R, Lund G, et al. Nonsurgical reconstruction of thoracic aortic dissection by stent-graft placement. *N Engl J Med.* 1999;340:1539–1545.
75. Dagenais F, Shetty R, Normand JP, Turcotte R, Mathieu P, Voisine P. Extended applications of thoracic aortic stent grafts. *Ann Thorac Surg.* 2006;82:567–572
76. Davies RR, Goldstein LJ, Coady MA, et al. Yearly rupture or dissection rates for thoracic aortic aneurysms: simple prediction based on size. *Ann Thorac Surg.* 2002;73:17–28.
77. Coady MA, Rizzo JA, Hammond GL, et al. What is the appropriate size criterion for resection of thoracic aortic aneurysms? *J Thorac Cardiovasc Surg.* 1997;113:476 –491.
78. Coady MA, Rizzo JA, Elefteriades JA. Developing surgical intervention criteria for thoracic aortic aneurysms. *Cardiol Clin.* 1999;17:827–839.
79. Loh YJ, Tay KH, Mathew S, Tan KL, Cheah FK, Sin YK. Endovascular stent graft treatment of leaking thoracic aortic tuberculous pseudoaneurysm. *Singapore Med J.* 2007;48(7):e193–195.
80. Kutty S, Greenberg RK, Fletcher S, Svensson LG, Latson LA. Endovascular stent grafts for large thoracic aneurysms after coarctation repair. *Ann Thorac Surg.* 2008;85(4):1332–1338.
81. Makaroun MS, Dillavou ED, Kee ST, et al. Endovascular treatment of thoracic aortic aneurysms: results of the phase II multicenter trial of the GORE TAG thoracic endoprosthesis. *J Vasc Surg.* 2005;41:1:9.

82. Cho JS, Haider SE, Makaroun MS. US multicenter trials of endoprostheses for the endovascular treatment of descending thoracic aneurysms. *J Vasc Surg*. 2006;43(supplA)12A:9A.
83. Coady MA, Rizzo JA, Goldstein LJ, Elefteriades JA. Natural history, pathogenesis, and etiology of thoracic aortic aneurysms and dissections. *Cardiol Clin*. 1999;17:615– 635;vii.
84. Cheng D, Martin J, et al. TEVAR versus open surgical repair of the descending aorta. *JACC*. 2010;55:987–1001.
85. LG Svensson, et al. Expert consensus document on the treatment of descending thoracic aortic disease using endovascular stent-grafts. *Ann Thorac Surg*. 2008;85:S1–41.
86. Glower DD, Fann JI, Speier RH, et al. Comparison of medical and surgical therapy for uncomplicated descending aortic dissection. *Circulation*. 1990;82:IV39–IV46.
87. Hausegger KA, Tiesenhausen K, Schedlbauer P, Oberwalder P, Tauss J, Rigler B. Cardiovasc treatment of acute aortic type B dissection with stent-grafts. *Intervent Radiol*. 2001;24(5):306–312.
88. Nienaber CA, Kische S, Akin I, et al. Strategies for subacute/chronic type B aortic dissection: the Investigation of Stent Grafts in Patients with type B Aortic Dissection (INSTEAD) trial 1-year outcome. *J Thorac Cardiovasc Surg*. 2010;140(6suppl):S101–S108; discussion S142–S146.
89. Elefteriades JA, Constantinos JL, Coady MA, et al. Management of descending aortic dissection. *Ann Thorac Surg*. 1999;67:2002–2005.
90. Masaaki K, Hong-zhi B, Kenji S, et al. Determining surgical indications for acute type b dissection based on enlargement of aortic diameter during the chronic phase. *Circulation*. 1995;92:107–112.
91. Erbel R, Oelert H, Meyer J, et al. Effect of medical and surgical therapy on aortic dissection evaluated by transesophageal echocardiography. Implications for prognosis and therapy. The European Cooperative Study Group on Echocardiography. *Circulation*. 1993;87:1604–1615.
92. Huptas S, Mehta RH, Kühl H, et al. Aortic remodeling in type B aortic dissection: effects of endovascular stent-graft repair and medical treatment on true and false lumen volumes. *J Endovasc Ther*. 2009;16:28–38.
93. Nienaber C, Rousseau H, Eggebrecht H, et al. Randomized comparison of strategies for type B aortic dissection: the INvestigation of STEnt grafts in Aortic Dissection (INSTEAD) trial. *Circulation*. 2009;120:2519–2528.
94. Umana JP, Lai DT, Mitchell RS, et al. Is medical therapy still the optimal treatment strategy for patients with acute type B aortic dissections? *J Thorac Cardiovasc Surg*. 2002;124:896–910.

9 Venous Intervention

Andrew B. McCann, MBBS,
and *Robert M. Schainfeld*, DO

CONTENTS

    CATHETER-DIRECTED THROMBOLYSIS
    PERCUTANEOUS MECHANICAL THROMBECTOMY
    ILIOFEMORAL DVT
    CHRONIC OBSTRUCTIVE LESIONS OF THE ILIAC VEIN
    IVC OBSTRUCTION
    IVC FILTERS
    SUPERIOR VENA CAVA FILTER PLACEMENT
    RETRIEVABLE IVC FILTERS
    AXILLOSUBCLAVIAN VEIN THROMBOSIS
    ALGORITHM FOR THE MANAGEMENT OF AXILLOSUBCLAVIAN
    SUPERIOR VENA CAVA SYNDROME
    REFERENCES

CATHETER-DIRECTED THROMBOLYSIS

Despite standard anticoagulant therapy, approximately 29–79% of patients with deep venous thrombosis (DVT) develop some symptomatic manifestations of post-thrombotic syndrome (PTS). The rapid and complete thrombus dissolution commonly achieved with thrombolytic therapy could potentially reduce the incidence of this dreaded complication. The benefits of early thrombus removal supported by experimental studies show that thrombolysis of acute DVT preserves valve and endothelial functions.

Catheter-directed thrombolysis (CDT) has emerged as a superior means of thrombolytic agent administration in the treatment of acute venous thromboembolic diseases. Direct infusion of thrombolytic agents into thrombosed segments can achieve high local concentrations of lytic agent that can theoretically accelerate thrombolysis, which increases the likelihood of a successful clinical outcome. Reducing the overall dose and duration of infusion of these agents has the potential to limit systemic bleeding risk when compared with systemic thrombolysis.

Pharmacologic thrombolysis is most likely to be successful when clot is fresh (<3 days old) and much less effective when presumed to be chronic, after 4 weeks *(1)*. A number of thrombolytic agents are available, differing in terms of their biological half-lives, fibrin affinity and specificity, time to clot lysis and dosing. These include alteplase, reteplase, tenectaplase, streptokinase and urokinase. None has specific FDA approval for use in DVT.

Large-scale randomized clinical trials evaluating the efficacy of CDT in venous thromboembolic disease have not been performed. Single-arm studies compared with historical controls suggest catheter-directed lysis could improve venous patency and preserve valvular function when compared with anticoagulation alone. Because of methodological flaws in small single center trials, it is not possible to draw definitive conclusions about the effects of thrombolytic therapy on the incidence of PTS. The largest published experience with CDT comes from the multicenter National Venous Thrombolysis Registry, a prospective, multi-center study, which evaluated CDT using urokinase in 303 limbs of 287 patients treated in both academic and community centers. Sixty-six percent had acute DVT, 16% had chronic DVT, and 19% had an acute episode superimposed upon a chronic condition. Iliofemoral (71%) and femoropopliteal DVT (25%) represented the anatomic distribution of thrombus in these patients. Phlebographic evaluation showed that complete lysis occurred in 31% and partial (50–99%) lysis in 52% of the cases. In 17% of the patients, less than 50% of the thrombus was dissolved. In the subgroup of patients with acute, first-time iliofemoral DVT, 65% of the patients achieved complete clot lysis. During follow-up, thrombosis-free survival was observed in 65% at 6 months and in 60% at 1 year. The degree of lysis was predictive of sustained vessel patency. In those with complete clot dissolution, vein patency at 1 year was 78% compared with only 37% of patients with only partial (<50%) lysis. Vein patency was associated with improved valvular function. Sixty-two percent of the patients with less than 50% clot lysis exhibited valvular incompetence, as compared to 72% of the patients who had complete lysis and resultant normal valve function ($p<0.02$). Importantly, in the sub-group of patients with acute, first-time iliofemoral DVT who had initial successful thrombolysis, 96% of the veins remained patent at 1 year. Major bleeding occurred in 11%, most commonly at venous access sites (39%) and 13% were retroperitoneal bleeds. Minor bleeding was reported in 16% of the cases. Intracranial hemorrhage occurred in 0.2%. Pulmonary embolism occurred during treatment in 1% of the patients, and two deaths were reported, with a mortality rate of 0.4% in the entire series *(2)*. More recent reports of CDT for DVT showed a reduction in major bleeding events by about half, possibly as a result of more careful patient selection *(3)*. These studies suggest that CDT for DVT achieves more rapid lysis, may reduce pain and edema, improves quality of life, preserves valvular competence, and completely restores vessel patency as compared with standard anticoagulation or systemic thrombolytic therapy, although at the expense of a higher rate of hemorrhagic complications.

At present, CDT should be reserved for exceptional circumstances, such as patients with limb-threatening ischemia caused by phlegmasia cerulea dolens, and in young patients with extensive iliofemoral/inferior vena caval (IVC) DVT where the risk–benefit ratio is favorable. Other candidates who potentially might benefit from CDT are those with multi-segment DVT, those with expected long-term survival and individuals who remain symptomatic despite therapeutic anticoagulation. Additional randomized trials are warranted to specifically address these issues.

In an era when all clinicians seek adherence to evidence-based guidelines, with few exceptions, patients with DVT or PE are treated similarly. Specifically, with regard to the role of adjunctive therapy with pharmacologic thrombolysis, the recently published American College of Chest Physician (3) guidelines is as follows:

- The routine use of systemic lytic therapy is not recommended in patients with DVT or PE (Grade 1A).
- The routine use of CDT is not recommended in patients with DVT (Grade 1C).
- In selected DVT patients with extensive acute proximal DVT (e.g., iliofemoral/IVC, symptoms <14 days, good functional status, life expectancy >1 year) who have a low risk of bleeding, CDT may be used to reduce symptoms and patient morbidity if appropriate expertise and resources are available (Grade 2B).
- After successful CDT in patients with acute DVT, correction of underlying venous lesions using balloon angioplasty and stents is recommended (Grade 2C).
- Pharmacomechanical thrombolysis (e.g., inclusion of thrombus fragmentation and/or aspiration) in preference to CDT alone to shorten treatment time if appropriate expertise and resources are available (Grade 2C).
- After successful CDT in patients with acute DVT, the same intensity and duration of anticoagulation treatment as for comparable patients who do not undergo CDT is recommended (Grade 1C).

A number of available infusion catheters exist. The EKOS Endowave (EKOS Corporation, Bothwell MA) is an FDA-approved thrombolytic infusion catheter that uses high-frequency, low-power ultrasound to accelerate clot dissolution by increasing the surface area of fibrin (Fig. 1). The theoretical attractions of this type of therapy include a shorter time to patency of the thrombosed vessel, increased safety due to a decreased dose of lytic agent, increased cost savings, shorter hospital stay and extension of lytic therapy offered to patients with sub-acute or chronic thrombosis. Contraindications to thrombolytic therapy are listed in Table 1.

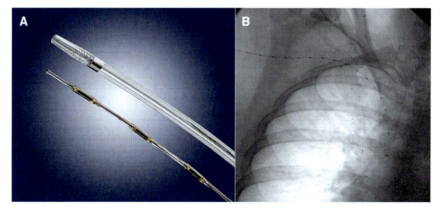

Fig. 1. (**A**) EKOS Endowave thrombolytic infusion catheter. (**B**) EKOS catheter traversing acutely thrombosed axillary-subclavian vein (Courtesy of EKOS Corporation, Bothwell, MA).

Table 1
Contraindications to Thrombolytic Therapy

Absolute
Stroke (<2 months)
Bleeding diathesis
Neurosurgery (intracranial, spinal) in past 12 months
Intracranial neoplasm
Recent (<3 months) intracranial trauma
Active or recent gastrointestinal tract bleeding
Relative
Uncontrolled hypertension (systolic >180 mmHg or diastolic >110 mmHg)
Major non-vascular surgery or trauma (<10 days)
Cardiopulmonary resuscitation (<10 days)
Puncture of a non-compressible vessel
Pregnancy
Bacterial endocarditis
Recent eye surgery

Technique of CDT (Key Points)

- Ultrasound-guided venous access with micropuncture needle via:
  - Common femoral vein
  - Popliteal vein
  - Tibial vein
  - Internal jugular vein
- Contrast venography to determine the extent and distribution of thrombus and treatment zone
- Thrombolytic infusion, e.g.,
  - Alteplase 0.5–2.0 mg/h
  - Reteplase 0.5–2.0 IU/h
  - Tenecteplase 0.25–1.0 mg/h
- Unfractionated heparin through the sheath side arm of the sheath at 200–400 U/h titrated to a PTT of 40–50 s
- Monitor fibrinogen q6 h: consider stopping or reducing lytic dose if fibrinogen <100 mg/dL

PERCUTANEOUS MECHANICAL THROMBECTOMY

Percutaneous mechanical thrombectomy (PMT) refers to a heterogeneous group of devices and techniques used to fragment, ablate or extract intravascular thrombus in an effort to produce more rapid and efficacious lysis. PMT has evolved as a possible alternative or adjunct to CDT to facilitate thrombus removal in peripheral vascular (arterial/venous) interventions. PMT has a number of advantages over CDT alone including more rapid restoration of flow in situations where limb viability is compromised (Table 2). Typically, complete thrombus removal requires a combination of both CDT and PMT.

A number of thrombectomy catheters with different mechanisms of action are commercially available. A detailed review of the individual characteristics of each of these catheters is beyond the scope of this discussion. Mechanisms of action generally fall

Table 2
Advantages and Limitations of Percutaneous Mechanical Thrombectomy
(PMT) Compared with Catheter-Directed Thrombolysis (CDT)

Advantages
Rapid thrombus removal; shorter procedural times
Less bleeding potential if no lytic agent administered
Power-pulse spray technique with Angiojet
Limitations
Hemolysis, renal failure or volume overload with rheolytic thrombectomy
Increased distal embolization risk
Less complete removal of thrombus from microvasculature
Risk of intimal/endothelial damage

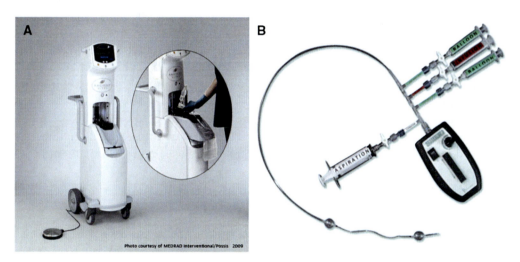

Fig. 2. (**A**) Angiojet rheolytic thrombectomy system. (**B**) Trellis-8 thrombolytic infusion and aspiration thrombectomy catheter system.

into one of the three categories (1) simple aspiration, (2) microfragmentation and (3) thrombo-aspiration (Venturi effect). Several of these catheters have the ability to co-administer thrombolytic agents to facilitate clot extraction. Randomized comparisons of different thrombectomy systems are not available.

The Angiojet rheolytic thrombectomy system (Medrad Possis, Minneapolis, MN) uses high-velocity saline jets to fragment and aspirate thrombus via a Venturi effect and is FDA approved for arterial and venous applications (Fig. 2A). It is 6 French compatible and a variety of catheter sizes exist to accommodate a wide range of vessel sizes. The benefits of local thrombolysis delivery with PMT may be combined using the power-pulse spray technique and the Angiojet 6F Xpeedior or DVX catheters. It has the potential advantage of diminishing the number and size of particles in addition to enhanced speed of clot lysis, whilst reducing the need for large quantities of thrombolytic agent. In this technique, the catheter outflow lumen is occluded and a high concentration of lytic infusion (e.g., 10–20 mg TPA in 50 mL saline) is pulsed outward from the distal catheter tip directly into the thrombus, theoretically maximizing lytic penetration. After 20–30 min dwell time, thrombectomy is then performed using the catheter in the normal thrombectomy mode. Active aspiration times need to be closely monitored as hemolysis may occur after 4 minutes of use. Anemia and renal dysfunction can occur as a result, albeit rarely. Adequate intravenous hydration is recommended and blood transfusion may be required as indicated.

The FDA-approved Trellis-8 catheter (Bacchus Vascular, Inc, Santa Clara, CA) combines the benefits of thrombolytic infusion and aspiration thrombectomy with embolic protection (Fig. 2B). The 8 French compatible catheter has proximal and distal balloons with drug infusion holes located between the two balloons. After placement of the catheter over a guidewire across the intended zone of treatment, the proximal and distal balloons are inflated, thus isolating the thrombotic segment. A thrombolytic agent (i.e., 4–6 mg rtPA) is then administered into the isolated segment and dispersion of the lytic drug is facilitated by catheter vibration by means of a central wire powered by an external drive unit. After 15–20 min, the proximal balloon can be deflated and thrombus aspirated from the distal port. The device has the theoretical potential to minimize both distal embolization and bleeding by reducing systemic absorption of lytic agent. The advantages of such a device include its ability to combine mechanical and pharmacologic therapies and treat patients who may possess traditional contraindications to thrombolytic therapy.

Experimental models suggest the greatest number and largest size of distal emboli occur with mechanical thrombectomy, and fewer with power-pulse spray thrombectomy combined with lytic therapy. CDT alone achieves the slowest reperfusion rate but with the fewest number of distal emboli *(4)*.

ILIOFEMORAL DVT

Venous thromboembolic disease remains a serious health problem with estimates suggesting that over 900,000 is cases occur annually in the United States *(5)*. It is associated with considerable morbidity and mortality. Up to 300,000 people die from pulmonary embolism annually. PTS estimated to occur in up to 30% of the patients with DVT after 8 years, is characterized by symptoms of leg edema, fatigue, venous claudication, pain and sometimes ulceration, all of which significantly impair quality of life. Venous hypertension secondary to a combination of residual venous obstruction and valvular incompetence is the primary mechanism for the development of PTS. Patients with more extensive DVT involving the iliac vein, inferior vena cava (IVC) and multi-segmental DVT are more likely to develop PTS than patients with infrainguinal DVT *(6)*. Up to 90% of these patients develop chronic venous insufficiency and 15% develop venous ulceration at 5 years *(7)*. Despite these compelling morbid observations, and the difference in thrombus burden between iliofemoral and infrainguinal DVT on clinical presentation, many clinicians treat them as if they were identical problems. Anticoagulation therapy with unfractionated heparin or low-molecular weight heparin bridged to warfarin is the mainstay of treatment for patients with DVT. This prevents thrombus propagation and embolization; however, does little to dissolve pre-existing thrombus.

Endovascular recanalization with CDT and PMT can improve patency in patients with iliofemoral DVT. Surgical intervention with operative venous thrombectomy and temporary arteriovenous fistula is an alternative to endovascular therapy. Compared with anticoagulation alone, operative intervention is associated with reduced leg swelling and ulceration with sustained patency rates of 65–85% in the long-term *(3)*. Owing to reduced procedural morbidity, endovascular approaches are recommended as first line treatment in most patients, but in patients deemed at high risk for bleeding on thrombolytic therapy, surgery may be considered where appropriate expertise and resources are available.

Indications for intervention include phlegmasia cerulea dolens and young patients with long life expectancy associated with iliofemoral/IVC or multi-segmental DVT.

A combination of CDT and PMT is usually required to achieve satisfactory dissolution of thrombus. Underlying residual stenoses often can be identified following pharmacomechanical thrombectomy and these lesions must be corrected to maintain vessel patency (Fig. 3). Response to percutaneous transluminal angioplasty (PTA) is often suboptimal and the placement of flexible self-expanding nitinol stents or stainless steel Wallstents (Boston Scientific, Natick, MA) is preferred to avoid potential stent compression (Fig. 4). Stents should be restricted to the iliac vein if possible. However, it is imperative to cover all areas of residual disease, so as to obviate restenosis of non-stented segments, even if this necessitates stenting into the common and/or femoral veins. Clinical and noninvasive imaging (e.g., duplex ultrasonography) is recommended post-procedure as a baseline, at 6- and 12-month intervals, and annually thereafter (Fig. 5). The reported 1-year patency rate is 79% in selected series *(2, 8)*. Despite the promise of CDT in the treatment of DVT, and its demonstrable excellent angiographic recanalization rates in highly selected patients, long-term follow-up results are not available.

Technique (Key Points)

- Ultrasound-guided venous access (popliteal vein preferred) with micropuncture needle
- CDT
- Percutaneous mechanical thrombectomy as required
- Consider retrievable IVC filter in select cases
  - Poor cardiopulmonary reserve
  - Free-floating iliocaval thrombus
- Venoplasty and stenting of all areas of residual stenoses
- Self-expanding stents (10–16 mm)

CHRONIC OBSTRUCTIVE LESIONS OF THE ILIAC VEIN

Anatomical abnormalities contribute to iliofemoral DVT in a significant number of patients. Left iliac vein compression from the right common iliac artery (May-Thurner syndrome, Cockett's or iliac vein compression syndrome) or non-occlusive iliac vein lesion (NIVL) is estimated to be present in 49–62% of cases of left lower extremity DVT (Fig. 6) *(9, 10)*. Review of CT scans obtained for unrelated purposes suggests that some degree of iliac vein compression probably represents a normal anatomical variant with almost 25% of the population having >50% compression of the iliac veins *(10)*. However, those who experience DVT, frequently have anatomically abnormal veins with spur formation and are at high risk of developing recurrent DVT and resultant PTS.

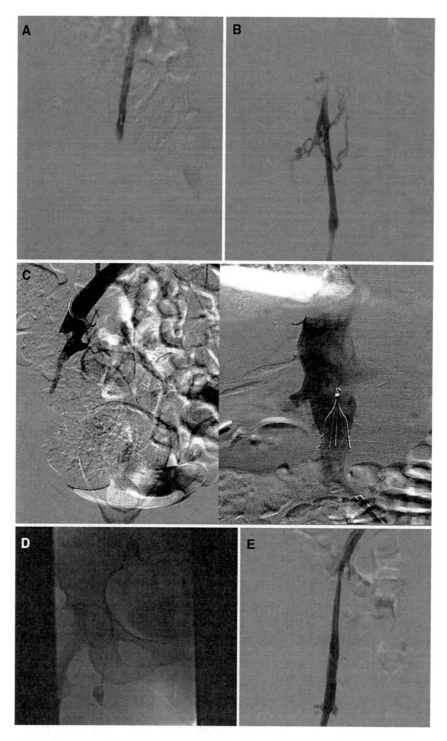

Fig. 3. (**A**, **B**) Venogram of thrombosed external iliac (EIV) and common femoral veins (CFV) post-balloon mitral valvuloplasty. (**C**) Venacavogram with Gunther-Tulip inferior vena cava (IVC) filter deployed due to CFV deep venous thrombosis being compressed by large groin hematoma and patent-foramen ovale. (**D**) Trellis infusion catheter inflated across thrombosed ilio-femoral veins. (**E**) Final venogram showing restored patency of stented EIV and CFV.

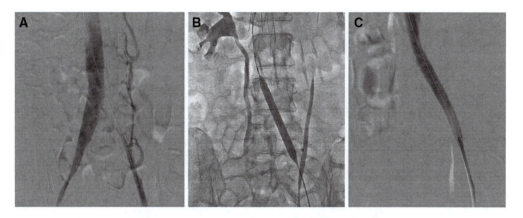

Fig. 4. (A) Iliocaval venogram after percutaneous mechanical thrombectomy, note IVC filter deployed after retinal hemorrhage during TPA. **(B)** Venoplasty of occluded left common iliac vein (CIV) presumed due to iliac vein compression (May-Thurner). **(C)** Wallstent deployed in IVC/CIV confluence restoring patent iliac vein.

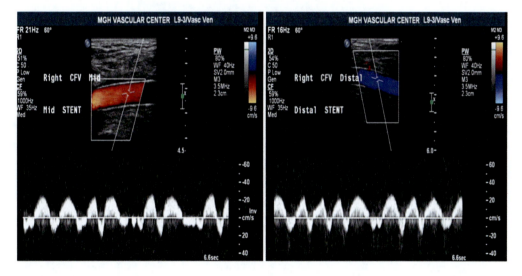

Fig. 5. Duplex ultrasound confirming patent stented CFV, with pulsatile Doppler waveform due to residual mitral valve stenosis (refer to case from Fig. 3).

Endovascular treatment of chronic iliac vein obstruction secondary to May-Thurner syndrome or NIVL has shown promising initial results, with high technical success and excellent primary-assisted and secondary patency rates. The stented limbs with NIVL fared better than those with thrombotic disease, with primary, assisted-primary and secondary cumulative patency rates of 79, 100 and 100%, and 57, 80 and 86% at 60 months, respectively (Fig. 7) *(11)*. The overall cumulative rate of instent restenosis (>50%) was seen in 5% of limbs and was higher in thrombotic (10%) as compared with 1% in NIVL limbs. Adequate coverage of the entire diseased segment as guided by intravascular ultrasound (IVUS) seems to provide best long-term results. This frequently necessitates placing the stent into the IVC to ensure full lesion coverage (Fig. 8) and, on occasions, extending the stents into the common femoral vein. The IVC

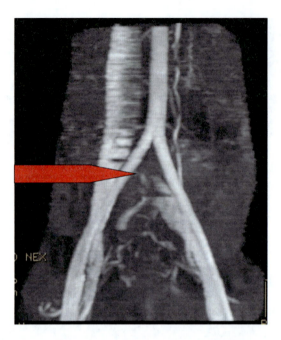

Fig. 6. Severe narrowing of left common iliac vein from overlying right common iliac artery (*arrow*) on coronal magnetic resonance venography, consistent with May-Thurner Syndrome or non-occlusive iliac vein lesion.

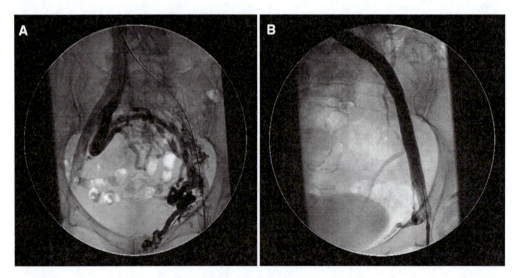

Fig. 7. (**A**) Ilio-femoral venogram with chronic (>8 years) left iliac vein occlusion. Robust cross-pelvic collaterals via right iliac veins draining into IVC. (**B**) Patent iliac veins following venoplasty and stenting with Wallstents. Notably absence of retrograde flow in internal iliac and collateral veins, confirming excellent hemodynamic result.

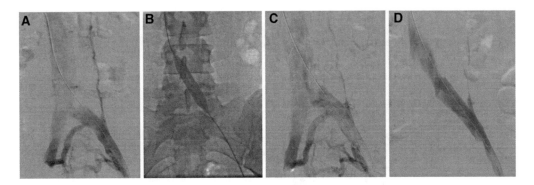

Fig. 8. (**A**) Venogram of severely stenotic iliac vein in 40-year old woman with significant edema and varicose veins of left thigh and calf. Retrograde filling of internal iliac vein with pelvic collaterals and ascending lumbar vein is seen. (**B**) Percutaneous transluminal angioplasty (PTA) of iliac vein. (**C**) Post-PTA venography with significant residual stenosis due to elastic recoil. (**D**) Venogram following successful revascularization of iliac vein with Wallstent extending into IVC.

placement raises concerns for risk of occlusion of the contralateral iliac vein; however, only a few rare cases of contralateral limb DVT (1%) have been reported and appear to be caused by recurrent thromboses from underlying prothrombotic risk factors.

Technique (Key Points)

- Access via common femoral vein if isolated iliac or IVC involvement. Popliteal vein if femoral vein thrombosed
- Liberal use of IVUS to define vessel reference diameter, lesion distribution and length
- Self-expanding stents sized to and placed into IVC (14–24 mm) to ensure entire lesion coverage

IVC OBSTRUCTION

Acute thrombotic occlusion of the IVC may occur as a consequence of propagation of iliofemoral DVT, hypercoagulable states, abdominal/pelvic malignancies (Fig. 9), retroperitoneal fibrosis (Fig. 10), caval filter thrombosis (Fig. 11), abdominal aortic aneurysms, congenital IVC anomalies and pregnancy. There is a high risk of pulmonary emboli despite anticoagulation and substantial risks of venous gangrene, renal vein thrombosis and renal dysfunction have been observed *(12)*. Other causes of IVC obstruction include extrinsic compression (e.g., right common iliac artery, large renal and hepatic cysts or masses (Fig. 12), hydronephrosis, and following liver transplantation, which can result from technical problems with vascular anastomoses).

Chronic obstruction of the IVC has a variable presentation. Most patients present with symptoms; however, 10% of the patients may remain entirely asymptomatic. Limb swelling is unilateral in two-thirds of the cases. This variable clinical presentation relates to the rich collateral pathways that may develop in these patients. Collateralization from the common iliac vein via the thoracolumbar vein is a particularly important collateral pathway and associated occlusion of the common iliac vein is particularly important in the development of symptoms *(13)*.

Previously, surgical thrombectomy with or without adjunctive temporary distal arteriovenous fistula creation had been performed for these patients *(14, 15)*. Endovascular

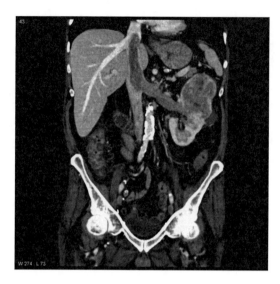

Fig. 9. Renal cell carcinoma with tumor and thrombus via left renal vein extending into suprarenal IVC by computed tomography.

therapy has become the preferred treatment modality owing to less procedure-related morbidity and mortality. In the largest reported series of endovascular therapy for IVC occlusion ($n = 120$), 82% of the lesions were infrarenal, with extension above the renal veins in 18% of the cases. Concurrent iliac vein obstruction was noted in 93% of the cases. IVC lesions were partial (>60% stenosis) in 86 and 14% of the cases were total occlusions. Procedural success rates of 100% for partial stenoses and 66% for total occlusions were achieved. No periprocedural mortality or late stent mortality was noted. Cumulative primary and assisted primary patency rates were 58 and 82% at 2 years, respectively *(13)*. Self-expanding stents are preferred for several reasons. These can be passively oversized to allow proper fixation and reduced migration risk in the highly compliant vein. The Wallstent has had the most clinical experience and are available in large enough sizes suitable for this type of intervention (Fig. 13). Advantages of nitinol stents include lack of foreshortening and better ability to conform to variable lumen diameters.

Technique

- CDT if thrombosis is acute and deemed to be an active component
  - Access via femoral vein at mid-thigh under ultrasound guidance
  - Large sheaths are required (9–14 F)
- Percutaneous mechanical thrombectomy as required
- High-pressure angioplasty and stenting for residual lesions
  - Wallstents preferred 14 mm (iliac) up to 24 mm (IVC), matched to reference diameter as measured by IVUS
  - Generous 3–4 mm overlap
  - Post dilatation
- Closure devices as indicated (Vasoseal, Datascope Corp., Montvale, NJ) because of mid-thigh access and large sheath size

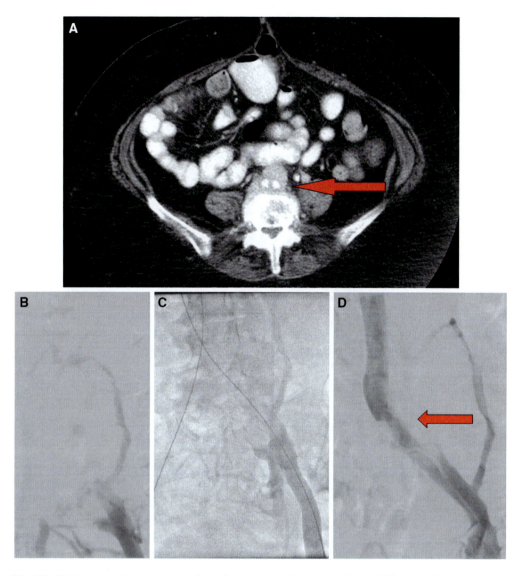

Fig. 10. (**A**) Computed tomography of pelvis demonstrating retroperitoneal fibrosis affecting the iliac veins (*arrow*). (**B**) Chronic left common iliac vein (CIV) occlusion due to retroperitoneal fibrosis. (**C**) Persistent iliac vein occlusion following PTA. (**D**) Successful stenting of chronically fibrosed vein with Wallstent restoring patency of vessel.

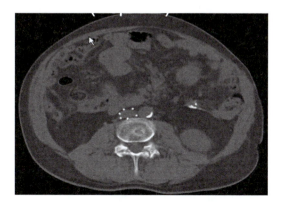

Fig. 11. Thrombosis of inferior vena cava and TrapEase filter by computed tomography.

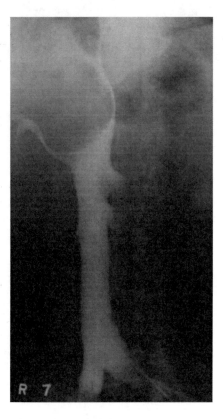

Fig. 12. Severe narrowing of intrahepatic inferior vena cava caused by ascites and liver mass.

IVC FILTERS

Interruption of the IVC to prevent pulmonary embolus (PE) was first suggested in 1868 by Trousseau. By the mid-1900s, a variety of surgical techniques were employed including ligation of the IVC (16) and several compartmentalization procedures resulting in partial IVC ligation (Fig. 14) *(17, 18)*. These procedures were associated with significant operative mortality rates. The transvenous placement of the Mobin-Uddin umbrella in 1967 heralded an important therapeutic option in selected patients with venous thromboembolic disease *(19)*. In 1973, Greenfield introduced his version of a conical filter inserted via venotomy (29.5 F), with the filter's apex positioned cephalad, which provided packing efficiency without flow disturbances *(20)*. The first percutaneous insertion of the Greenfield filter was reported in 1984. Currently, eleven devices that are FDA approved are commercially available *(21)*.

The ideal caval filter would have properties as outlined below *(22)*:

- Secure fixation
- Biocompatible, nonthrombogenic, infinite implant lifetime performance
- High filtering efficiency with no impedance of flow
- Ease of percutaneous insertion

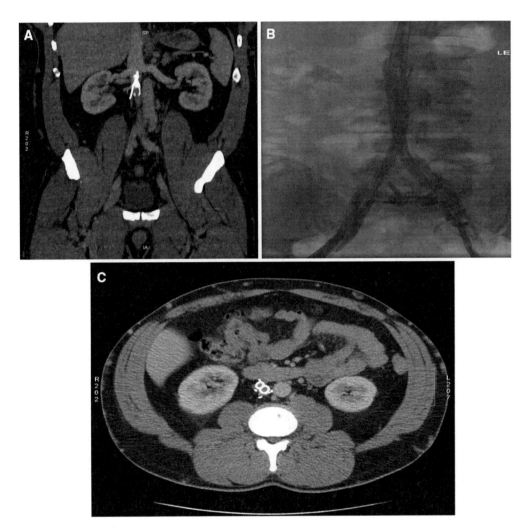

Fig. 13. (A) Computed tomography showing a chronically thrombosed G2 Express filter. (B) Venogram of patent IVC after "kissing stents" (Wallstents) adjacent to contracted filter. (C) Confirmation of patent IVC stents across IVC filter by computed tomography.

  – small caliber delivery system
  – simple release mechanism and control
  – able to be repositioned
- MR compatible
- Inexpensive
- Low access site thrombosis
- Able to be readily retrieved

Important attributes would include ease of insertion and the ability to capture thromboemboli while preserving patency of the IVC with secure fixation. The long-term performance of an IVC filter is particularly important in patients considered for prophylactic filter insertion. Despite the recent major advances in technology, the ideal device is yet to be designed.

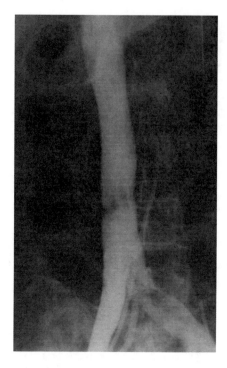

Fig. 14. Surgically placed clip for inferior vena cava interruption resulting in caval lumen deformity.

One of the largest trials of IVC filters randomized 400 patients with proximal DVT to anticoagulation alone or anticoagulation plus IVC filter placement. At 2 weeks, patients with an IVC filter had significantly fewer PE (1 vs. 5%) *(23)*. At follow-up to 8 years, an overall higher incidence of DVT was noted in the filter arm (35 vs. 27%) albeit, with less symptomatic PE (6 vs. 15%) *(24)*. Despite theoretical benefits of IVC filter implantation, there has not been a single randomized trial evaluating the efficacy of IVC filter placement in patients who cannot be anticoagulated. Prospective randomized data comparing filters to anticoagulation alone do not exist.

Indications

Classic indications for IVC filter placement include patients with documented PE or proximal DVT with a contraindication to anticoagulation, a complication of anticoagulation necessitating cessation of therapy, and progression of DVT or recurrent PE on therapeutic anticoagulation therapy. Massive pulmonary embolus with poor cardiopulmonary reserve, large free-floating proximal DVT and poor compliance with anticoagulation medications constitute other settings where filter placement may be considered. IVC filter placement has been used prophylactically in settings where patients are at high risk of VTE but cannot receive effective prophylaxis (such as the trauma patient). There is no consensus of routine placement during DVT thrombolysis but some authors have suggested its utility (Fig. 4) (Table 3) *(25)*.

Table 3
Indications and Contraindications for Inferior Vena Cava (IVC) Filter Insertion

Classic indications (proven venous thromboembolism)
Contraindication to anticoagulation
Recurrent VTE despite therapeutic anticoagulation
Complication of anticoagulation
Inability to achieve effective anticoagulation
Other potential indications
VTE with limited cardiopulmonary reserve
Large, free-floating iliofemoral/caval thrombus
Poor compliance with anticoagulation medications
Chronic thromboembolic disease (undergoing pulmonary thromboendarterectomy)
High risk of anticoagulation complication (e.g., ataxia/fall risk)
Recurrent PE with filter in place
DVT thrombolysis
Prophylactic indications
   Severe trauma with high risk of VTE
   History of VTE requiring high-risk surgery (e.g., bariatric or orthopedic)
Contraindications
Complete thrombosis of the IVC
Bacteremia or septic emboli
Uncorrectable, severe coagulopathy

Available Filter Types

A number of different filters are available for use in the United States (Fig. 15). These differ substantially in design, materials, profile, introducer size and potential for retrievability (Table 4). No randomized controlled trials have been performed comparing the safety and efficacy of different filter designs; hence filter choice is dictated more by local expertise and availability.

The American College of Chest Physicians (ACCP) guidelines for IVC filter placement are as follows *(3)*:

1. For patients with DVT or PE, the routine use of IVC filter in addition to anticoagulation is not recommended (Grade 1A).
2. For patients with acute proximal DVT or PE if anticoagulation therapy is not possible because of risk of bleeding, placement of IVC filter is indicated (Grade 1C).
3. For patients with acute DVT or PE, who have an IVC filter inserted as an alternative to anticoagulation, the recommendations are that they should receive a conventional course of anticoagulation if their risk of bleeding resolves (Grade 1C).

Technique of IVC Filter Insertion

Pre-procedural imaging should be reviewed to identify the presence of thrombosis at venous access sites. The most common access site for IVC filter placement is the right common femoral vein, which allows direct entry to the vena cava and results in less tilting of the filter as compared with the left common femoral vein. Other potential access sites include the left common femoral vein and the right or left internal jugular

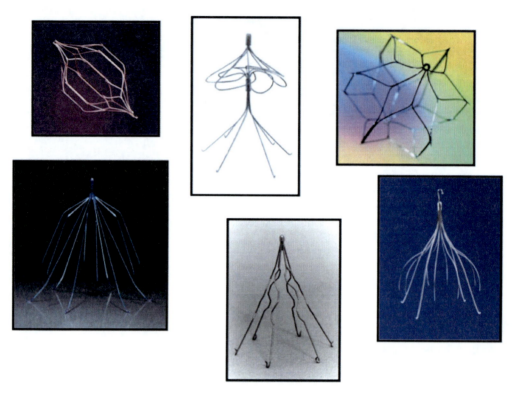

Fig. 15. Designs of various inferior vena caval filters.

veins. Occasionally the antecubital, subclavian and popliteal veins may be used depending on the clinical scenario and introducer sheath size requirements.

Venacavography is performed with a pigtail catheter placed at the distal IVC bifurcation to determine the diameter and length of the infrarenal cava, the level of the renal veins and the presence of caval thrombus. The normal IVC diameter is usually < 28 mm, but "megacava" (above 30 mm in diameter) may be identified in 2–3% of cases *(26)*. This may be found in patients with right-sided heart failure. The bird's nest filter (Cook, Bloomington, IN), which can accommodate a vena cava up to 40 mm in diameter, can be used in these instances or alternatively bilateral iliac vein filters deployed. Venography may identify IVC anomalies that have implications for IVC filter placement. Duplication of the IVC, occurring in 1–2% of the population *(27)*, is characterized by a left-sided IVC draining into a normally located left renal vein, which then joins the right IVC to form a common suprarenal cava (Fig. 16). Suprarenal filter placement or placement of a filter in both the right and left IVC is required to reliably prevent PE in this instance. IVC transposition occurs in 0.5% of the individuals. In this anomaly, the left IVC usually joins the suprarenal IVC at or just inferior to the left renal vein.

Placement of IVC filter should follow specific manufacturer's recommendations. In general, the apex of the filter should be at or just below the level of the renal veins, at the site of high flow, to reduce the risk of filter thrombosis. After deployment, repeat venacavography is performed to ensure appropriate device placement, wall apposition and to exclude caval wall disruption (Fig. 17).

Table 4
Types and Features of IVC Filters

Device	Date of Introduction	Indication	Material	Max IVC size (mm)	Introducer size (outer diameter) (F)		MRI compatible
Bird's Nest	1982	Permanent	Stainless Steel	40	14	Fem/Jug	Yes
VenaTech (LGM)	1989	Permanent	Phynox	28	12	Fem/Jug	Yes
Simon nitinol	1988	Permanent	Nitinol	24–28	7	Fem/Jug	Yes
Greenfield	1989	Permanent	Titanium	28	12	Fem/Jug	Yes
Greenfield	1994	Permanent	Stainless Steel	28	14	Fem/Jug	Yes
TrapEase	2000	Permanent	Nitinol	30	6	Fem/Jug	Yes
OptEase	2002	Optional	Nitinol	30	6	Fem/jug	Yes
VenaTech LP	2001	Permanent	Phynox	28	7	Fem/Jug	Yes
Günther-Tulip	2000	Optional	Conichrome	30	8.5	Fem/Jug	Yes
Celect	2008	Optional	Conichrome	30	8.5	Fem/Jug	Yes
Option	2009	Optional	Nitinol	28	6.5	Fem/Jug	Yes
G2/G2X, Eclipse	2005–2010	Optional	Nitinol	28	9	Fem/Jug	Yes
Recovery	2002	Optional	Nitinol	28	9	Fem/Jug	Yes

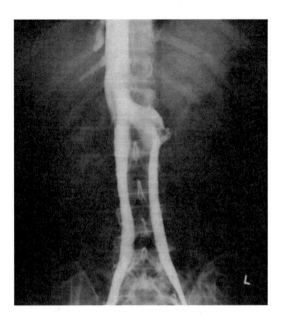

Fig. 16. Duplicated inferior vena cava. Left IVC communicates with the right IVC and drains into left renal vein.

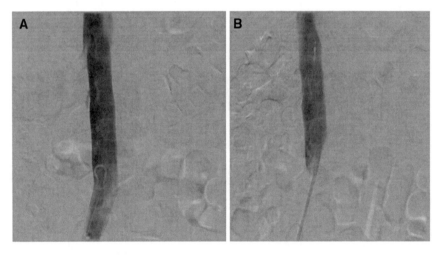

Fig. 17. (**A**) Pre-filter inferior venacavogram with Omni diagnostic catheter at distal IVC. (**B**) Post-deployment of Gunther-Tulip filter with apex positioned at confluence of renal veins.

Intravascular ultrasound and surface ultrasound-guided filter placement has been described and allows filter placement at the bedside in critically ill patients when fluoroscopy is unavailable *(28)*.

Post-procedural Care

Patients can usually be discharged the same day of the procedure, however, owing to other medical issues, patients frequently need to remain in hospital. There is no consensus regarding the need for re-introduction of anticoagulation in patients whose contraindication resolves. Owing to an increase risk of subsequent DVT in one study, we recommend re-introduction of anticoagulation when deemed safe *(23, 24)*. Annual follow-up to assess patency of the IVC and mechanical stability of the filter should be performed. Physical examination and abdominal X-ray suffices in most cases, supplemented with either duplex ultrasonography or CT venography if concerns arise based on clinical grounds. Venography should be reserved for patients in whom these modalities are not helpful.

Complications

Most complications are minor and the risk of serious complications is low. Procedure-related complications include access site hematoma and thrombosis, contrast agent reaction, air embolization and pneumothorax (particularly with internal jugular access). Uncommon, potentially serious complications include filter migration and malposition (Fig. 18), IVC penetration with perforation of vascular/gastrointestinal structures (Fig. 19), IVC thrombosis (*see* Figs. 11 and 13) with potential to progress towards phlegmasia cerulea dolens, device fracture and guidewire entrapment during central venous catheterization *(29)*. A small increased incidence of DVT is noted following IVC filter placement (Fig. 20) *(25)*. Recurrent pulmonary embolism is noted in 2–5% of the cases *(26)*.

Technique Summary

- Venacavography to identify caval size, renal veins location and exclude IVC anomalies
- Anticoagulation once contraindications resolve
- Annual surveillance to assess caval patency and filter stability

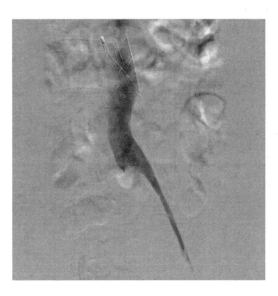

Fig. 18. Malpositioned IVC filter: Simon-Nitinol filter deployed in left common iliac vein.

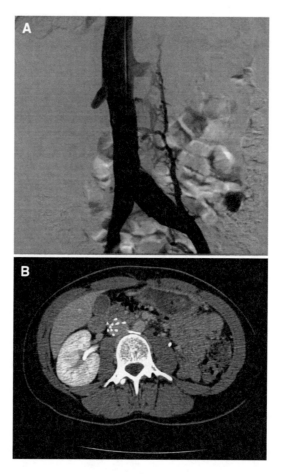

Fig. 19. (**A**) Excessive tilting and perforation of a G2 filter outside wall of IVC as depicted on venacavogram. (**B**) Computerized tomography confirming IVC perforation and stent strut in close proximity to adjacent aorta.

Suprarenal IVC Filter Placement

Suprarenal IVC filter placement should be considered in patients with an indication for IVC filter placement in the following circumstances (1) infrarenal vena caval thrombosis; (2) renal vein thrombosis; (3) gonadal vein thrombosis; (4) pregnancy and women of childbearing age who may become pregnant; (5) certain anatomical variants such as low insertion of the renal veins and duplicated IVC; (6) thrombus propagation proximal to a previously placed infrarenal IVC filter; (7) malposition or migration of a prior filter above the renal veins; and (8) recurrent PE following infrarenal IVC filter placement, preferably after an upper extremity emboli source has been ruled out *(30)*. Compared with infrarenal filter placement, suprarenal placement is not associated with an increased risk of complications such as renal dysfunction, filter migration, recurrent pulmonary emboli or caval thrombosis *(31)*. The optimal choice for suprarenal filters is either a titanium Greenfield or over-the-wire guided stainless steel Greenfield filter *(32, 33)*.

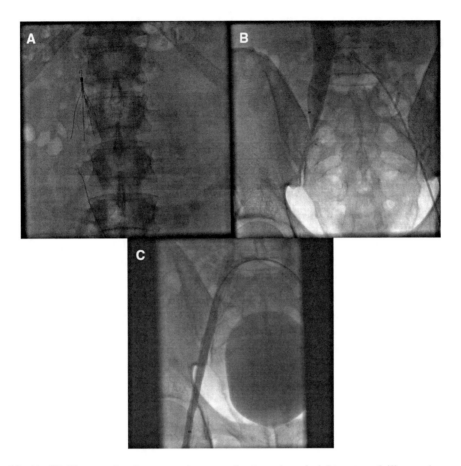

Fig. 20. (**A, B**) Venography demonstrating acutely thrombosed right external iliac and common femoral veins after Celect filter deployed via right CFV. (**C**) Post-stenting venogram with restoration of patent ilio-femoral veins at time of filter retrieval.

SUPERIOR VENA CAVA FILTER PLACEMENT

Upper extremity DVT (UEDVT) is associated with pulmonary embolism in approximately 12% of the cases. Superior vena cava (SVC) filter placement has been proposed in patients with UEDVT with contraindications to anticoagulation, failed anticoagulation with PE due to UEDVT despite therapeutic anticoagulation and complications of anticoagulation *(34)*. The stainless steel Greenfield filter generally is believed to be an ideal choice for SVC filtration due to its short length, alternating hook design and being over-the-wire, allowing tracking and precise positioning. Limited data suggest SVC filter placement is both safe and effective with a low incidence of serious complications. SVC perforation has been reported as a rare complication. Guidewire entrapment is more prone to occur with SVC filter placement *(35)*.

Technique Summary

- Access via internal jugular or femoral veins under ultrasound guidance.
- Perform venacavography – ensure proper orientation by reversing the filter.
- Do not place filter if SVC > 28 mm in diameter.

- Deploy proximal to innominate vein confluence.
- Most experience with titanium or stainless steel Greenfield filters.

RETRIEVABLE IVC FILTERS

Retrievable IVC filters have been developed on the premise that contraindications to anticoagulation are usually temporary, and subsequent filter removal can potentially avoid complications associated with long-term filter implantation. Approved filters for retrieval by FDA in United States include the OptEase (Cordis, Miami Lakes, FL), Recovery, G2, G2X and Eclipse (Bard Peripheral Vascular, Tempe, AZ), Günther-Tulip (Cook, Bloomington, IN) and the Option IVC filters (Angiotech Pharmaceuticals, Vancouver, British Columbia). Most of the optional retrievable filters are relatively new and thus limited data are available on their long-term performance when used as permanent devices. Although most retrievable filters are placed in patients with a well-defined risk to anticoagulation, less than 50% of the filters are eventually removed *(21)*. Patients with a favorable life expectancy with a retrievable filter in situ, who can safely resume anticoagulation, should be considered for filter retrieval. Absolute contraindications to attempted filter retrieval are filter thrombosis and failure to tolerate anticoagulation in a patient with ongoing risk of venous thromboembolism. Relative contraindications include a dwell time beyond the manufacturer's recommendations.

These generally can be retrieved with either proprietary retrieval equipment, or any commercially available snare and an appropriate sized sheath. An example of retrieval of a Gunther-Tulip filter is depicted in Fig. 21.

Failure to successfully retrieve usually is due to (1) excessive tilting of the filter impairing engagement of the nose-cone with snare equipment (Fig. 22), and (2)

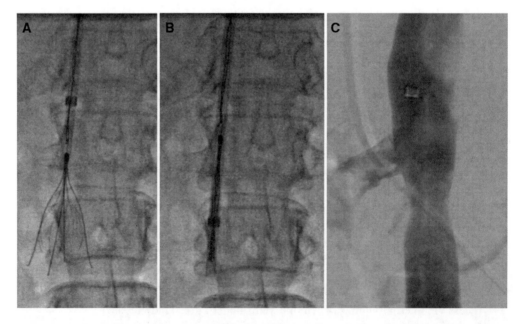

Fig. 21. (**A**) Retrieval of Gunther-Tulip IVC filter with snaring of hook. (**B**) Filter being collapsed within sheath during retrieval. (**C**) Post-filter retrieval venacavogram with mild spasm at site of previous filter.

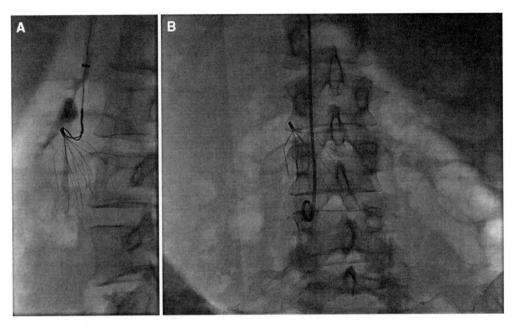

Fig. 22. (A) Failure to snare hook of filter due to excessive tilting of device (*see* Fig. 19a). (B) Attempts to reposition filter with pigtail catheter to facilitate retrieval.

excessive device endothelialization *(36, 37)*. A variety of other techniques including the use of rigid endobronchial biopsy forceps to free the tip of the filter from the caval wall may be employed in these cases *(38)*.

AXILLOSUBCLAVIAN VEIN THROMBOSIS

Axillosubclavian vein thrombosis (ASVT) accounts for approximately 2–4% of all cases of DVT *(39)*. Despite traditionally being regarded as more benign than lower extremity DVT, it is recognized that pulmonary emboli may occur in approximately 12% (range 11–36%) of the patients and disabling PTS may occur in some patients (13%). It is useful to categorize etiology into primary and secondary forms, in lieu of the fact that severity of symptoms and treatment management strategies do differ between both groups.

Secondary ASVT occurs due to indwelling vascular devices (e.g., central venous or tunneled catheters, pacemaker leads (Fig. 23)), implantable cardiac defibrillators (Fig. 24), thromphophilia or a combination of both accounts for the majority of cases of ASVT. Symptoms range from asymptomatic to severe, but are frequently mild. Significant comorbidities are often present in the majority of patients with upper extremity DVT. Patients can be managed with short-term anticoagulation for 3 months with or without catheter removal in most cases. The ideal solution is removal of the catheter, if feasible, and anticoagulation for a minimum of 4 weeks. In cases when a functioning catheter is of medical necessity, it is acceptable to anticoagulate the patient and upon eventual removal of the catheter, continue an additional 4-week course of anticoagulation, as tolerated. Favorable clinical outcomes albeit in small patient series

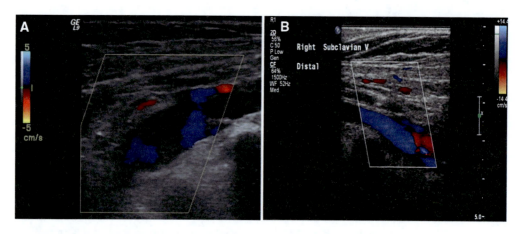

Fig. 23. (**A**) Sonography of an acutely thrombosed subclavian vein (SCV) after pacemaker insertion. (**B**) Widely patent subclavian vein after 3 months of anticoagulation.

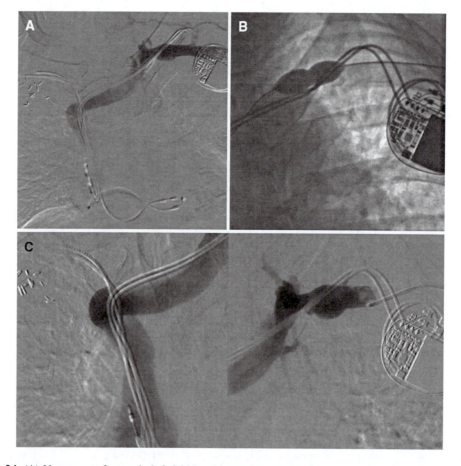

Fig. 24. (**A**) Venogram of stenotic left SCV and innominate vein presenting with symptoms of superior vena cava (SVC) syndrome due to contralateral SCV and innominate vein occlusion. (**B**) Balloon catheter (12 mm) dilation with waist at high-pressure inflations confirming stenosis. (**C**) Postvenoplasty of both lesions demonstrating patent veins. Clinically at 4-week follow-up, total resolution of symptoms and sonography confirming patent veins.

support this conservative strategy. CDT may be considered when symptoms are severe or when maintenance of future vascular access is jeopardized and preservation of the vein is judged to be at a premium.

Primary ASVT (Paget-Schroetter syndrome), though much less common, tends to affect otherwise young healthy individuals and can lead to chronic disabling symptoms. Repetitive activity in the setting of an underlying abnormality of the thoracic outlet predisposes afflicted individuals to axillosubclavian vein thrombosis. Compression of the subclavian vein between the first rib and a hypertrophied scalene muscle and subclavius tendon is the usual anatomic abnormality. Perivenous fibrous and venous web formation may develop in chronic cases. Arm pain, swelling and fatigue in the involved extremity following a history of trauma or strenuous use of the arm are common presentations. When treated with anticoagulation alone patients frequently experience chronic disabling symptoms and severe PTS develops in 13% of the cases *(40)*. The severity of symptoms correlate closely with the degree of obstruction and establishing venous patency early becomes paramount *(41)*. The optimal strategy has not been subject to a randomized multicenter trial. However, literature suggests patients fare better when venous patency is achieved expeditiously. Controversy exists regarding the optimal approach, but we recommend early CDT to establish venous patency (Fig. 25), followed by in-hospital surgical decompression with first rib resection, via a transaxillary approach. If residual stenosis exists after surgical decompression or persistent symptoms prevail, PTA and stenting may be required to prevent rethrombosis of the diseased vein. Elective evaluation of the contralateral arm is recommended as the anatomical abnormality is frequently bilateral,

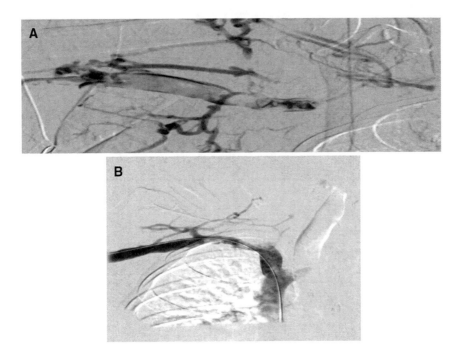

Fig. 25. (A) Venogram of right arm via basilic vein access depicting acute thrombus involving axillary and SCV. **(B)** Post-lysis (4 h TPA) venography showing patency of axillary and SCV, albeit with residual stenosis at proximal SCV (pre-first rib resection).

which has been reported in 61% of the patients. During venography, images should be acquired both in the neutral position as well as during thoracic outlet maneuvers (Figs. 26 and 27). As for treating the asymptomatic contralateral vein, elective repair should be reserved for those individuals where the compression of vein involves the dominant arm and their occupation exposes them to increased risk for thrombosis *(42)*.

Results of Treatment

The results of first rib resection in the context of the proposed algorithm, as outlined below, have been very favorable. In Machleder's initial series, 50 consecutive patients were entered into a sequential treatment program for spontaneous axillary-subclavian vein thrombosis.

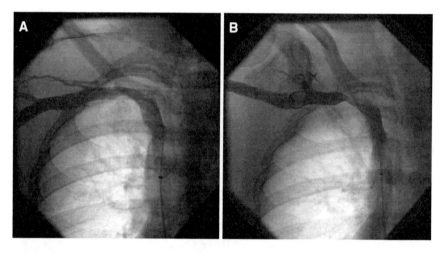

Fig. 26. (**A**) Follow-up venogram, 3-weeks after transaxillary first rib resection illustrating patent axillary-SCV in neutral position. (**B**) Venogram of right arm with thoracic outlet maneuvers (TOS) revealing severe narrowing of SCV.

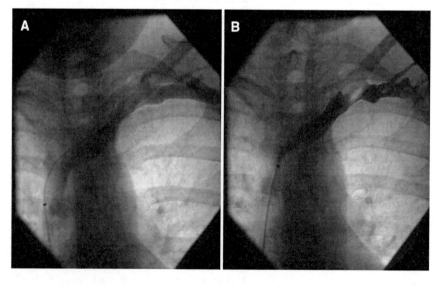

Fig. 27. (**A**) Contralateral left arm venography revealing a widely patent axillary-SCV in neutral position. (**B**) Venography with TOS maneuvers resulting in compression of SCV.

Forty-three underwent initial thrombolytic or anticoagulatant therapy followed by long-term warfarin treatment. Thirty-six (72%) had first-rib resection of the underlying structural abnormality, and nine patients had post-operative balloon venoplasty. Pain-free status was achieved in 93% of the patients with a patent vein as well as 64% of patients whose vein was occluded. No episodes of recurrent thrombosis after surgical correction at a mean follow-up period of 3.1 years were observed. The results of this small series may have been limited by the fact that the surgical strategy employed at the time antedated the evolution of a treatment algorithm wherein the first rib resection is performed immediately following or soon after thrombolysis. Urschel and Patel *(43)* reported that in their large series of 626 patients with Paget-Schroetter syndrome spanning 50 years of experience, 506 of them received thrombolytic therapy within 6 weeks of symptom onset followed by prompt first rib resection. Excellent or good results were experienced in 486 patients, defined as complete or almost complete pain relief, with return to full employment. Forty-two extremities were not seen until after 6 weeks after venous occlusion. Patients were treated with thrombolytic therapy, although none could be completely opened, all were treated with prompt surgery, and 24 subsequently recanalized or developed sufficient collateral circulation to report good results later, whereas 9 had only fair results. Five patients manifested symptoms of severe PTS.

ALGORITHM FOR THE MANAGEMENT OF AXILLOSUBCLAVIAN

Venous Thrombosis *(43)*

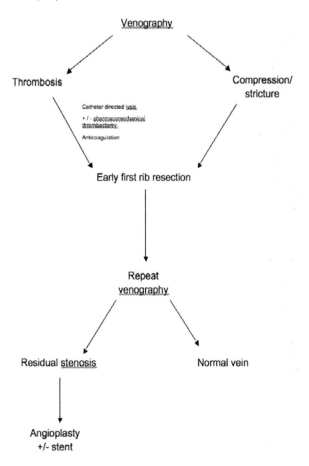

Technique Summary (Key Points)

- Basilic (preferable) or cephalic vein access.
- CDT.
- Adjunctive percutaneous mechanical thrombectomy with CDT as required.
- Repeat venography at 6–24 h to ensure patency.
- Early (in-hospital) first rib surgical resection via transaxillary approach.
- Repeat venography at 4 weeks and PTA +/−stenting if residual stenosis. Contralateral venography in neutral and with active thoracic outlet syndrome maneuvers to exclude asymptomatic disease.

SUPERIOR VENA CAVA SYNDROME

Superior vena cava (SVC) syndrome is the constellation of clinical symptoms resulting from the obstruction of blood flow through the SVC. Annual estimates as to the incidence in the United State approach 19,000 cases, with an increasing frequency attributed to the prevalence of central venous catheters. Obstruction of the SVC results in venous hypertension of the head, neck, upper thorax and extremities of varying severity. A wide variety of etiologies may result in SVC syndrome (Table 5). Intrathoracic malignancy accounts for 60–85% of the cases (44). Obstruction of malignant etiologies may result from a combination of extrinsic SVC compression and direct tumor invasion. Indwelling catheter-related stenosis, radiation fibrosis and concomitant thrombosis may contribute. Benign causes are re-emerging as common causes of SVC obstruction with increasing use of cardiac pacemakers/defibrillators and long-term indwelling catheters.

Common symptoms include dyspnea, cough, chest discomfort, dysphagia, hoarseness and head fullness. Headaches, confusional state and coma suggest associated cerebral edema, although rarely seen in <10% of the cases. Signs include facial and upper extremity swelling, jugular venous distension, all of which may be aggravated by lying supine or bending forward, in addition to the development of prominent chest wall collateral veins (Fig. 28). Airway compromise secondary to laryngeal edema is uncommon. Most patients develop symptoms progressively over several weeks or longer, but modest improvement may be seen with collateral pathway recruitment.

The severity of symptoms depends upon the rapidity of onset and relationship of obstruction to the origin of the azygous vein. Well-described venous collateral pathways

Table 5
Causes of SVC Syndrome

Malignancy
Bronchogenic carcinoma
Non-Hodgkin's lymphoma
Benign causes
Indwelling central venous catheters
Pacemakers/ Implantable cardiac defibrillators
Granulomatous infection (e.g., tuberculosis)
Fibrosing mediastinitis
Thoracic aortic-aneurysm related compression (e.g., syphilis)
Post surgical (e.g., post cardiac or cardiac-lung transplant)

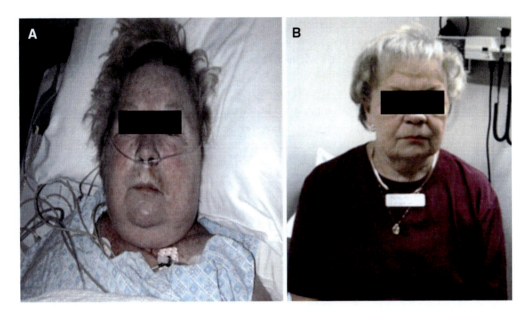

Fig. 28. (A) Photograph of woman with metastatic colon cancer manifesting features of SVC syndrome. (B) Photo of same woman 48-h after pharmacologic thrombolysis and stenting of thrombosed SVC.

(via azygous, internal mammary, paraspinous, lateral thoracic and esophageal venous systems) may take weeks to become well established. As such, obstructions below the level of the azygous vein insertion tend to be more severe.

Diagnosis

Patients with clinical suspicion of SVC syndrome should undergo contrast-enhanced chest CT. The level and extent of occlusion and degree of collateral development can be determined. CT scan may also detect thoracic malignancy and alterative diagnoses such as pericardial effusion and pulmonary embolus that may co-exist in the cancer patient. Magnetic resonance venography is an alternative in patients with iodinated contrast allergy, but should be avoided in cases of severe renal impairment due to the reported association with nephrogenic systemic fibrosis *(45)*. Duplex ultrasonography may be used to exclude thrombosis of the axillary, subclavian and innominate veins and assess patency of upper extremity veins (e.g., basilic, cephalic) to plan for interventional procedures, but cannot reliably determine patency of the SVC due to lack of an adequate acoustic window. Venographic confirmation is done at the time of endovascular intervention.

Treatment

Treatment is directed towards relief of symptoms and treatment of the underlying cause (e.g., malignancy). The etiology of the obstruction, the presence of co-existent SVC thrombosis, the severity of symptoms and the patient's life expectancy all influence management and treatment options. General measures include head elevation to reduce central venous pressure and administration of diuretics which may have a limited salutary role in reducing venous pressure. In mild cases this may allow sufficient resolution of symptoms whilst venous collaterals develop. Anticoagulation is recommended to reduce the risk of thrombus formation or subsequent propagation, preserve venous collateral patency and reduce the risk of pulmonary embolus. Glucocorticoid therapy may be useful in steroid responsive malignancies (e.g., lymphoma) or in patients with laryngeal edema and impending airway collapse.

Revascularization should be considered in the presence of significant symptoms. The treatment goals are different in malignancy-related SVC obstruction as compared to those cases due to benign disease. In malignancy, life expectancy is usually about 6 months, and palliation of symptoms is the main goal of therapy. Long-term patency is less of an issue. In benign disease, patients are often younger, and thus durability assumes greater importance as does maintaining venous access.

Randomized trials have not been performed comparing endovascular and surgical approaches. Surgical options include bypass grafting from the jugular or innominate vein to the right atrial appendage or SVC. Autologous vein (spiral saphenous or femoral) is the conduit of choice, but polytetrafluoroethylene (ePTFE) and human allograft may be used if venous conduit is unavailable. In benign disease, 1-year primary and secondary patency rates of 61 and 83% are noted. Five-year primary, assisted-primary and secondary patency rates of 45, 68 and 75%, respectively, have been reported *(46, 47)*. Results for endovascular intervention for benign SVC syndrome remain to be determined. Limited data show high technical success of 88% with reported primary patency of 44% and primary-assisted and secondary patency rates of 96% at 36 months but with a need for frequent repeat interventions to maintain patency at 3 years *(48, 49)*. The technical success of SVC stenting for malignant disease is excellent, reportedly 95–100%. The majority of patients experience immediate clinical relief of symptoms within hours to days following successful recanalization of occluded SVC. Primary and secondary patency rates are 85 and 93%, respectively, at 3 months, employing endovascular stenting, with no long-term data available due to the dismal life expectancy of these patients *(50)*.

Thrombolysis may be used in cases with associated caval thrombosis as an adjunct to PTA and stenting to reduce the likelihood of PE. It is most effective when the acuity of the thrombus is felt to be fresh. After the procedure, patients are treated with either unfractionated heparin or low-molecular weight heparin with transition to warfarin therapy depending upon the clinical scenario.

Endovascular Techniques

Successful SVC endovascular therapy begins with bilateral upper extremity contrast venography to define the extent and location of stenosis/occlusion and presence of thrombus. Focal SVC stenoses may be approached via the femoral vein but with more complex occlusive disease involving the brachiocephalic and axillo-subclavian venous system, access from the basilic or internal jugular veins may be required. Heparin is administered during the intervention to avoid thrombosis. A variety of wires and catheter combinations may be required to traverse the occlusions/lesions. In the presence of significant thrombus, CDT should be initially undertaken. Careful screening for contraindications is required (Table 9.1) and screening for intracranial metastatic disease is recommended in malignant SVC syndrome before employing thrombolytic agents.

Residual stenoses and thrombus are treated with balloon angioplasty. Balloon sizes ranging from 8 to16 mm typically are required. Lesions tend to be fibrotic and stent placement usually is recommended to avoid restenosis from elastic recoil. The diameter of a stent should be oversized by approximately 10–20% compared to the normal vein in an attempt to avoid stent migration. The type of stents employed is determined by the diameter, length and location of the diseased segment. In focal lesions, Palmaz /Genesis balloon-expandable stents (Cordis Corporation, Warren, NJ) are preferred due to their superior performance of high radial strength and precise positioning, although they are inflexible and short in length. Larger diameter self-expanding stents, such as the Gianturco Z-stents (Cook Medical, Bloomington, IN) may be required if the SVC is extremely capacious, but have wide gaps between the struts, predisposing to restenosis due to tumor ingrowth. Wallstents (Boston Scientific, Natick, MA) are composed of stainless steel with less radial strength but are flexible and available in long lengths. Nitinol stents although flexible and able to be accurately placed are limited by their available maximum diameters of only 14 mm, which may be too small to accommodate most SVCs. Indwelling catheters or recently implanted pacemakers, if deemed to be at risk for compromised function and can be safely removed, should be repositioned following successful stenting (Fig. 29). If pacing lead extraction is not feasible or difficult, stenting across pacemaker leads appears to be safe without adverse consequence *(51)*. In cases of obstruction of the confluence of the brachiocephalic veins with SVC, unilateral stenting usually is sufficient to relieve symptoms as collaterals provide adequate drainage from the contralateral side. However, in younger patients with anticipated long life expectancy where maintenance of vascular access assumes importance, bilateral revascularization with "kissing stent" implantation should be considered (Fig. 30) *(53)*. There is no consensus as to the type or duration of antithrombotic regimen post procedure. In cases without thrombosis, combination antiplatelet therapy with aspirin and clopidogrel until stent endothelialization occurs is often sufficient. Anticoagulation should be strongly considered in the presence of significant SVC obstruction or malignancy when thrombus appears to have a punitive role.

Post procedural upper duplex ultrasound is performed to serve as a baseline for future comparison. Follow-up contrast venography or CT venography is performed at 3–6 months in selected cases or as appropriate when the clinical scenario suggests restenosis or rethrombosis.

Complications

Complications are infrequent (3.2–7.8%) and include minor complications (puncture site hematoma, epistaxis, and chest pain) and major complications (SVC rupture, pulmonary embolus, pericardial tamponade, stent migration and hemorrhage) *(52)*. Pulmonary edema may occur with the postulated mechanism due to increased venous return to the heart.

SVC syndrome is a disease with shifting etiologies and expanding treatment options fueled by the increased use of central venous catheters and the associated incidence of intraluminal thrombosis. Endovascular therapy is an appropriate primary intervention in benign SVC obstruction. It is less invasive with lower morbidity, equal efficacy and mid-term patency as compared to surgery. However, the long-term results are not yet known.

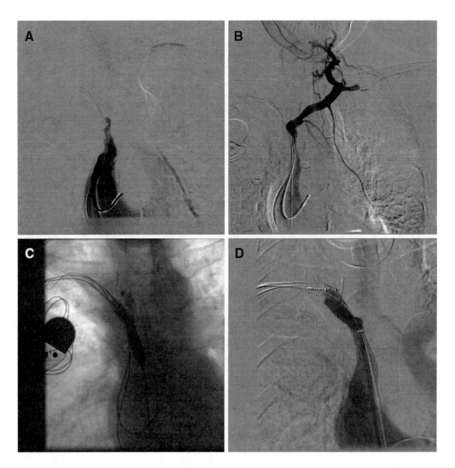

Fig. 29. (**A**) Sub-total occlusion of SVC in woman with metastatic lung cancer and permanent pacemaker via right SCV. (**B**) Left innominate vein demonstrated to be patent with severe SVC stenosis. (**C**) Balloon dilation of SVC with 12 mm high-pressure catheter, note the deflection of pacemaker wires. (**D**) Final venacavogram post-stenting (Genesis) of SVC after pulling pacer wires out of position and reimplanting after successful stent deployment.

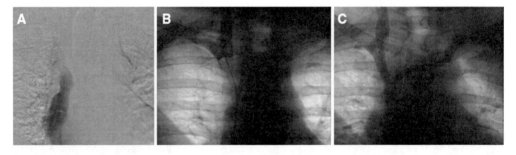

Fig. 30. (**A**) Venacavogram with occlusion of SVC and bilateral innominate venous stents in young male with implantable cardiac defibrillator-induced SVC thrombosis. (**B**) Post-mechanical thrombectomy of SVC with persistent occlusion. (**C**) Venography following reconstruction of innominate vein confluence with "kissing-stents" and SVC stenting.

Surgical therapy is an acceptable option in selected patients with benign SVC syndrome, who are not suitable or who fail endovascular therapy. Despite the lack of available trials, evidence suggests endovascular therapy is reasonable as the first line therapy for patients with malignancy. Although multiple interventions are the norm, endovascular therapy is minimally invasive, safe and efficacious with high assisted primary and secondary patency rates achieved.

Technique Summary (Key Points)

- Pre-procedural CT with contrast via bilateral veins.
- Bilateral upper extremity venography (via basilic veins) using ultrasound guidance.
- CDT if thrombus present.
- Percutaneous mechanical thrombectomy combined with CDT as indicated
- PTA/stenting
- Stents
    - Palmaz/Genesis (12–14 mm),
    - Nitinol (10–14 mm),
    - Wallstents (14–24 mm),
- Individualized antiplatelet and anticoagulant therapy.

REFERENCES

1. Theiss W, Wirtzfeld A, Fink U, Maubach P. The success rate of fibrinolytic therapy in fresh and old thrombosis of the iliac and femoral veins. *Angiology.* 1983;34(1):61–69.
2. Mewissen MW, Seabrook GR, Meissner MH, Cynamon J, Labropoulos N, Haughton SH. Catheter-directed thrombolysis for lower extremity deep venous thrombosis: report of a national multicenter registry. *Radiology.* 1999;211(1):39–49.
3. Kearon C, Kahn SR, Agnelli G, Goldhaber S, Raskob GE, Comerota AJ. Antithrombotic therapy for venous thromboembolic disease: American College of Chest Physicians Evidence-Based Clinical Practice Guidelines (8th Edition). *Chest.* 2008;133(6 Suppl):454 S–545 S.
4. Greenberg RK, Ouriel K, Srivastava S, et al. Mechanical versus chemical thrombolysis: an in vitro differentiation of thrombolytic mechanisms. *J Vasc Interv Radiol.* 2000;11(2Pt1):199–205.
5. Heit JA, Cohen AT, Anderson FJ. Estimated annual number of incident and recurrent, non-fatal venous thromboembolism (VTE) in the US. *Blood.* 2005;106:267A.
6. Prandoni P, Lensing AW, Prins MR. Long-term outcomes after deep venous thrombosis of the lower extremities. *Vasc Med.* 1998;3(1):57–60.
7. Akesson H, Brudin L, Dahlstrom JA, Eklof B, Ohlin P, Plate G. Venous function assessed during a 5 year period after acute ilio-femoral venous thrombosis treated with anticoagulation. *Eur J Vasc Surg.* 1990;4(1):43–48.
8. Juhan C, Cornillon B, Tobiana F, Schlama S, Barthelemy P, Denjean-Massia JP. Patency after iliofemoral and iliocaval venous thrombectomy. *Ann Vasc Surg.* 1987;1(5):529–533.
9. Kibbe MR, Ujiki M, Goodwin AL, Eskandari M, Yao J, Matsumura J. Iliac vein compression in an asymptomatic patient population. *J Vasc Surg.* 2004;39(5):937.
10. Mickley V, Schwagierek R, Rilinger N, Gorich J, Sunder-Plassmann L. Left iliac venous thrombosis caused by venous spur: treatment with thrombectomy and stent implantation. *J Vasc Surg.* 1998;28(3):492–497.
11. Neglén, P, Hollis, KC, Olivier, J, Raju, S. Stenting of the venous outfow in chronic venous disease: Long-term stent-related outcome, clinical, and hemodynamic result. *J Vasc Surg.* 2007;46:979–990.
12. Radomski JS, Jarrell BE, Carabasi RA, Yang SL, Koolpe H. Risk of pulmonary embolus with inferior vena cava thrombosis. *Am Surg.* 1987;53(2):97–101.
13. Raju S, Hollis K, Neglen P. Obstructive lesions of the inferior vena cava: clinical features and endovenous treatment. *J Vasc Surg.* 2006;44(4):820–827.

14. Neglen P, Nazzal MM, al-Hassan HK, Christenson JT, Eklof B. Surgical removal of an inferior vena cava thrombus. *Eur J Vasc Surg.* 1992;6(1):78–82.
15. Meissner AJ, Huszcza S. Surgical strategy for management of deep venous thrombosis of the lower extremities. *World J Surg.* 1996;20(9):1149–1155.
16. Amador E, Li TK, Crane C. Ligation of inferior vena cava for thromboembolism. Clinical and autopsy correlations in 119 cases. *JAMA.* 1968;206(8):1758–1760.
17. Miles RM. Prevention of pulmonary embolism by the use of a plastic vena caval clip. *Ann Surg.* 1966;163(2):192–198.
18. Moretz WH, Rhode CM, Shepherd MH. Prevention of pulmonary emboli by partial occlusion of the inferior vena cava. *Am Surg.* 1959;25:617–626.
19. Mobin-Uddin K, Callard GM, Bolooki H, Rubinson R, Michie D, Jude JR. Transvenous caval interruption with umbrella filter. *N Engl J Med.* 1972;286(2):55–58.
20. Greenfield LJ, McCrudy JR, Brown PP,Elkins RC. A vena cava filter for the prevention of pulmonary embolus. *Surgery.* 1973:599–605.
21. Rectenwald JE. Vena cava filters: uses and abuses. *Semin Vasc Surg.* 2005;18:166–175.
22. Kinney TB. Update on inferior vena cava filters. *J Vasc Interv Radiol.* 2003;(4):425–440.
23. Decousus H, Leizorovicz A, Parent F, et al. A clinical trial of vena caval filters in the prevention of pulmonary embolism in patients with proximal deep-vein thrombosis. Prevention du Risque d'Embolie Pulmonaire par Interruption Cave Study Group. *N Engl J Med.* 1998;338(7):409–415.
24. Eight-year follow-up of patients with permanent vena cava filters in the prevention of pulmonary embolism: the PREPIC (Prevention du Risque d'Embolie Pulmonaire par Interruption Cave) randomized study. *Circulation.* 2005;112(3):416–422.
25. Yamagami T, Yoshimatsu R, Matsumoto T, Nishimura T. Prophylactic implantation of inferior vena cava filter during endovascular therapies for deep venous thrombosis of the lower extremity: is it necessary? *Acta Radiol.* 2008;49(4):391–397.
26. Reed RA, Teitelbaum GP, Taylor FC, Pentecost MJ, Roehm JO. Use of the bird's nest filter in oversized inferior venae cavae. *J Vasc Interv Radiol.* 1991;2(4):447–450.
27. Athanasoulis CA, Kaufman JA, Halpern EF, Waltman AC, Geller SC, Fan CM. Inferior vena caval filters: review of a 26-year single-center clinical experience. *Radiology.* 2000;216(1):54–66.
28. Passman MA, Dattilo JB, Guzman RJ, Naslund TC. Bedside placement of inferior vena cava filters by using transabdominal duplex ultrasonography and intravascular ultrasound imaging. *J Vasc Surg.* 2005;42(5):1027–1032.
29. Grassi CJ, Swan TL, Cardella JF, et al. Quality improvement guidelines for percutaneous permanent inferior vena cava filter placement for the prevention of pulmonary embolism. *J Vasc Interv Radiol.* 2003;14(9Pt2):S271–S275.
30. Kalva SP, Chlapoutaki C, Wicky S, Greenfield AJ, Waltman AC, Athanasoulis CA. Suprarenal inferior vena cava filters: a 20-year single-center experience. *J Vasc Interv Radiol.* 2008;19(7):1041–1047.
31. Sharafuddin MJ, Sun S, Hoballah JJ. Endovascular management of venous thrombotic diseases of the upper torso and extremities. *J Vasc Interv Radiol.* 2002;13(10):975–990.
32. Greenfield LJ, Proctor MC. Supra-renal filter placement. *J Vasc Surg.* 1998;28:432–438.
33. Matchett WJ, Jones MP, McFarland DR, Ferris EJ. Suprarenal caval filter placement: Follow-up of four filter types in 22 patients. *J Vasc Inter Radiol.* 1998;9:588–593.
34. Owe EJ, Schoettle GJ, Harrington OB. Placement of a Greenfiled filter in the superior vena cava. *Ann Thorac Surg.* 1992;53:896–897.
35. Usoh F, Hingorani A, Ascher E, et al. Long-term follow-up for superior vena cava filter placement. *Ann Vasc Surg.* 2009;23(3):350–354.
36. Millward SF, Oliva VL, Bell SD, et al. Gunther tulip retrievable vena cava filter: results from the Registry of the Canadian Interventional Radiology Association. *J Vasc Interv Radiol.* 2001;12(9):1053–1058.
37. Binkert CA, Bansal A, Gates JD. Inferior vena cava filter removal after 317-day implantation. *J Vasc Interv Radiol.* 2005;16(3):395-398.
38. Stavropoulos SW, Solomon JA, Trerotola SO. Wall-embedded recovery inferior vena cava filters: imaging features and technique for removal. *J Vasc Interv Radiol.* 2006;17(2Pt1):379–382.

39. Joffe HV, Kucher N, Tapson VF, Goldhaber SZ. Upper-extremity deep vein thrombosis: a prospective registry of 592 patients. *Circulation.* 2004;110(12):1605–1611.
40. Lee JT, Karwowski JK, Harris EJ, Haukoos JS, Olcott Ct. Long-term thrombotic recurrence after nonoperative management of Paget-Schroetter syndrome. *J Vasc Surg.* 2006;43(6):1236–1243.
41. Sevestre MA, Kalka C, Irwin WT, Ahari HK, Schainfeld RM. Paget-Schroetter syndrome: what to do? *Catheter Cardiovasc Interv.* 2003;59(1):71–76.
42. Machleder HI. Evaluation of a new treatment strategy for Paget-Schroetter syndrome: spontaneous thrombosis of the axillary-subclavian vein. *J Vasc Surg.* 1993;17:305–315.
43. Urschel HC, Patel AM. Surgery remains the most effective treatment for
44. Paget-Schroetter syndrome: 50 years' experience. *Ann Thorac Surg.* 2008;86:254–260.
45. Rice TW, Rodriguez RM, Light RW. The superior vena cava syndrome: clinical characteristics and evolving etiology. *Medicine.* 2006;85(1):37–42.
46. Lin J, Zhou KR, Chen ZW, Wang JH, Yan ZP, Wang YX. Vena cava 3D contrast-enhanced MR venography: a pictorial review. *Cardiovasc Intervent Radiol.* 2005;28(6):795–805.
47. Alimi YS, Gloviczki P, Vrtiska TJ, et al. Reconstruction of the superior vena cava: benefits of postoperative surveillance and secondary endovascular interventions. *J Vasc Surg.* 1998;27(2):287–299.
48. Kalra M, Gloviczki P, Andrews JC, et al. Open surgical and endovascular treatment of superior vena cava syndrome caused by nonmalignant disease. *J Vasc Surg.* 2003;38(2):215–223.
49. Bornak A, Wicky S, Ris HB, Probst H, Milesi I, Corpataux JM. Endovascular treatment of stenoses in the superior vena cava syndrome caused by non-tumoral lesions. *Eur Radiol.* 2003;13(5):950–956.
50. Rizvi AZ, Kalra M, Bjarnason H, et al., Benign superior vena cava syndrome: stenting is now the first line of treatment. *J Vasc Surg.* 2008;47:372–380.
51. Nagata T, Makutani S, Uchida H, et al. Follow-up results of 71 patients undergoing metallic stent placement for the treatment of a malignant obstruction of the superior vena cava. *Cardiovasc Intervent Radiol.* 2007;30:959–967.
52. Slonim SM, Semba CP, Sze DY, Dake MD. Placement of SVC stents over pacemaker wires for the treatment of SVC syndrome. *J Vasc Interv Radiol.* 2000;11(2Pt1):215–219.
53. Ganeshan A, Quen Hon L, Warakaulle DR, Morgan R, Uberoi R. Superior vena caval stenting for SVC obstruction: Current status. *Eur J Radiol.* 2009;71(2):343–349. Epub 2008 Jun 12.

Index

A
Abdominal aortic aneurysms (AAAs)
  contraindications, 163–164
  definition of, 160
  diagnosis, 160
  EVAR
    advantage, 175
    anatomical considerations, 167–170
    characteristics, CT angiogram, 166
    components, 164
    endoleaks, 170–175
    Gore Excluder, 165
    Medtronic Endurant stent graft, 166
    vs. open surgical, 176
    patient selection, 177
    surveillance, 175–176
    Zenith FLEX AAA endograft, 165
  intervention indications
    asymptomatic aneurysm, 163
    symptomatic aneurysm, 162–163
  screening for, 160–162
  USPSTF, 161–162
Acculink for Revascularization of Carotids in High Risk Patient (ARCHeR) trial, 121
Acute mesenteric ischemia (AMI)
  diagnosis and treatment, 87–88
  incidence and prevalence, 86–87
Acute stroke interventions
  imaging, 151–152
  Merci device, 153
  technical aspects, 153
  treatment, MCA occlusions, 152–153
AMI. *See* Acute mesenteric ischemia (AMI)
Angiojet rheolytic thrombectomy system, 195–196
Angiosculpt balloon, 55
Ankle brachial index (ABI)
  LEAD, 7
  PAD, 25
Ankle Brachial pressures (ABI), 44
Anticoagulation therapy
  mesenteric artery intervention, 93
  renal artery intervention, 84
Antiplatelet therapy
  mesenteric artery intervention, 92
  renal artery intervention, 84
Arterial duplex ultrasonograms, 44–45
ASVT. *See* Axillosubclavian vein thrombosis (ASVT)
Asymptomatic abdominal aortic aneurysms, 163
Asymptomatic Carotid Atherosclerosis Study (ACAS), 116, 118
Asymptomatic Carotid Surgery Trial, 11
Atherogenesis, 1
Atherosclerosis
  distribution, in LEAD, 3
  management of, 9–10
  noncoronary arteries, 3
  polyvascular, 4
Axillosubclavian vein thrombosis (ASVT)
  algorithm, management, 219
  etiology and symptoms, 215
  key points, 220
  venogram, first rib resection, 218

B
Balloon angioplasty, 92
Balloon expandable stents, 59
Balloon-mounted stents, ICAD, 147, 148
BASIL. *See* Bypass Versus Angioplasty in Severe Ischemia of the Leg (BASIL)

From: *Peripheral and Cerebrovascular Intervention*, Contemporary Cardiology
Edited by: D. L. Bhatt, DOI 10.1007/978-1-60327-965-9
© Springer Science+Business Media, LLC 2012

Bowel ischemia, 93
Bypass Versus Angioplasty in Severe
   Ischemia of the Leg (BASIL), 42

C
Carotid and Vertebral Artery Transluminal
   Angioplasty Study (CAVATAS)
   trial, 120
Carotid artery stenosis
   CAS
      ACT–1 clinical trial, 125
      aortic arches, 126–129
      ARCHeR trial, 121
      CAVATAS trial, 120
      vs. CEA, 125
      complications, 130
      contraindications, 125
      CREST trial, 123–124
      EVA–3S trial, 121–122
      ICSS trial, 122–123
      neuroprotection, 130
      SAPPHIRE trial, 120–121
      schema, carotid stenting trials, 120
      SPACE trial, 122
      stents, 129
   CEA
      ACAS, 116, 118
      anatomical criteria, 118
      complications, 119
      vs. medical therapy, 117
      NASCET, 116
      recommendations, 119
   management of, 10–11
   risk of stroke, 6
Carotid artery stenting (CAS)
   ACT–1 clinical trial, 125
   aortic arches, 126–129
   ARCHeR trial, 121
   CAVATAS trial, 120
   vs. CEA, 125
   complications, 130
   contraindications, 125
   CREST trial, 123–124
   EVA–3S trial, 121–122
   ICSS trial, 122–123
   neuroprotection, 130
   SAPPHIRE trial, 120–121
   schema, carotid stenting trials, 120
   SPACE trial, 122
   stents, 129
Carotid atherosclerosis
   management of, 9–10
   prevalence of, 3–4
Carotid endarterectomy (CEA)
   ACAS, 116, 118
   anatomical criteria, 118
   complications, 119
   vs. medical therapy, 117
   NASCET, 116
   recommendations, 119
Carotid intima media thickness (C-IMT), 8
Carotid Revascularization Endarterectomy
   versus Stenting Trial (CREST), 123
Carotid-subclavian bypass, 106
Catheter-directed thrombolysis (CDT)
   American College of Chest Physician
      guidelines, 193
   contraindications, thrombolytic therapy,
      194
   efficacy evaluation, 192–193
   EKOS Endowave thrombolytic infusion
      catheter, 193
   key points, techniques, 194
   vs. PMT, 195
   thrombolytic agents, 192
Cerebral aneurysms
   coil embolization technique
      complications of, 150–151
      narrow and wide necked aneurysms, 150
      pre-procedure and post-procedure
         images, 149
   incidence of, 148
   risk of rupture study, 148–149
Cerebrovascular anatomy
   Circle of Willis, 144
   internal carotid artery (ICA)
      anterior cerebral artery (ACA), 143
      middle cerebral artery (MCA), 142–143
      segments, 141–142
      posterior cerebral arteries (PCA), 144
      vertebral arteries, 143–144
Chronic intestinal ischemia, 2–3
Chronic mesenteric ischemia (CMI)
   diagnostic approach, 88
   incidence and prevalence, 87
   treatment of, 88–91
Chronic total occlusions (CTO) crossing, CLI
   adjunctive tools, 52–54
   atherectomy devices, 56–58

Index

reconstruction
    atherectomy devices, 56–58
    balloons, 54–56
    stents, 58–60
    subintimal dissection method of Bolia, 48–52
    wires and catheters, 52
Cilostazol, 23
CLI. *See* Critical limb ischemia (CLI)
CMI. *See* Chronic mesenteric ischemia (CMI)
Computed tomography
    AAAs, 160
    acute stroke, 151
    IVC filter, 205
    occlusive AMI, 87
    retroperitoneal fibrosis, 203
    SVC syndrome, 221
Cook Zenith thoracic stent graft, 179
Coronary-subclavian steal, 104, 105
Critical limb ischemia (CLI)
    BASIL, 42
    clinical evaluation
        ABI and PVR, 44
        arterial duplex ultrasonograms, 44–45
        diagnosis tests, 44
        invasive testing, 46–47
        noninvasive testing, 44–46
        PV-CTA, 46–47
    clinical symptoms of
        gangrene, 44
        nonhealing wounds, 44
        rest pain, 43
        ulcerated lesions, 43
    contraindications, 25–26
    endovascular interventions, 60–75
    endovascular therapy, 42
    epidemiology, 42
    indications, lower extremity intervention, 21
    multivessel/multisegment disease, 41
    POBA, 54
    revascularization procedure, 23–24
    risk factors, 44
    TASC definition, 41
    treatment of
        endovascular techniques, 48–60
        revascularization and limb amputation, 48
CROSSER catheter, 52, 53
Cryoplasty procedure, 55
Cutting balloon, 55

D

Deep venous thrombosis (DVT)
    ASVT
        algorithm, management, 219
        etiology and symptoms, 215
        key points, 220
        venogram, first rib resection, 218
    CDT
        American College of Chest Physician guidelines, 193
        contraindications, thrombolytic therapy, 194
        efficacy evaluation, 192–193
        EKOS Endowave thrombolytic infusion catheter, 193
        key points, techniques, 194
        vs. PMT, 195
        thrombolytic agents, 192
    chronic obstructive lesions, iliac vein, 197
    iliofemoral DVT, 196–197
    IVC filter
        American College of Chest Physicians (ACCP) guidelines, 207
        computed tomography, 205
        designs of, 208
        indications and contraindications, 207
        insertion technique, 207–208
        malpositioned filter, 211
        obstruction of, 201–202
        properties, 204–205
        retrievable filters, 214–215
        retroperitoneal fibrosis, 203
        suprarenal IVC filter placement, 212–213
        surgically placed clip, 206
        types and features of, 209
        venacavography, 210
    IVC obstruction, 201–204
    PMT
        Angiojet rheolytic thrombectomy system, 195–196
        vs. CDT, 195
        mechanisms of action, 194–195
        Trellis–8 thrombolytic infusion and aspiration thrombectomy catheter system, 195–196
    SVC syndrome
        causes of, 220

Deep venous thrombosis (DVT) (continued)
  complications, 223–225
  diagnosis, 221
  endovascular techniques, 222–223
  key points, 225
  post-mechanical thrombectomy, 224
  symptoms, 220–221
  treatment, 221–222
  venacavogram, 224
Descending thoracic aortic aneurysm (DTAA), 178–179
Diagnosis
  AAAs, 160
  AMI, 87–88
  CMI, 88
  RAS, 81–82
  subclavian artery stenosis, 102–103
  SVC syndrome, 221
Diamondback 360°, 56–57
Disabling claudation
  contraindications, 25–26
  indications, lower extremity intervention, 20
  therapy for
    antiplatelet therapy, 21–22
    diabetes and blood pressure, 22
    pentoxifylline and cilostazol, 23
    smoking cessation and regular exercise, 21
  weighted mean prevalence, 2
Distal EPDs, 130
Drug eluting balloons, 56
Drug-eluting stents (DES)
  ICAD, 147–148
  renal artery stenosis, 86
Duplex ultrasonography
  CLI, 44–45
  RAS, 81
  SVC syndrome, 221
Dutch Randomized Endovascular Aneurysm Management trial (DREAM), 176

E
EKOS Endowave thrombolytic infusion catheter, 193
Embolic protection devices (EPDs)
  carotid stenosis, 130
  renal artery stenosis, 85

Endarterectomy *versus* Angioplasty in Patients with Symptomatic Severe Carotid Stenosis (EVA–3S) trial, 121–122
Endotension, 175
Endovascular aortic repair (EVAR)
  advantage, 175
  anatomical considerations
    access arteries, 169–170
    aortic side branches, 170
    distal attachment site, 169
    proximal attachment site, 167–169
  characteristics, CT angiogram, 166
  components, 164
  endoleaks
    endotension, 175
    type 1, 171–172
    type 2, 172–173
    type 3, 173, 174
    type 4, 174
  Gore Excluder, 165
  Medtronic Endurant stent graft, 166
  vs. open surgical, 176
  patient selection, 177
  surveillance, 175–176
  Zenith FLEX AAA endograft, 165
Endovascular techniques
  CLI, 48–60
  SVC syndrome, 222–223
  vertebral artery stenosis
    arterial and radial accesses, 133
    complications, 136
    diagnostic aortic arch angiography, 133–134
    embolic protection devices, 135–136
    patients follow-up, 136
    selective angiography, 134
    telescoping technique, 134–135
EPDs. *See* Embolic protection devices (EPDs)
EVAR. *See* Endovascular aortic repair (EVAR)
Excimer laser atherectomy, 58, 59
EXCIMER LASER catheter, 53

F
Femoro-popliteal disease
  atherectomy and cryoplasty, 33
  interventional therapy results, 30

occlusion images, 32
setting of, 31
stenotic lesions, 31, 32
TASC classification, 29
treatment approaches, 28
FRONTRUNNER catheter, 53

G
Gore Excluder, 165
Gore TAG thoracic stent graft, 178
Gunther-Tulip IVC filter, 214

H
Hypogastric artery (HA), 170

I
ICAD. *See* Intracranial atherosclerotic disease (ICAD)
Iliac artery disease
    angioplasty and stenting results, 34
    balloon expandable and covered stents, 28
    contralateral and transbrachial approaches, 27–28
    ipsilateral femoral access approach, 26–28
    occlusion images, 31
    TASC classification, 29
Iliofemoral DVT, 196–197
IMA. *See* Internal mammary artery (IMA)
Incidence and prevalence
    AMI, 86–87
    CMI, 87
    RAS, 79–80
Inferior vena cava (IVC) filter
    American College of Chest Physicians (ACCP) guidelines, 207
    computed tomography, 205
    designs of, 208
    indications and contraindications, 207
    insertion technique, 207–208
    malpositioned filter, 211
    obstruction of, 201–202
    properties, 204–205
    retrievable filters, 214–215
    retroperitoneal fibrosis, 203
    suprarenal IVC filter placement, 212–213
    surgically placed clip, 206
    types and features of, 209
    venacavography, 210
In-stent restenosis (ISR), 86
Internal mammary artery (IMA), 104
International Carotid Stenting (ICSS) trial, 122–123
Intracranial atherosclerotic disease (ICAD)
    angioplasty and stenting, 146–147
    endovascular management, 145–146
    medical management of, 145
    natural history, 144
    stent designs
        balloon-mounted stents, 147, 148
        drug-eluting stents (DES), 147–148
        self-expanding stents, 147
Intracranial endovascular interventions
    acute stroke interventions
        imaging, 151–152
        Merci device, 153
        technical aspects, 153
        treatment, MCA occlusions, 152–153
    cerebral aneurysms
        coil embolization technique, 149–151
        incidence of, 148
        risk of rupture study, 148–149
    cerebrovascular anatomy
        Circle of Willis, 144
        internal carotid artery (ICA), 141–143
        posterior cerebral arteries (PCA), 144
        vertebral arteries, 143–144
    ICAD
        angioplasty and stenting, 146–147
        endovascular management, 145–146
        medical management of, 145
        natural history, 144
        stent designs, 147–148
Intravascular ultrasound (IVUS)
    IVC, 199
    PIONEER CATHETER, 54
    renal artery intervention, 84
The Investigation of Stent grafts in patients with type B Aortic Dissection trial (INSTEAD), 180
IVC filter. *See* Inferior vena cava (IVC) filter

L
Large artery occlusions. *See* Acute stroke interventions
LEAD. *See* Lower extremity arterial disease (LEAD)

Lower extremity arterial disease (LEAD)
   vs. malignancies, 6
   prevalence of, 2
   REACH registry, 5
   revascularization, 10
   screening for, 7–8
Lower extremity intervention, indications
   critical limb ischemia, 21
   disabling claudation, 20

M

Magnetic resonance venography, SVC syndrome, 221
Medtronic Captiva thoracic stent graft, 178
Medtronic Endurant stent graft, 166
Mesenteric aortogram, 89
Mesenteric artery intervention
   adjunctive therapies
      anticoagulation therapy, 93
      antiplatelet therapy, 92
   complications, 93
   percutaneous modalities, 92
   postintervention care, 93
   technical aspects
      interventional wires, 92
      sheath and guide selection, 91
      sheath/guide engagement, 91–92
      vacular access, 91
Multivessel/multisegment disease, 41

N

Nonocclusive AMI, 87–88
North American Symptomatic Carotid Endarterectomy Trial (NASCET), 116

O

Occlusive AMI, 87
OUTBACK LTD catheter, 54

P

PAD Awareness, Risk, and Treatment: New Resources for Survival (PARTNERS) program, 11
Paget-Schroetter syndrome. *See* Primary ASVT
Pentoxifylline, 23

Percutaneous mechanical thrombectomy (PMT)
   Angiojet rheolytic thrombectomy system, 195–196
   vs. CDT, 195
   mechanisms of action, 194–195
   Trellis–8 thrombolytic infusion and aspiration thrombectomy catheter system, 195–196
Peripheral arterial disease (PAD)
   clinical evaluation (*see* Critical limb ischemia (CLI))
   contraindications, 25–26
   intervention factors, 26
   postprocedural care and follow-up, 33, 35
   screening tests, 24–25
   therapy for
      antiplatelet therapy, 21–22
      diabetes and blood pressure, 22
      pentoxifylline and cilostazol, 23
      revascularization procedure, 23–24
      smoking cessation and regular exercise, 21
   treatment methods
      femoro-popliteal disease, 28, 31–33
      iliac artery system, 26–28
Peripheral vascular CTA (PV-CTA), 46–47
PIONEER catheter, 54
Plain old balloon angioplasty (POBA), 54
PMT. *See* Percutaneous mechanical thrombectomy (PMT)
POBA. *See* Plain old balloon angioplasty (POBA)
PolarCath Peripheral Dilatation System, 55
Primary ASVT, 218
Proximal EPDs, 130
Pulse volume recordings (PVR), 44
PV-CTA. *See* Peripheral vascular CTA (PV-CTA)

R

RAS. *See* Renal artery stenosis (RAS)
Renal artery fibromuscular dysplasia, 80
Renal artery intervention
   access and guidewires, 83
   adjunctive therapies
      anticoagulation therapy, 84
      antiplatelet therapy, 84
      EPD, 85

Index 235

complications, 85
percutaneous modalities, 84
postintervention care and follow up, 85
restenosis, 86
sheath and guide selection and
  engagement, 83
Renal artery stenosis (RAS)
  clinical outcomes, 83
  diagnosis, 81–82
  indications, 80–81
  intervention (*see* Renal artery intervention)
  prevalence of, 3, 79–80
  revascularization, 81–82
  screening, 81
  treatment, 82
Retrievable IVC filters, 214–215
Revascularization and limb amputation, 48

S

Self-expanding stents
  CLI, 59–60
  ICAD, 147
SilverHawk Plaque Excision System, 57–58
Stenting and Angioplasty with Protection in
  Patients at High Risk for
  Endarterectomy (SAPPHIRE) trial,
  120–121
Stent-Supported Percutaneous Angioplasty of
  the Carotid Artery *versus*
  Endarterectomy (SPACE) trial, 122
Subclavian artery stenosis
  angiographic evaluation, 107
  aortic arch anatomy, 99–102
  carotid-subclavian bypass, 106
  case examples, 111–113
  complications, 110
  diagnosis, 102–103
  etiology, 102
  intervention indications
    claudication, 104
    coronary-subclavian steal, 104, 105
    IMA, 104
    subclavian steal syndrome, 105–106
  noninvasive testing, 103–104
  stroke prevention, 110–111
  subclavian to carotid artery transposition,
    106–107
  technical success rates, 107
  thoracic outlet syndrome, 102

Subclavian steal syndrome, 105–106
Superior vena cava filter placement, 213–214
Superior vena cava (SVC) syndrome
  causes of, 220
  complications, 223–225
  diagnosis, 221
  endovascular techniques, 222–223
  key points, 225
  post-mechanical thrombectomy, 224
  symptoms, 220–221
  treatment, 221–222
  venacavogram, 224
Symptomatic abdominal aortic aneurysms,
  162–163

T

Thoracic endovascular aortic repair (TEVAR)
  acute type B aortic dissection, 180
  aortic arch anatomy, 181
  CASE study, 183–185
  chronic type B aortic dissection, 180
  complications, 182
  contraindications, 182
  Cook Zenith thoracic stent graft, 179
  discharge and follow-up, 183
  Gore TAG thoracic stent graft, 178
  indications, 177, 179
  left subclavian artery coverage and
    revascularization, 181
  Medtronic Captiva thoracic stent graft, 178
  post-implant care, 183
  procedural steps, 182–183
  spinal drainage, 181
  vascular access, 182
TransAtlantic Inter-Society Consensus
  (TASC), 41
Transcutaneous oxygen tension
  (TcPO2), 46
Treatment
  AMI, 87–88
  ASVT, 218–219
  CMI, 88–91
  RAS, 82
  SVC syndrome, 221–222
Trellis–8 thrombolytic infusion and aspiration
  thrombectomy catheter system,
  195–196
TurboHawk peripheral plaque excision
  system, 58

U

United States Preventive Services Task Force (USPSTF), 161–162
Upper extremity arterial stenosis. *See* Subclavian artery stenosis
Upper extremity DVT (UEDVT), 213
U.S. Open *versus* Endovascular Repair trial (OVER), 176
USPSTF. *See* United States Preventive Services Task Force (USPSTF)

V

VASCUTRAK balloon, 54–55
Vertebral artery stenosis
  anatomy regions, 131, 132
  endovascular technique
    arterial and radial accesses, 133
    complications, 136
    diagnostic aortic arch angiography, 133–134
    embolic protection devices, 135–136
    patients follow-up, 136
    selective angiography, 134
    telescoping technique, 134–135
  etiology of, 131
  symptoms, VBI, 131–132
  therapy
    endovascular treatment, 132–133
    registries, vertebral artery stenting, 133
Vertebrobasilar insufficiency (VBI), 131–132
Veterans Administration Asymptomatic Carotid Stenosis Study, 11

W

Warfarin *vs.* Aspirin for Symptomatic Intracranial Disease (WASID) trial, 144

Z

Zenith FLEX AAA endograft, 165